Table of Contents

Partnering for Success

Partnering for Success

Chapter 1

A Program That's Made for You

Congratulations on taking the first step towards a healthier, better you!

You've made the right choice. The doctors and health coaches at the PreDiabetes Centers are here to help you avoid or delay a diabetes diagnosis and reach your dreams of living a long, happy and healthy life.

Diabetes is a serious medical condition that can put you at risk for long-term health problems. It's the seventh-leading cause of death in the U.S. and affects more than 25 million children and adults. Another 79 million Americans have prediabetes, defined as blood sugar that is higher than normal but not yet in the diabetes range. A prediabetes diagnosis means that your body is starting to develop type 2 diabetes, the condition that occurs when the body does not produce enough insulin or resists the effects of insulin.

Remember, there is no "quick fix" for prediabetes. It has taken years for your body to develop the cascade of negative processes now affecting your health. By enrolling in this program, you have come to terms with the fact that you can no longer continue to do nothing.

You are finally taking control of your health. Reversing your prediabetic state won't be easy, but you will be provided with the tools and support you need to ensure success.

The skills you learn and treatment you receive at PreDiabetes Centers will change how you live and how you feel. Commitment to your personalized treatment plan will stop prediabetes in its tracks.

Defeating prediabetes means not only avoiding type 2 diabetes but reducing the harmful effects caused by associated conditions.

How Did I Develop Prediabetes?

Prediabetes is a true medical condition caused by many factors, and it's not just about your lifestyle or your weight. Your genetic makeup may have put you at an increased risk for the condition. Or, you could have a hormonal imbalance that's causing your body to become resistant to insulin, a hormone produced in the pancreas. Harmful associated conditions, such as high blood pressure or abnormal cholesterol levels, also contribute to the development of prediabetes.

Prediabetes develops as a result of the complex interplay between hormones produced by abdominal fat—known as visceral fat—and hormonal effects on cells in the body. As abdominal fat cells grow, they produce ever-increasing amounts of inflammation-promoting hormones. This has destructive effects on the body, specifically the body's ability to use insulin. This leads to an increase in blood sugar (glucose) levels. When the pancreas doesn't make enough insulin or your cells become insulin resistant, the body is unable to properly convert blood sugar to energy for cells, which means cells are starved of energy. This causes rising levels of cortisol, the hormone that signals to the brain that the body is hungry, which will cause you to eat more, leading to increased production of fat cells, further exacerbating the dysfunctional cycle. This negative process can also cause the development of hypertension and atherosclerosis (hardening of the arteries).

And it's not just overweight or obese people who carry abdominal fat—thinner people can have it too. "Bad" fat storage can be affected by poor dietary choices or even genetics, and it will produce the same destructive cycle that leads to the development of diabetes.

Reducing the amount of abdominal fat on the body can help reduce the amount of pro-inflammatory, insulin-desensitizing fat cells in the body and increase the production of a "good" fat hormone called adiponectin, which helps regulate blood sugar levels. These changes can prevent the onset of diabetes.

Partnering for Better Health

You've been fighting this disease on your own with limited success. Or perhaps you had no idea you were developing prediabetes and you are just now beginning to tackle the problem. Still, without proper guidance and support, defeating prediabetes is nearly impossible.

You probably have consulted the Internet for health advice. The problem is, it's filled with conflicting information from people who are unfamiliar with your individual risk factors and special circumstances. Similarly, diet and exercise programs advertised on TV may sound enticing, but they don't take into account many important factors, including your medical background and hidden issues that can be uncovered in our extensive, comprehensive analysis.

The PreDiabetes Centers PATHFinder Program is customized to fit your needs. You'll have in-depth consultations with a physician and health coach. Treating prediabetes and developing effective, customized treatment plans to avoid type 2 diabetes is all they do. Throughout your 12-month program you will receive consistent support both one-on-one in the Center and in scheduled telephonic sessions. Additionally, your health coach will guide you and answer questions about medications, nutrition, supplements, exercise and any adverse effects you may experience.

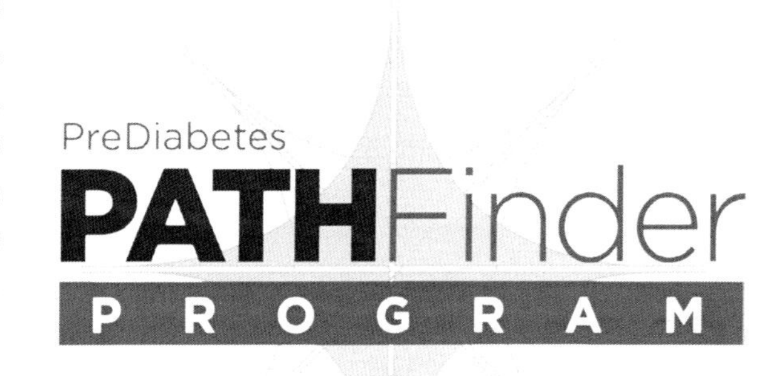

It's normal to feel overwhelmed or unsure about changing your lifestyle and many of the habits you've had for years. Don't worry: You now have a partner to help you navigate the treatment plan and manage your health. We understand how challenging this can be, especially while juggling work, family and other responsibilities. Prediabetes is a complex, confusing condition that is difficult to understand, let alone treat.

PreDiabetes Centers is honored to stand by your side as you forge a path to a brand-new you. Let the team at PreDiabetes Centers guide and inspire you. Together with your experienced, knowledgeable team, you can prevent the onset of diabetes.

A Personalized Approach

A one-size-fits-all strategy to defeat diabetes doesn't work. Without knowing what exactly is happening inside your body, treatment will be experimental and ineffective.

There may be unique negative processes occurring in your body that require targeted action. Some people have low levels of vitamin D. Others may be at increased risk for cardiovascular disease. Perhaps you have a health condition that makes it difficult to perform certain exercises, or you take medications that need to be carefully monitored.

One very important piece of this complex puzzle called prediabetes is understanding how to correctly and thoroughly assess the condition. In addition to your detailed history and comprehensive physical exam, we have the ability to assess your health with comprehensive biomarker blood testing. Your physician and health coach will continually monitor biomarkers in your body associated with prediabetic conditions to measure the effect of your treatment. With biomarker testing, the team at PreDiabetes Centers can isolate your areas of need and develop and consistently adjust a treatment program specifically for you.

Five times over the course of the program, your blood will be comprehensively analyzed for biomarkers that indicate disease or poor functioning. After each test, your health coach and physician will adjust your treatment plan to continuously move you closer to a long-term positive outcome.

Together, your progress will be reviewed and you will be able to see real results at each consultation.

Consistent and comprehensive re-evaluation is essential to the PreDiabetes Centers PATHFinder Program. Without it, you won't know if your health is improving and you're successfully reversing the diabetes process.

Why the Program Works

The PreDiabetes Centers yearlong treatment program is based on clinically proven practices and scientific research for the treatment of prediabetes and the prevention of diabetes. Advanced medical treatment is combined with a holistic approach to create a personalized, flexible treatment plan just for you.

Your physician and health coach will customize your treatment based on five measures of your health:

- **Insulin dynamics.** An evaluation of how well your pancreas is functioning and how your body is responding to insulin.
- **Hormone balance.** How your hormones are affecting your metabolism, if they are causing inflammation and their status of optimization.
- **Inflammation.** Tests examine whether there is excessive inflammation in your body. Too much can eventually lead to diabetes and cardiovascular disease.
- **Vascular integrity.** Evaluating the vascular status, which includes good and back cholesterol, triglycerides and other abnormal markers that contribute to diabetes and other associated conditions. If you are prediabetic, your vascular health may already be damaged.
- **Core influencers.** How much sleep, stress, relaxation, social support and education are affecting your condition.

Research shows that focusing on these areas can prevent or reduce risk for diabetes and diabetes-related complications. The goal of your treatment is to optimize these areas of function.

Armed with in-depth knowledge of processes occurring inside your body and clinically proven methods of treatment, PreDiabetes Centers can provide you with the care you need.

"What Happens if I Don't Complete the Program?"

Diabetes can be reversed—if you catch it early enough. It may take as many as 10 years for prediabetes to develop into diabetes, or as few as three. Once diabetes progresses, it becomes a chronic disease that requires lifelong care.

Diabetes puts you at risk for several other health problems such as heart disease, stroke, kidney failure and other conditions.

Here are a few quick facts about diabetes and its related complications from the American Diabetes Association (ADA):

- People with diabetes are twice as likely to die from heart disease, the first-leading cause of death in the U.S.
- People with diabetes are twice as likely to suffer a stroke.
- Diabetes is the leading cause of blindness in adults.
- Diabetes is the leading cause of kidney failure.
- About 60%-70% of diabetics have nervous system damage.
- More than 60% of nontraumatic lower-limb amputations occur in people with diabetes.
- People with advanced diabetes must constantly monitor their blood sugar and inject themselves with insulin.

Another factor to consider: Diabetes is costly! People with diabetes spend more than twice as much on health care compared to people without the disease. The national cost of diabetes in the U.S. exceeds more than $174 billion a year, according to the latest estimate.

There is still time to prevent the deadly complications of diabetes and the accompanying financial burden. PreDiabetes Centers will help you reverse the diabetes process, boost your health and energy level, and enhance your quality of life.

You Can Do It!

Don't let anything stand between you and the healthy lifestyle you've always dreamed of.

Before you get started, remind yourself of all your reasons for becoming healthy, whatever they may be: To achieve better health, set a good example for your kids or live a longer life. Remember to take care of yourself so that you are better able to reach your personal health goals.

Here are a few suggestions on how to approach the program:

✓ **Use this book.** It is filled with valuable tips, recipes, information and strategies to prevent diabetes.

✓ **Use your health coach.** He or she is a wonderful resource of information and has experience fighting diabetes. If you have any questions about the program—or if you need extra motivation—your health coach is there to help you.

✓ **Use your time with the doctor wisely.** You will have a lot of face time with a PreDiabetes Centers doctor. Ask your doctor tough questions and don't worry about appearing uninformed—prediabetes is a complex disorder.

✓ **Throw yourself into the program.** Don't be afraid to fail. The only way you are going to beat diabetes is to push yourself past your comfort zone. After a while, you will see and feel the results.

Make a commitment to improving your quality of life. Diabetes is a deadly disease, but you still have time to defeat it.

Chapter 2

Client Stories

You will encounter many challenges on your journey to a life free of prediabetes. However, you will experience life-altering triumphs.

Many people don't know what to expect when they begin the program. They are unsure of how their day-to-day lives are going to change and how difficult it will be to reshape the habits they've developed over a lifetime.

Your health coach will offer guidance and assistance to ensure that you become more comfortable and are able to adhere to your new health regimen. Like most of our clients, you likely will see a difference in your health and daily functioning in the first couple of months.

It's helpful to know how people just like you navigated the first few months of the program. To give you a better understanding, we rounded up a few real-life stories from our clients.

We hope their stories comfort and inspire you, and that you know that many others have succeeded in the program... which means you can too!

True Story: "I've Changed My Habits and Expectations"

Marc

Age: 53

Hometown: Raceland, LA

Interests: Work, family, fishing, tennis, eating

Health conditions: High blood pressure, high cholesterol

Q: Why did you get tested for prediabetes?

A: When I was younger, I always worried about being thin. I used to work outside in a physically demanding job, and I got enough exercise to balance out the bad foods I was eating. When I started working in an office, everything changed. I started eating worse and I got a lot heavier.

For 20 years I suspected that my health was deteriorating. I had high blood pressure for 15 years and high cholesterol too. After a while, it seemed like my blood pressure and cholesterol meds weren't working anymore. My doctor would tell me to cut carbs and start exercising, but he was really passive about it.

I finally put the pieces together and started looking around on the Internet for answers. I liked the focus on [biomarker] numbers at PreDiabetes Centers, so I got tested and went from there.

Q: What do you like about the program?

A: The health coaches and doctors have a can-do attitude and realistic approach. I like that they are genuinely concerned and dedicated to making a positive impact on people with prediabetes. The education I've received has been a wake-up call.

Q: How has your lifestyle changed since you've been in the program?

A: I walk a lot now, and my diet has drastically changed. I've been surprised at how full I feel on a much smaller amount of food. It's funny, when I cheat and have a cheeseburger po'boy—I'm from Louisiana—I can't eat the whole thing, and I immediately feel bad. My body is now accustomed to good food, and when I eat the bad stuff my body rejects it.

I went to a nice restaurant with my family just before I entered the program and was served a really small portion. I almost lost my mind. "Where's the rest of my food?" I wondered. Most people today are gluttonous animals—we go out to eat, pig out as fast as we can and then go home and belch on the couch for the rest of the night.

Now I go to restaurants with an entirely different mindset. I look at the menu. I take time to make good choices and ask the staff what exactly is in each dish. I look at these meals as a social event where I can spend time with my family. I've really changed my habits and expectations.

Q: How are you feeling now?

A: I feel really good. I've lost 25 pounds. My blood pressure went from 135/80 to 111/57 and I don't have to take as much medication. I like the way I'm living and eating right now. I haven't taken an antacid in three months! I struggled with fast-paced walking at first, but now I walk every day.

Q: What advice would you give to people entering the program?

A: It's really about overcoming human nature. It's easy to get couch-potato syndrome. With work and family stress, you may feel too tired to do something about your health. I've been unselfish all my life, focusing on my wife, kids, dogs, even birds, but I was neglecting me. You have to take time for yourself.

Q: What are your future goals?

A: I want to keep losing weight and get off cholesterol and blood pressure medicine. I want to live as long as I can and just enjoy life. I still love eating—I just eat better food these days!

True Story: "I Have More Willpower Than I Thought"

Q: Why did you decide to be screened for prediabetes? Was the diagnosis a surprise?

A: I have several friends who have diabetes. They always asked me, "How do you not have diabetes?"

I knew my eating habits were the same as theirs, so I thought it would be a good idea to get tested.

Q: Have you previously tried changing your diet or sought any kind of health treatment?

A: I have been able to start diet and exercise programs for short periods of time, but I can't stay on them. I'd go on vacation or out to dinner, and all of sudden I'd have to start all over again. Without support and proper education, starting down this path is like trying to climb Mount Everest without climbing gear.

Nate

Age: 46

Hometown: Austin, TX

Interests: Proud father and grandfather, soon-to-be law student

Health conditions: High blood pressure, high cholesterol

Q: What has been the most rewarding aspect of treatment?

A: The realization that I could eat healthy foods and still be satisfied. I also like seeing how my body responds to what I put in it. I feel so much better!

Q: Has it been easy to incorporate the program into your everyday life?

A: The challenge before was making choices when the fridge was empty or when I went out to eat. Now I walk into a grocery store and know "I can get that, I can't get that." When you remove the decision-making process, it becomes easy.

Q: Have you discovered anything about yourself during treatment?

A: I discovered I had more willpower than I thought I had. I also learned that I know very little about choosing proper foods. My friends and family have definitely noticed a difference. I've lost 25 pounds. They notice the weight loss and how I select foods with a purpose, not just because they look good.

Q: If you could give one piece of advice to someone entering the program, what would it be?

A: Take it seriously. Your regular doctor may not identify prediabetes as a serious problem, but it's important to work on correcting it before it becomes diabetes.

Q: What are your future goals?

A: I want to spend quality time with my family. I'm about to enroll in law school and hope to have a happy and productive life.

True Story: "I Go One Meal at a Time, but I Can See Results"

Q: Has managing your prediabetes been a challenge?

A: I seem to have a disability when it comes to creating a nutritionally balanced diet. When I hit the right balance, I have more energy and feel better. When I don't hit the right balance, I'm irritable and tired.

Q: Were you surprised by your diagnosis?

A: I was a little surprised at the diagnosis because I had been tested by my regular physician for years. However, my brother was diagnosed as prediabetic, so I had family history of the disease.

Ellen

Age: 55

Hometown: Chicago, IL

Interests: Playing games (especially poker), watching movies, hanging out with friends

Health conditions: High cholesterol, GERD, aches and pains

Q: What do you think of the program?

A: Several aspects of the program are extraordinary! My health coach responds quickly and with detailed suggestions every time I reach out. The health coaches are competent in their knowledge of food and the medical aspects of the program. They're friendly, motivational, educational and affirming.

Q: Have there been any surprises?

A: I was amazed that my doctor called me on the phone!

Q: What has been the most rewarding aspect of the program?

A: The weight loss. I have lost 10 pounds since I started the program. My friends and family have noticed a difference.

Q: If you could give one piece of advice to someone entering the program, what would it be?

A: Be gentle with yourself. You are changing a lifetime of behaviors. If you get stuck, ask for help.

Q: How are you feeling now?

I hate to cook and hate numbers even more. Therefore, figuring out how much to eat of different nutrients, such as proteins and fats, and then planning, shopping and preparing meals three times a day has been hard. I am still struggling with how to prepare a balanced diet for each and every meal. Right now, I am going one meal at a time in hopes of more stability in mood and energy.

True Story: "I Need Structure in My Health Regimen"

Q: Do you have any health conditions in addition to prediabetes?

A: Along with being overweight, I have low thyroid and have struggled for years with joint and muscle pains.

Q: Have you ever tried to change your diet or sought treatment for your health?

A: I have tried many different diets and programs that I thought would help me lose weight, reduce joint pain and improve my health. I tried the Zone, Jenny Craig, eDiets, Weight Watchers, and even a personal chef.

None of these were successful.

Q: Why did you decide to get tested?

A: Since the testing was free at PreDiabetes Centers, I decided to go for it. I was overweight and not eating well, and knew that one of my grandparents had diabetes.

It wasn't a surprise to learn I was at risk.

Q: What do you like most about the program?

A: I like the information and support I have received at PreDiabetes Centers, and the structure has helped me a lot. I need to feel like I am accountable to someone.

Gail

Age: 53

Hometown: Houston, TX

Interests: Swimming, kayaking, boating, spending time with her dog

Health conditions: Low thyroid, joint and muscle pain, insulin resistance, migraines, mild depression

Q: What has been the most rewarding aspect of the treatment?

A: People have noticed a difference in how I look. They say, "Wow, you look like you are losing weight," or "You look healthy!" It feels great to get that feedback. I lost 10 pounds in 8 weeks and I felt better than I had in 10 years. I feel confident I can lose more weight and get back to a healthier and more active lifestyle.

It's easy to pretend that you don't have a problem until you see the numbers. Knowing I can actually change those numbers has been the most rewarding part of the program.

Q: How are you feeling now?

A: I feel hopeful.

PreDiabetes Centers Health Coach: Tanja Burkinshaw, RN

As a health coach at PreDiabetes Centers, I provide education and encouragement to clients while managing their care plan. I am a clinic nurse, teacher, motivator and sometimes a counselor.

Our program strives to educate clients on healthy eating. In our society, we eat with our eyes and our taste buds, but not for our health. I help people cut through the clutter of strange and unhealthy diets and educate them on what is truly good.

A lot of people think if they simply lose weight, they will "fix" their health. Although weight loss is a helpful component for many clients, there are many other factors that take part in a client's journey to better health. Depending on an individual's health picture, we use both pharmaceutical approaches as well as holistic medicinal approaches to manage their care.

We do not measure success with a scale. We measure success objectively with lab results that show how much harmful sugar has been removed from your circulatory system, or if your pancreas has been allowed to rest.

To see people's hemoglobin A1c results drop over the course of the program is an exciting thing! The excitement and relief on their faces as they see their hard work paying off is wonderful. It means that they are prolonging and protecting beta islet cells in their pancreas, which will keep them from suffering the ills of diabetes.

It takes education, time and patience to replace unhealthy habits with good ones. I often remind my clients to be patient, because they are typically hard on themselves. This is one of the reasons our program lasts a year: It's a marathon, not a sprint.

We revisit our approach based on lab results, which gives us the opportunity to adjust your plan step by step. Trying to change everything all at once often produces only fleeting results.

How do you eat an elephant? One bite at a time.

PreDiabetes Centers Physician: Alan Hopkins, MD

As a physician at PreDiabetes Centers, I am solely focused on prediabetes and its associated conditions. Since this is all I do, I'm able to provide patients with a specialized, personalized approach. A PreDiabetes Centers physician leads the team that takes care of you. This team will spend the time with you and help you understand prediabetes, its treatment and your individualized care plan.

Many patients have seen their primary care doctor and have been told they have prediabetes. They have been instructed to watch their diet and exercise. Naturally, a patient will ask, "What does that mean?" "What diet?" "How much exercise?" "What else should I do?" It is easy to fail when you are lost and don't have access to the support you need to overcome prediabetes.

The value of our program is that we treat the individual and not just the disease. For example, many patients with prediabetes are overweight, but some aren't. While losing weight might improve the obese patient, it clearly is not going to help the person who may need to gain weight. Treatments can also be differentiated based on biomarkers. Each person's body functions in a unique way, and biomarkers reflect this uniqueness. There are many reasons why a person develops prediabetes and both the patient and care team must uncover these reasons together.

I often tell overweight patients that a side effect of treating prediabetes is weight loss. If you have high blood pressure, that may come down. If you have cholesterol problems, they will probably improve significantly. Our body is interconnected so that if one system of the body fails, it affects other systems. Once patients really understand this concept they realize that our program can address multiple conditions that they may have suffered with for years.

Our first step in the process begins with a comprehensive exam and review of nearly 100 unique biomarkers. With this information, we initiate an aggressive treatment plan with a strong emphasis on nutrition, supplements and pharmaceutical protocols. Our patients actively participate in the individual design of their program. We find out their likes and dislikes and form a connection that will be the basis of the ongoing support they will receive.

By our second visit together, patients typically see substantial progress in their biomarkers and biometrics. The treatment team will begin to address their physical function. The patient undergoes consultation with a personal trainer and is motivated to exercise to build endurance and muscle tone. The team will encourage participation in activities that the patient has wanted be active in for years but hasn't had the strength or endurance to enjoy. We are also careful to evaluate and optimize sleep, as we know this has enormous metabolic effects on our energy and performance.

In the third visit, we review biomarkers again and address any setbacks that may have occurred and optimize metabolism and physical function. The phase II evaluation by the personal trainer is scheduled at this visit to increase your strength and endurance. We also focus on stress at this visit with an evaluation of contributing issues such as smoking or lack of family support. We educate the patient in stress-lowering techniques and provide supplements that have been shown to support proper release of stress hormones. When needed, we initiate our various smoking-cessation protocols. In support of family, we offer to meet with the family on the patient's behalf, with the intent to educate and offer insight into helpful family-support dynamics.

At the fourth visit, we begin to wean patients off any medications that we may have employed to combat their disease processes if the repeat biomarkers suggest we are able to do so. There is an emphasis on creating a sustainable plan to be free of prediabetes and live in optimal health. Because patients are much healthier at this time, we usually are able to eliminate or drastically reduce medicines that they may have been taking and move them to natural supplements if necessary.

The fifth visit is our opportunity to make sure we got it right. We review a full comprehensive set of biomarkers and assess the patient's overall health status. We make any final recommendations and transition the patient to a new life free of prediabetes.

We believe strongly that knowledge is power. The first step to healing is accepting the disease and understanding how you can beat it. With comprehensive treatment, prediabetes can be reversed for most patients. However, the PreDiabetes Centers program is not easy and everyone will have a different starting point. The healing process takes time, and each patient will have different individual goals and distinctive ways to accomplish them. Consistency, education and commitment are so important to the process because we are not shooting just for success over the year—we are looking for success that will last a lifetime!

Chapter 3

"I'm Committed, What's Next?"

You've taken the first step and joined the program. Committing to a diabetes-free life will require you to rethink many of the behaviors and attitudes you hold about nutrition, exercise, sleep and stress.

You've probably considered for years that you needed to be healthier, seek more medical expertise, and that your lifestyle habits may need improvement. You may have been frustrated with our health care system and also tried to change some of your ways, but then lost the willpower and gave up on a new healthy regimen. Were there times when you told yourself that you're too weak to take control of your health? Have you had times of feeling defeated? Lacked motivation?

Don't let these negative thoughts sabotage your health.

Remember, you aren't going to beat diabetes in a few weeks. It's going to take dedication and flexibility to incorporate new therapies and healthy behaviors into your life. You may backslide from time to time, but this is no reason to quit trying.

Take pride in the fact that you are actively taking control of your health. PreDiabetes Centers has a proven, scientific method to treat, manage and reverse prediabetes. Since the program is customized just for you, there is no reason you can't succeed.

Hit the "reset" button on how you think about your health. Let PreDiabetes Centers show you a new path to healthy living.

Before you begin, remember this...

You are not here simply because of your food choices and weight gain. Reaching this point is a culmination of many contributing factors, many of which you had little to no control over. Your genetics, hormone imbalances, stressors and sleep disorders are just a few of the factors that brought you into the diabetes spectrum.

We understand this and we support your proactive decision to stop this disease in its tracks.

Consider Core Physical Imbalances

Because there are factors outside of your control that may have brought you to this point today, you need to consider that you might have underlying medical issues that contribute to your condition or are caused by prediabetes. There are effective methods to treat these issues that will be considered as your physician develops your personalized treatment plan.

Your physician will work very closely with you to determine the initial priorities within your treatment plan, which also includes the fundamentals of basic nutrition.

Changing How You Think About Food

Changing your relationship with food is one of the most challenging parts of the program.

Start to think about eating as a way to supply nourishment—nutrient-dense food—and not just as a way to seek comfort or quickly satisfy hunger. This will guide you in the right direction.

This doesn't mean that you have to eat bland food. It means you will have to begin learning about the food you put into your body.

Here are some of the reasons you may be struggling with nutrition:

A family history of poor eating habits.

If you were raised eating fast food, microwave meals or nutrient-poor food, you may be unfamiliar with healthy meal preparation. As you go through the program, you will learn how to monitor what goes into your body. You will also learn new food preparation skills that will help you adapt to a new healthy eating regimen.

Acknowledge that the comfort foods and eating habits you've relied on have led you down the path of prediabetes. Continuing down this path will lead to the onset of diabetes. Be prepared to change some family recipes and to try new items at your favorite restaurant. The goal of the program is to find comfort in how you feel, not what you eat.

You don't have time to eat nutritiously.
Fast food is convenient. Cooking takes time. If you work or have a family, finding time to prepare healthy meals can be difficult. After a long day at work, 15 minutes in the kitchen may feel like too much to bear, and the only restaurant near your work is a greasy drive-through.

Whether it's waking up 10 minutes early every morning to prepare lunch (so you can avoid that greasy fast food restaurant!) or learning recipes that can be prepared for dinner in less than 15 minutes, it's essential that you set aside time to focus on healthful eating.

By managing your schedule, you can manage your health. The program will teach you the skills you need to eat healthy at home and monitor the food you eat at restaurants, but you will have to budget extra time in your schedule until your new eating habits become second nature.

Practice the recipes. Memorize your nutrition requirements. The extra time you spend now will save you time later. You'll be surprised at how easy meal preparation gets over time.

An unsupportive environment.
Do you prepare meals for a spouse or children who have poor eating habits? You may find that members of your family aren't as dedicated to a healthy lifestyle as you are and may be resistant to any change in the family's diet.

Remember, you enrolled in this program to improve your health. If you cook for the whole family, you may encounter hostility or discouragement from those in your household. You should remind them that family history of this condition is one of the strongest predictors of developing prediabetes.

Since every family is different, find a compromise that works for both you and them. Your family may not understand just how serious prediabetes is, and how much worse you'll be if it develops into diabetes.

Friends who you frequently dine out with may also be surprised or unsupportive of your new nutrition plan. It's important to prepare yourself to make healthy meal choices–no matter who you are with.

If it gets tough, reach out to your health coach and people who want to see you succeed. Their optimism and positive attitude will motivate you and healthy food choices will become much easier.

Your social life revolves around food.
Do you dine out with friends and coworkers? Perhaps you enjoy cooking big celebratory meals at home. Happy hours and food-centered gatherings may be an important part of your social life, and monitoring your nutrition may seem impossible... but it's not!

Eating health-smart foods at restaurants and home is easier than ever. Most restaurants have healthier options on their menu. Plus, there are many websites that offer calorie and nutritional information on popular dishes.

Be sure to read nutritional labels at the grocery store. Our health coaches will teach you how to read these labels and utilize them in your meal planning.

Don't worry that your new diet will prevent you from dining with friends and family. The program will equip you with the skills and technology necessary to deal with these situations.

Introducing Exercise into Your Life

Living a sedentary life is no longer an option. Your metabolism isn't functioning properly and your cells are becoming insulin resistant. This sets off a chain reaction in your body that causes your blood sugar to rise, your pancreas to work overtime, and your overall health to plummet. If you're overweight, other health conditions are likely interfering with your ability to fully participate in life.

Here's how to approach the program's personalized fitness plan:

Manage your expectations.
Though you will probably lose weight, this is not a weight-loss program. The goal of exercise is to increase insulin sensitivity in your body, build muscle and improve mobility.

If you have been sedentary for a long time, exercise will be difficult at first. Your body needs time, and your physician will integrate a number of interventions at the time of your first consultation. Before your second consultation, your body needs to begin responding and rebuilding energy stores. The physical demands will grow easier over time. When you and your physician meet again, together you will determine if you are ready to start your fitness plan. You will meet with a personal trainer and start phase I of the fitness regimen. For many, this maybe a walking program. For others interested in a more aggressive approach, you may move to phase II much quicker, if approved by your physician.

Make a plan.
You have probably tried exercise regimens before and achieved limited success. Since this program is customized just for you, have confidence that you can successfully reach the fitness goals set for you by the PreDiabetes Centers health coach and personal trainer.

An extensive physical and continuous biomarker blood testing will identify which parts of your health need attention, and whether or not there are any specific medical conditions that will limit your exercise regimen.

Your personal trainer will customize a plan tailored to fit your needs and will be available to address concerns and difficulties as you progress in the program.

Find physical activities you enjoy.
Exercise is essential, but not always fun. If you can stimulate your mind or accomplish other tasks while you exercise, it will seem like less of a burden. Here's a tip: Coordinate your regimen with a favorite TV show, or exercise outdoors or in an environment that inspires you.

Set aside time to exercise.
Don't let life's distractions prevent you from exercising. Set aside time for your workouts and keep

your appointment. It's easy to procrastinate, but every time you let yourself slide, you're one step closer to falling back into the old habits that led to prediabetes in the first place.

Find your motivation.

Don't let a few failures provide an excuse to give up on exercise. Exercise is hard! Finding the motivation and persistence to keep exercising is even more difficult. Remind yourself why you decided to finally a make a change in your life and let it serve as your inspiration.

Stop Smoking

Kicking a tobacco habit may be difficult, but it's imperative for good health. Your PreDiabetes Center team will address tobacco addiction. There are many tools for smoking cessation, including nicotine gums, lozenges and patches that can be an effective aid for some. There are also a number of medications that can help you quit smoking. Your physician will work closely with you to determine your best options.

Remedies for Sleep, Stress and Other Health Problems

In addition to nutrition and exercise, there are other factors in your life that will require attention, maybe for the first time. Poor sleep and stress are important co-factors in the development of diabetes. If you haven't considered these factors before, take time to consider how they are affecting both your health and quality of life.

Sleep

Sleep is important. Lack of quality sleep can affect the level of insulin in your body and cause you to become more hungry, creating one more obstacle on the road to wellness. Depending on the severity of this issue for you, your physician may wait to address this issue a little later in the program, allowing time for your body to adjust to the medical and lifestyle changes and determine how those may affect your sleep.

Stress

The hormone cortisol, also known as hydrocortisone, increases with stress. The main function of cortisol is to increase sugar in your blood. If you are prediabetic, it makes sense to avoid stress to regulate blood sugar levels.

Whether you choose yoga, pilates, cardiovascular exercise, classical music or some other relaxation technique, it's important to find a way to reduce the amount of stress in your life. Reducing stress will allow you to focus on the program.

Sleep and stress are discussed in much greater detail in other chapters of this book.

Improving Your Health with Supplements and Medication

There are a ton of supplements on the market. It can be difficult to know which are right for you and if they are actually helping. With biomarker testing, we will be able to determine your specific areas of need and address them with targeted supplements you can trust. With repeated testing, you'll be able to learn if the supplements are helping. Supplements are an effective tool in diabetes prevention and will most likely be a part of your personalized program.

In addition to the medications that you normally take, it's possible that your PreDiabetes Centers physician will prescribe medication to combat specific prediabetes-related health problems. Your treatment aims to use the least amount of medication needed to keep you on track with your health goals.

Getting Started

Beating diabetes won't be easy, but if you stay committed to the program, there is no reason why you can't succeed.

Your treatment planned will be paced to ensure your ability to remain compliant and for you to see long-term benefits. Don't get discouraged if you experience setbacks. They happen, and they're an important part of the learning process. Your health coach and doctor are here to make sure you succeed and they are an excellent information resource.

If you find that you are having trouble with a particular part of the program, let your doctor or health coach know. They have years of experience fighting diabetes and can teach you skills and strategies that will help you stick with the program and reverse the diabetes process.

Chapter 4

Your Personalized Treatment Plan

The PreDiabetes Centers PATHFinder program is a comprehensive, 12-month plan to halt your progression to type 2 diabetes and minimize the serious complications that are already occurring in your body. It requires aggressive treatment that encompasses all areas of your life, including dietary planning, nutritional supplementation, hormone optimization, medication support, sleep hygiene support, personalized fitness planning, and stress modulation. You can expect your health team to evaluate, re-evaluate and adjust your treatment plan throughout the 12 months in order to achieve your health goals and reverse the progression to diabetes.

Remember, treatment is an ongoing, positive process. If you follow the treatment plan designed by your physician and health coach, you will be on the path to a diabetes-free life!

Treatment Overview

Your treatment plan will be based on the results of a comprehensive assessment that includes a detailed medical and family history, physical examination and analysis of advanced biomarkers. Your health team will also perform nutritional and hormonal screening to identify underlying hormone imbalances, nutritional deficiencies, vascular abnormalities and inflammation.

You must be committed to remaining on schedule for your consultations with the physician and health coach. Five focused consultations are scheduled with your team that will average at least

30 minutes of dedicated one-on-one time with the physician. Each appointment will also include dedicated one-on-one time with your health coach that will range from 20 minutes to 1 hour, depending on the type of consultation. The timing of these consultations is important to ensure adequate time for you to begin treatment, for your body to show response to that treatment, to assess your response, and to adjust your prescribed therapy if necessary.

In addition, you will have the opportunity to work with a personal trainer who will conduct a fitness evaluation and develop a personalized fitness plan for you. The initial evaluation by the personal trainer will be scheduled after your first follow-up appointment, usually around the fourth month of treatment. During this consultation, you and your personal trainer will agree upon phase I of your fitness plan. You will be re-evaluated approximately 90 days later to determine if you are ready to begin phase II of the fitness plan. Each consultation will last one hour.

Before your first fitness consultation, start to think about how you will incorporate a new exercise regimen into your lifestyle that will keep you motivated and energized.

Your Health Coach

We understand there are many challenges on your path to avoid diabetes, and we plan on supporting you every step of the way. Your health coach is an invaluable partner in your journey to reverse the diabetes process.

The health coach will communicate with you continuously throughout the program, offering support, education, encouragement and guidance. We're focused on moving you to a healthier state as quickly as possible, and we understand that this may not be easy for you. Your treatment plan requires multiple changes, many of which need to occur simultaneously and immediately. Remember, many of your core issues are connected. Addressing only one area at a time will not produce the long-term benefits you need that are available in this program.

You will have scheduled telephone sessions with your health coach, and they will likely be more frequent and lengthier during the early phase of your program. This is the time when you will require more intense education, support and guidance until you achieve a level of success and confidence... one step at a time.

Here's how to prepare for your health coach teleconferences:

- ✓ Write down your questions before the call.
- ✓ Identify challenges and barriers you face and be prepared to freely discuss them with your health coach.
- ✓ Review your treatment plan and ask questions.
- ✓ Be prepared to discuss food shopping, meal preparation, physical activity, sleep, stress and energy levels.
- ✓ Discuss any issues you may have adhering to your medication or supplement regimen.
- ✓ Have your calendar in front of you to schedule your next teleconference and confirm your next scheduled blood draw and visit.

Stay Connected at Your Convenience

We offer a private Client Portal that you may access through a login on our website where you can review educational materials and communicate with your PreDiabetes Center team. Think of the portal as a private room where you can address questions or issues and learn more about your health. Based on your specific concerns or goals, your health coach may upload educational materials and recommend that you view them through the Client Portal. You also may view your lab work after reviewing with your physician, log your dietary intake and workout sessions, schedule an appointment, and order nutraceuticals or prescription refills. We have made all of these activities as convenient and seamless as possible.

Have a question for your health coach or physician? Through the portal you have the opportunity to send an email directly to your health coach, ensuring timely response to meet your needs.

We will add informative articles to the portal to help you on your treatment journey. We also offer a library of three-minute educational videos that cover a variety of topics, including:

- Food preparation techniques
- Biomarker discussions
- Tips and strategies to succeed
- Sleep hygiene tips
- Stress management techniques

... And more!

Your Outcomes and Long-Term Success

The PreDiabetes Center will monitor your progress by measuring changes in key biomarkers and other metrics. This is accomplished at every visit. Together, you and your physician will determine your response to therapy and examine whether adjustments are required to achieve your health goals. Many adjustments may need to be made throughout the 12 months. This is expected in order to achieve long-term, sustainable health goals.

Additionally, clients have the option of entering a maintenance program at the program's end in order to maintain good health. As you age or experience major life changes, or perhaps fail to maintain good habits, you may find yourself at risk of diabetes once again. If life events alter your health pathway and you are in need of assistance, you're not alone. Support, guidance and encouragement from a partner—a specialized medical team—help tremendously. We're your partner for life if necessary.

Chapter 5

Managing Expectations and Goals

Your personalized treatment plan is based on a proactive treatment and disease prevention program with objective, measurable outcomes. It is based on proven clinical guidelines and emerging scientific knowledge. This program is not designed to be a quick fix; it has taken many years to develop prediabetes and reversing where you are will not happen overnight.

You will need to be vigilant to avoid diabetes and its long-term complications. You must also be prepared to work hard to achieve lifelong health.

Setting Your Expectations

Your personalized treatment plan will include both short- and long-term goals. Your PreDiabetes Centers physician and health coach will spend much time, especially in the beginning, reviewing your test results, physical assessments and personal goals when building your personalized treatment plan. They will also work one-on-one with you throughout the 12-month program to educate you about insulin dynamics, hormonal imbalances, inflammation, vascular integrity and other core influencers, and how each affects your health.

You will most likely have many questions regarding the program and what you need to do. Your health coach will be available to answer these questions, and he or she also will reach out to you directly between your appointments. Some telephonic coaching calls will be scheduled so that you and your health coach can manage time effectively. Additional sessions at the PreDiabetes Center may also be scheduled.

Short-term goals are based on the results of your medical history, fitness and nutritional background, initial comprehensive exam, and comprehensive blood tests. Your physician will review this data and determine your supplementation and possible medication needs. Your health coach will look at this data and, based on your preferences and personal schedule, determine your specific program needs.

Improving your health and blood results is first on the agenda. It's your responsibility to keep your appointments, complete any forms, logs or questionnaires, and review material given to you to better understand how all the core elements affect your current health.

You will need to set up new routines and healthy habits that have been discussed with your health coach. This includes the intermittent use of a client-monitoring device that is provided to you to help monitor your activity level and food intake. *We ask that you make every effort to succeed even when setbacks occur or when you think the results are not happening fast enough.*

Your health coach will work with you to help you better understand the nutrition and fitness components of your program, and make sure you have all the tools and information you need to follow the PURE and VITALITY nutrition plans. The PreDiabetes Centers personal trainer will work with you one-on-one to design a customized fitness program specifically based on your individual needs and preferences.

Long-term goals are focused on integrating all components of your PreDiabetes Centers personalized program to address the factors contributing to your metabolic imbalance. This includes continued biomarker measurement and comparison to previous results, office consultations with your physician and health coach, and ongoing medication, supplemental and nutritional support. You and your health care team will also work to enhance core influencers such as stress reduction and sleep efficiency, and your personal trainer will continue to review your fitness program progress.

Lifelong good health is your ultimate goal. To achieve this, you must commit to the health plan that is created for you. This will take discipline and perseverance. Changing unhealthy habits can be difficult and disruptive, so focusing on long-term success will be critical. Count on having setbacks. Recognize this and commit to doing the work required to attain your healthiest self possible.

Anticipate significant changes to your current lifestyle, but with these changes comes substantial rewards! Becoming and staying healthy in today's world takes enormous effort. We understand this and are here to guide you through the entire process to ensure your success.

Learn How to Manage Change

Any change can be stressful. It pushes us out of our comfort zone and makes us confront our fears. Change also generates uncertainty, which can mean a loss of control and loss of predictability. How you manage change determines whether or not you are successful with it. If you view change as an opportunity for improvement with benefits that outweigh the cost of not changing, then you are much more likely to incorporate that change into your life.

A lifestyle change is a major event that impacts every aspect of who you are–your physical, mental and emotional well-being. By planning for major changes and understanding and analyzing the obstacles, you are more likely to succeed.

Think about your decision to commit to the PreDiabetes Centers PATHFinder program. What prompted this? Often, it's having seen first-hand the reality of living with diabetes. Watching a family member or friend check blood sugar multiple times throughout the day, or perhaps suffer the loss of a limb due to diabetic complications, can be a strong catalyst for change.

The next step is to prepare for change. This necessitates an understanding of all that will need to be done to implement the change. It requires not only tending to the physical issues, but also the self-awareness and understanding of potential emotional barriers that may need to be resolved. Understanding what may be holding you back is essential at this juncture.

You've decided to address your prediabetes. Perhaps you have tried to eat better in the past, but found nutrition confusing and somewhat overwhelming. You may even have felt frustrated that you failed at past attempts. Your health coach will work closely with you on nutritional education and provide you with PURE and VITALITY meal planning guidelines and resources to ensure your success with Concierge Nutrition.

From here, action is taken. Studies show that changing a habit takes approximately 45 days. If the change is too overwhelming or if you are not well prepared, the desired change can fail. An important concept during the action phase is to remember to take small, incremental steps to increase the odds of success.

Actively participate in your change. Visualize what you want to become, how you will look, how you will act, and how you will feel with this change.

The last stage in managing change is learning how to maintain it. This is when you practice your behavior every day and recognize it as a new part of who you are. Remember, change is dynamic, and even when you are successful in making a change, that change is never complete or over.

As you near the 12-month mark of the program, you should recognize significant improvements in your health. You will feel better and have positive blood results, greater muscle mass, and healthier nutrition and daily habits. All of these outcomes are based on your success in managing change.

Setting Your Goals

As part of the process of regaining control over your health, it's vital that realistic goals are determined. These goals should be specific, measurable and achievable, and shouldn't be in conflict with other aspirations. Your health coach will work with you to determine your personal program goals. It's important that these goals meet not only the program objectives, but are also your desired goals.

The health coach offers a fresh perspective and can teach you more effective ways of thinking about your desired outcomes. He or she is your center of support and will assist you along your journey.

Be sure to create a personal support system that can provide you with the emotional support and understanding to help you feel good about the changes you are making. The people you choose for your support system should encourage you, especially during difficult stages or setbacks. Their support helps you maintain your changes and keeps you on track to a healthier lifestyle. Some may feel threatened by your new habits, so sharing your goals with close friends and family is essential.

Goals for each objective will be broken down into smaller, short-term goals to make them more manageable. Each short-term goal will have action steps associated with it so that you know exactly what you need to do in order to succeed. An example of this is the PURE nutrition plan that you will adopt at the start of the program. To begin your nutritional transformation, your goal will be to eat only foods from this plan for 10 days. The PURE nutrition plan consists of whole, nutrient-dense foods that will re-nourish your body. Menus, recipes, food choices and substitutes will be provided. You will also be given tips on how to shop for groceries and stock your pantry.

As you progress through the year, it will be important to keep the momentum and excitement of the first few months going. Feedback in the form of positive biomarker results, inevitable weight loss and greater stamina will help maintain your continued efforts.

It's also important to give yourself a pat on the back as you meet your smaller objectives. Be kind to yourself and allow small celebrations along the way. This may be treating yourself to flowers, a massage or a night at the movies to acknowledge your success.

Evaluation of your predetermined goals is critical. Where do you stand three, six or nine months into the program? Are your biomarkers trending in a positive direction? What can be done to augment your results? How do you feel physically? Are you eating foods that are satisfying? Does your personalized exercise plan still meet your needs?

Often, we lose sight of where we started and how we felt in the beginning. It's important to step back and evaluate your progress throughout the year. Focus on the journey and not the final result. Try to make your new habits an enjoyable process as you assimilate them into your everyday life.

Understanding Challenges

Inevitably, there will be setbacks throughout the year. It's important to recognize that this will happen and it does not mean you are a failure. Treat setbacks as a means to learn from your mistakes. With the help of your health coach, you can analyze what went wrong, alter your strategies and get back on track. Having a setback actually can be a good thing–it teaches you perseverance and commitment. By challenging yourself, taking chances and trying new things, you may risk failure. But the overall reward of optimal health is much greater.

Understand the big picture of what you are trying to accomplish. Small setbacks during major life changes are just that—minor setbacks. Diabetes is not inevitable. You are taking the steps to avoid diabetes and chronic disease, and you will be successful in the long run.

Maintaining Your Results

Once you complete the 12-month PreDiabetes PATHFinder program you will begin a maintenance period that can be just as important, if not more, in sustaining your results.

Your success ultimately resides with you. We offer you the comprehensive, dynamic solution to a fuller, healthier life, but you are responsible for making this life change and sustaining it. It's your lifelong plan for health and wellness.

Methods to maintain your success include:

- ✓ **Close monitoring** of your biomarkers and responding early and quickly to negative trending results
- ✓ **Quarterly** physician consultations
- ✓ **Health coach outreach** on a regular basis to provide education and support
- ✓ **Ongoing** online and group education on a variety of topics
- ✓ **Continued use** of a patient-tracking device to monitor your activity and nutrition
- ✓ **Participation** in a support group
- ✓ **Continued access** to your medical record through our Client Portal

Chapter **6**

Understanding Your Medical Evaluation

The PreDiabetes Centers PATHFinder program begins with a comprehensive medical evaluation by a PreDiabetes Center physician. The physician will assess your overall health and identify any deficiencies or risk factors for disease progression. Based on results from the initial evaluation, the physician will formulate your personalized health plan. Subsequent follow-up visits will help your physician and health coach monitor your progress and adjust treatment based on your response.

During the initial medical evaluation, the physician will perform a comprehensive physical examination and review your medical history, noting your current health conditions, medications (prescription and over-the-counter), drug allergies and prior immunizations. Your physician will want to know if you:

- Have had prior surgeries or hospitalizations, especially hysterectomy or prostatectomy
- Take any vitamins or supplements
- Smoke cigarettes
- Drink alcohol or caffeine

Your physician also will assess family medical history, with attention to a history of diabetes and other medical conditions. Research shows that having a family history of diabetes significantly increases risk for prediabetes and diabetes. Also, a family history of high cholesterol may have predisposed you to high cholesterol and other cardiovascular risks, which are associated conditions of prediabetes. Your personalized treatment plan will incorporate treatment of these conditions.

Your physician will conduct a review of your organ systems in a physical assessment and biomarker assessment. Symptoms that you would want to discuss with your physician include numbness in feet or hands, vision changes and increased thirst or urination. To understand the complexity of the symptom evaluation, consider your energy level. For many, a decreased energy level may be thought of as nothing more than a sign of age, exhaustion, increased weight, or poor diet. While all of these can be contributing factors, we consider other core issues such as an improperly functioning thyroid gland, a condition that could affect your energy levels. Hormones are produced by the thyroid and other glands, so a thorough hormone system evaluation will be conducted.

An organ systems evaluation is critical, as one dysfunctional system in the body often affects other organ systems. For example, your adrenal glands or pituitary gland may affect how your body responds to stress. They also have a direct effect on how your body uses sugar (glucose) and fat for energy. Reporting symptoms that you are experiencing is helpful for the physician to pinpoint the cause of illness.

Next, the physician will perform a physical examination to check for signs of heart, liver, kidney and lung diseases. Elevated blood pressure will be followed closely as this is a common condition among prediabetics and raises the risk for complications such as kidney disease and cardiovascular disease. The physician also will administer a neurological examination to check for nerve damage, or diabetic neuropathy, a common problem among diabetics that may be developing in a person with prediabetes. The physician will pay special attention to the eyes using an opthalmoscope, which examines small blood vessels in the eye and damage that can result from prolonged elevation of blood sugar. The physician will measure whether the patient has lost nerve function in the extremities. Examination of the skin may reveal wounds that have been slow to heal, which can be related to elevated blood sugars.

Additionally, baseline weight and waist circumference will be measured. The use of waist circumference has become an important biometric to follow since abdominal fat loss is one goal of the PreDiabetes Centers treatment plan.

Biomarkers: What Do They Say About My Health?

PreDiabetes Centers understands that a complex disease like prediabetes requires comprehensive assessments. To get a more holistic, upstream view of your health status and diabetes risk, PreDiabetes Centers uses an advanced analysis of biomarkers, which are proteins, chemicals and other substances found in the bloodstream that can be measured and used to indicate disease or other aspects of health.

Some biomarkers that you may recognize include cholesterol, estrogen and glucose. Biomarkers are usually evaluated as groups of tests, or panels, associated with different health conditions. There are cardiovascular panels, metabolic panels, liver panels and more. With mainstream medical practice, typically a panel or two of these blood tests are ordered and maybe some additional biomarkers. PreDiabetes Centers has a more comprehensive approach: We monitor dozens of biomarkers associated with prediabetic conditions, such as C-peptide, leptin and adiponectin.

Your initial comprehensive biomarker panel allows you and your doctor to recognize negative processes in the body–early signs of disease–that may be symptomless and aren't yet detectable in traditional screenings. Identifying these problems early on will help your physician effectively treat and reverse prediabetic processes before they progress to advanced levels.

Biomarker levels often change in a predictable pattern and at predictable levels when a person heads down the path to diabetes. By measuring these levels, PreDiabetes Centers will be able to customize a treatment plan for you and your unique metabolic functioning. We will monitor how your body is responding to lifestyle changes and medical treatment implemented in the program.

As mentioned before, the treatment plan will measure and optimize these areas of function:

- **Insulin dynamics.** An evaluation of how well your pancreas is functioning and how your body is responding to insulin.

- **Hormone balance.** How your hormones are affecting your metabolism, if they are causing inflammation and their status of optimization.

- **Inflammation.** Examines whether there is excessive inflammation in your body. Too much can eventually lead to diabetes and cardiovascular disease.

- **Vascular integrity.** Evaluating the vascular status including good and bad cholesterol, triglycerides and other abnormal markers that contribute to diabetes and associated conditions. If you are prediabetic, your vascular health may already be damaged.

- **Core influencers.** How sleep, stress, relaxation, social support and education are affecting your condition.

Think of your comprehensive initial lab testing as a snapshot of your body's biomarkers at the start of your journey towards wellness. This initial testing and follow-up testing will serve as a roadmap that enables you and your health care team to assess your progress throughout the program.

Your Guide to Biomarker Tests

The biomarkers included in the initial panel cover a wide array of body processes and organ systems. Some of the most important markers we measure are those that are linked to your body's management of and response to glucose–what we call "insulin dynamics." Additional tests help us monitor biomarkers associated with prediabetic conditions, including other endocrine disorders (diseases related to endocrine glands, which produce the majority of hormones) and cardiovascular disease.

Insulin Dynamics

The biomarker tests that measure your insulin dynamics will yield the most critical information in understanding your pancreatic function and how your body is responding to insulin and glucose. The results of these tests help your physician monitor prediabetic conditions in your body, including insulin resistance and metabolic syndrome, which is a group of risk factors related to obesity that occur together and increase risk for type 2 diabetes.

Insulin Dynamic Biomarker	Why Is It Important?
Glucose	A type of sugar that serves as a major source of energy for most of the body's cells. High or low levels of glucose can cause health problems. It's important to keep blood glucose levels steady.
Hemoglobin A1c	Hemoglobin A1c identifies the average amount of glucose in the blood for the past 2-3 months. High levels indicate your metabolism is not functioning effectively.
Insulin	A hormone that helps glucose get into the body's cells where it can be used for energy. High levels after fasting overnight indicate that your body is not processing glucose effectively.
C-peptide	A byproduct produced in the pancreas in equal amounts to insulin. A C-peptide test can determine how much insulin the body is producing.
Proinsulin	Elevated levels of proinsulin indicate that the pancreas is working extra hard to control blood sugar.
Proinsulin-to-insulin ratio	Proinsulin-to-insulin ratio helps identify people who are more insulin resistant. A high ratio is a risk factor for type 2 diabetes and also indicates faster progression to type 2 diabetes.

Vascular Integrity

Your insulin dynamics, especially increased blood glucose levels, affect your cardiovascular health. Individuals with diabetes are at least twice as likely to have heart disease or a stroke, compared to people without diabetes. Diabetics with cardiovascular disease have a higher risk for serious health problems, including:

- Strokes at an earlier age
- More extensive coronary artery disease, a narrowing of the blood vessels that supply blood and oxygen to the heart
- A higher rate of death and disability following a heart attack or stroke, the most common causes of death in both men and women with diabetes

Over time, high levels of blood glucose can result in the accumulation of fatty materials on the insides of blood vessel walls. These deposits slow blood flow, increasing the chance of clogging and hardening of blood vessels (atherosclerosis).

Weight gain around the abdominal area, high blood pressure and tobacco use can also worsen blood vessel health in people with diabetes.

People with diabetes have elevated levels of inflammation in the body, including their arterial walls, which results in blood vessel changes leading to heart disease. Many of the disorders afflicting people with prediabetes–such as central obesity, insulin resistance, cardiovascular disease, and metabolic syndrome–are associated with a pro-inflammatory state.

The biomarker tests measure multiple cardiovascular biomarkers to give you a better picture of your risk of atherosclerosis–which, in turn, affects vessels of the kidney, brain and almost every other organ.

"Good" and "Bad" Cholesterol

Cholesterol is a lipid that is found in food and also produced by the liver. It's needed to make hormones, build cell walls and help digest fat. Some types of cholesterol boost heart health, such as "good" high-density lipoprotein (HDL) cholesterol. Others are not so good, such as "bad" low-density lipoprotein (LDL) cholesterol and triglycerides.

Typical lipid lab panels administered at your doctor's office check HDL levels. However, much more information is gleaned by looking at components and types of HDL, LDL and very low-density lipoprotein (VLDL).

Vascular Integrity Biomarker	Why Is It Important?
Total HDL	Total HDL refers to all of the HDL cholesterol in the blood. HDL helps protect against heart disease, so high levels are desirable.
High-density lipoprotein-2 (HDL_2)	This is the most protective form of HDL cholesterol. The higher the level, the more protection against cardiovascular disease.
High-density lipoprotein-3 (HDL_3)	This type of cholesterol has slightly less protective power than HDL_2. High levels of HDL_3 are desirable.
Apolipoprotein A1 (Apo A1)	Apo A1 helps to clear cholesterol from the body. Low levels are a better indicator of cardiovascular risk than HDL cholesterol.
Total LDL	Total LDL is the unhealthy cholesterol that promotes cardiovascular disease. Low levels are desirable.
Lipoprotein(a) (Lp(a))	Lp(a) is a form of unhealthy cholesterol that's 10 times worse than LDL cholesterol. High levels increase risk of heart attack at a younger age. Aggressive treatment is necessary to decrease risk.
Intermediate density lipoprotein (IDL)	People with diabetes and prediabetes may have higher levels of IDL, a type of cholesterol that can promote atherosclerosis, a hardening of the arteries.

Vascular Integrity Biomarker	Why Is It Important?
LDL pattern	LDL pattern indicates how large or small your LDL cholesterol particles are. If most are small, you are at higher risk for cardiovascular disease. Pattern B people have small, sticky LDL cholesterol that attaches easily to arteries, promoting cardiovascular disease. Pattern A, with larger, less sticky LDL cholesterol, is desired.
Apolipoprotein B100 (Apo B100)	Apo B100 is a part of unhealthy LDL cholesterol. Low levels are desirable.
ApoB100/ApoA1 ratio	This ratio helps to understand whether healthy or unhealthy cholesterol is dominant. A high level is associated with increased risk for cardiovascular disease, metabolic syndrome and insulin resistance.
Very low-density lipoprotein (VLDL)	VLDL is one of the major classes of cholesterol. It contains the most triglyceride (fat) and increases risk for cardiovascular disease. Low levels are desirable.
Remnant lipoproteins	High levels of remnant lipoproteins are seen in people with diabetes and are an early sign of the shift to smaller cholesterol particles and increased risk for heart attack and stroke.
Non-HDL cholesterol	The total amount of all bad forms of cholesterol (LDL and VLDL). Non-HDL cholesterol is a risk factor for cardiovascular disease, so low levels are desired.
Triglycerides	Triglycerides are measured as a reflection of fat ingestion and metabolism. People with prediabetes and diabetes are more prone to high triglyceride levels, which increases cardiovascular disease risk.

Hormone Balance

Glands make up your endocrine system, producing hormones that are released into your bloodstream that help the body's organs perform their particular jobs, such as regulating metabolism and overseeing the reproductive process. Checking these biomarkers helps recognize if your hormones are working with you or against you. The metabolic glands we assess in the initial lab panel include:

- Pancreas
- Adrenal glands
- Thyroid gland
- Reproductive glands (ovaries and testes)

The pancreas and its hormones, insulin and C-peptide, are critical in the evaluation of hormonal biomarkers. Other biomarkers measured include fat-related biomarkers, adrenal biomarkers, thyroid biomarkers and sex-hormone biomarkers.

Fat-Related Biomarkers

Most people who want to lose weight would like to lose subcutaneous fat, which lies under the skin and is often referred to as "love handles" or "saddlebags." Subcutaneous fat isn't harmful. What's really dangerous is fat that lies deep in the abdomen next to your organs, also known as visceral fat. This deep abdominal fat puts pressure on the kidneys, which are already suffering from the damaging effects of prediabetes.

Fat cells release the hormone leptin, a biomarker that plays a key role in appetite and metabolism. Leptin sends signals to the brain that you're full and should stop eating. However, with obese individuals, their bodies don't receive or respond to leptin signals. This is called "leptin resistance," which is similar to insulin resistance.

Adiponectin is a hormone secreted from fat cells that contributes to a healthy metabolism. Low levels are a risk factor for metabolic syndrome and type 2 diabetes. Adiponectin has many protective, health-promoting effects including making the body more sensitive to insulin, protecting blood vessels, helping with weight loss and controlling energy metabolism.

Adrenal Biomarkers

Another important biomarker we measure is cortisol, called the "stress hormone." When you experience physical and emotional stress, you release high amounts of cortisol due to this overstimulation of the adrenal glands. Elevated levels of cortisol may hurt your metabolism and cause insulin resistance and inflammation. But like other harmful processes occurring in your body, it can be stopped with proper lifestyle changes, including stress reduction and improved sleep.

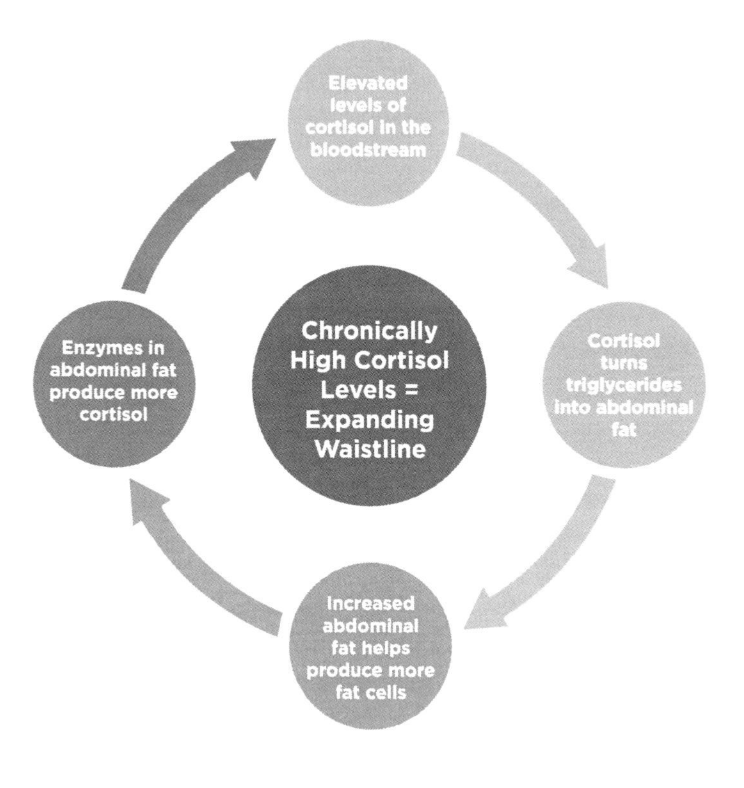

Thyroid Biomarkers

The thyroid is the organ that helps set your metabolism and regulates how quickly or slowly you burn energy. If your thyroid produces an excess of these hormones, your metabolism revs too high, leading to a condition called hyperthyroidism. Too few of the thyroid hormones can cause you to burn energy too slowly and may result in hypothyroidism, which can contribute to weight gain. When initiating a weight-loss program, it's important to assess for metabolic causes of weight gain, like hypothyroidism.

Thyroid disease, like diabetes, is a metabolic disorder. Testing for thyroid dysfunction in people with prediabetes is important because the two conditions are often present together.

Sex Hormone Biomarkers

Puberty, hot flashes, menopause... these life events are caused by changes in the levels and balance of sex hormones. There are "male" and "female" sex hormones that every person has, but levels of these hormones differ between genders. Levels will also vary if a woman is experiencing pre-, peri- and postmenopause. Understanding the normal variations in hormone levels is helpful in understanding your results. Sex hormone biomarkers not only impact your sex organs, they have far-reaching effects that impact your response to insulin and glucose metabolism.

One of the most common causes of obesity in women is polycystic ovary syndrome (PCOS), characterized by elevated levels of androgens, particularly testosterone. Increased levels of testosterone are produced by the ovaries in response to higher circulating levels of insulin in the blood. Subsequently, the testosterone is converted to estrogens in the fat tissue, leading to symptoms of estrogen dominance and progesterone deficiency. Women with PCOS are at higher risk of diabetes, metabolic syndrome, heart disease, high blood pressure, and uterine cancer.

Testosterone is an important biomarker measured in men and women, Men have higher levels of testosterone, and levels tend to decrease with age in both genders. Decreased levels are associated with muscle and bone loss and increased fat storage, which raises the risk for diabetes.

Insulin resistance can lead to high insulin levels and reduce the amount of available testosterone, which may affect libido and sexual performance. To treat sexual dysfunction, you must first identify contributing factors, like low testosterone levels.

Hormone Balance Biomarker	Why Is It Important?
Leptin	A hormone released by healthy fat cells that helps to control appetite. Chronically high leptin levels can cause the body to stop responding to its effects, which can cause overeating and weight gain.
Adiponectin	This hormone helps break down lipids and glucose and fights inflammation in blood vessels. People who are overweight have low levels of this hormone.
Resistin	As fat cells become unhealthy, they release more of this hormone. Resistin promotes inflammation and insulin resistance. Low levels are desirable.

Hormone Balance Biomarker	Why Is It Important?
Cortisol	A hormone released in the body in response to stress. It works against insulin, increasing blood sugar levels.
Triiodothyronine (T3) and thyroxine (T4)	T3 and T4 are produced by the thyroid and help set your metabolism. An excess of these hormones causes your metabolism to rev too high, leading to a condition called hyperthyroidism. Too few of the thyroid hormones causes you to burn energy too slowly, resulting in hypothyroidism.
Thyroid stimulating hormone (TSH)	Produced in the pituitary gland, TSH indicates how well your thyroid is functioning.
Thyroid microsomal antibody	Elevated levels of this antibody, also known as the thyroid perioxidase antibody (TPO), could indicate that the body's own immune system is harming the thyroid gland.
Total testosterone	Total testosterone is all testosterone in the blood.
Free testosterone	This is testosterone available for immediate use.
Sex hormone binding globulin (SHBG)	SHBG binds with both testosterone and estrogen (estradiol) and carries them through the bloodstream. Reduced levels of testosterone in combination with low levels of SHBG can put you at risk for metabolic syndrome.
Estradiol	Estradiol is a type of estrogen produced by the body. In women, estrogen is produced by visceral fat cells, so overweight women may have high levels. Overweight men may also have high levels because testosterone converts to estradiol. This can result in low testosterone levels and feminizing effects in men.

Hormone Balance Biomarker	Why Is It Important?
Luteinizing hormone (LH) and follicle-stimulating hormone (FSH)	LH and FSH are produced by the pituitary gland. In women, they promote ovulation and stimulate secretion of estradiol and progesterone from the ovaries. Increased levels of LH and FSH are associated with menopause or a decrease in ovarian function. High levels of LH, when compared to FSH, may be indicative of PCOS.
Total prostate-specific antigen (PSA)	Total PSA is not a sex hormone, rather it's a protein produced by cells of the prostate gland. Levels of this biomarker may be increased in prostate cancer, benign prostatic hyperplasia (BPH) and prostatitis (inflammation of the prostate).

Inflammation Biomarkers

The immune system is constantly defending against infectious diseases, autoimmune disorders, atherosclerosis and other diseases. More evidence points to chronic activation of the immune system (also known as chronic inflammation) as the cause of a host of diseases, including cardiovascular disease, diabetes and metabolic syndrome. Assessing for elevated levels of certain biomarkers can help identify the presence and degree of inflammation in your body.

High-sensitivity C-reactive protein (CRP) is an important biomarker. High levels of CRP indicate inflammation. Insulin resistance may also spur the release of CRP. Research shows that elevated levels of CRP doubles the risk of developing diabetes, compared to those with normal CRP levels, and is an important predictor of cardiovascular risk.

Inflammation Biomarker	Why Is It Important?
High-sensitivity C-reactive protein (CRP)	High levels of CRP indicate inflammation.
Tumor necrosis factor alpha (TNF-alpha)	TNF-alpha measures inflammation and may be elevated in some people with prediabetes. Studies show a link between TNF-alpha and the development of type 2 diabetes in insulin-resistant people.
Interleukin-6 (IL-6)	IL-6 is an immune system protein that may be elevated in prediabetes, cardiovascular disease and obesity.
Interleukin-8 (IL-8)	IL-8 is an immune system protein that may be elevated in prediabetes, cardiovascular disease and obesity.
Plasminogen activator inhibitor type 1 (PAI-1)	PAI-1 is an enzyme that prevents the breakdown of blood clots. These levels are increased in obesity, insulin resistance, smoking and metabolic syndrome, and are associated with increased blood clotting in people with these conditions.
Homocysteine	An amino acid found in the blood that's affected by both diet and genetics. Elevated levels are a risk factor for heart disease, stroke and other diseases involving plaque formation to the arteries.

Other Important Biomarkers

Hematology Biomarkers
Hematology biomarkers are measured in a complete blood count (CBC) panel. Abnormal lab results can reflect conditions such as anemia, infection, dehydration, and problems with blood clotting. When people suffer from significantly high levels of blood glucose, dehydration can result.

Nutritional Biomarkers
Nutritional biomarkers provide valuable information about whether you're getting enough (or too much) vital nutrients. Some nutritional deficiencies, like vitamin D, have close ties to prediabetes.

Many people have an iron deficiency, especially women in the years leading up to menopause. Anemia is the fallout from iron deficiency and is usually identified by looking at a person's hemoglobin and hematocrit. Both low and high levels of iron are a problem.

Uric acid is created by our bodies when we eat proteins and foods containing a compound called purine, found in red meat, organ meats, asparagus, mushrooms and many other food sources. It's not uncommon for people with prediabetes to have high levels of uric acid. Fructose (think high fructose corn syrup) in your diet can also cause elevations in uric acid levels. Having high levels of uric acid may lead to kidney stones and a related condition of diabetes called gout, a type of arthritis.

There are strong ties between elevated uric acid levels, obesity and metabolic syndrome. Excess uric acid also can promote chronic, low-level inflammation in your blood vessels, causing the vessels to narrow.

Kidney Biomarkers
Prediabetes makes the kidneys vulnerable and can eventually lead to kidney failure. This happens because high blood glucose levels damage the small blood vessels in the kidneys, the vital organs that filter waste and water from the bloodstream and excrete them as urine.

Liver Biomarkers
The liver's main job is to break down and remove harmful substances, such as alcohol and other

chemicals. Liver biomarkers are used to detect disease or damage to the liver or bile ducts, which carry digestive fluid from the liver. If a duct becomes blocked–by a gallstone, for example–waste can build up in the bile duct system and bloodstream.

Fat accumulation in the liver is dangerous. Fatty liver or non-alcoholic steatorrhea (NASH) impairs the liver's function. NASH often shows up in overweight individuals with high cholesterol or triglycerides who have insulin resistance. The fat that accumulates can cause inflammation and scarring in the liver, which can lead to permanent liver damage. In fact, NASH is one of the leading causes of cirrhosis.

Other Important Biomarker	Why Is It Important?
Hematology biomarker **Complete blood count (CBC)**	CBC looks at your red blood cells, white blood cells and platelets. Abnormalities can indicate a variety of diseases including infection and anemia. Anemia is important to correct before starting an exercise program.
Hematology biomarker **White blood cell (WBC)**	WBC count evaluates your body's immune system response.
Hematology biomarker **WBC differential**	A WBC differential analyzes the amounts of each type of WBC (neutrophils, monocytes, basophils, lymphocytes, and eosinophils). Elevated levels of WBCs are typically seen in response to a sudden onset of infection, trauma or inflammation. People with diabetes or prediabetes may be more susceptible to infections, cuts and bruises, and tend to heal slower.
Hematology biomarker **Platelet count**	Platelets are a type of blood cell involved in blood clotting. Individuals with prediabetes are at an increased risk for developing blood clots, and an elevated platelet count can raise this risk.

Other Important Biomarker	Why Is It Important?
Nutritional biomarker **Uric acid**	Uric acid levels can be elevated in people with prediabetes and can lead to gout, an arthritic condition.
Nutritional biomarker **Vitamin D**	Vitamin D is stored in fat tissues, making it difficult for the body to access and use the vitamin. Obesity combined with vitamin D deficiency puts people at even higher risk for insulin resistance.
Nutritional biomarker **Calcium**	Low levels of calcium in your blood can coincide with low vitamin D.
Nutritional biomarker **Vitamin B12**	Vitamin B12 helps protect against nerve damage, a complication of diabetes. Low levels can cause homocysteine levels to rise, increasing risk for cardiovascular disease. Low levels contribute to depression and anemia.
Kidney biomarker **Blood urea nitrogen (BUN)**	BUN indicates how well the kidneys are removing waste from the body. Kidney damage is a complication of prediabetes.
Kidney biomarker **Creatinine**	Creatinine helps you to understand how well the kidneys are removing waste from the body. Kidney damage is a complication of prediabetes.
Kidney biomarker **Estimated glomerular filtration rate (EGFR)**	EGFR can indicate kidney disease, an associated condition of diabetes. The lower EGFR rate, the more severe the disease.
Kidney biomarker **Chloride (Cl)**	Chloride is important in water distribution and general cell function.

Other Important Biomarker	Why Is It Important?
Kidney biomarker **Potassium (K)**	Potassium levels are tightly controlled and play a role in the electrical conduction in nerve, muscle and heart tissues.
Kidney biomarker **Sodium (Na)**	Sodium works with other electrolytes in the body to help regulate the amount of fluid in the body. When you're dehydrated, it means you have increased sodium levels and excess fluid in the body.
Kidney biomarker **Carbon dioxide (CO2)**	CO2 is good indicator of how much acid versus base is in your body. Lower-than-normal levels are common in acidosis (including diabetic ketoacidosis, kidney disease and severe diarrhea) or breathing disorders.
Liver biomarker **Alanine aminotransferase (ALT), aspartate aminotransferase (AST) and alkaline phosphatase (ALP)**	High levels of ALT, AST and ALP may indicate that your liver tissue is experiencing inflammation.
Liver biomarker **Bilirubin**	Elevelated levels of bilirubin can indicate liver disease.
Liver biomarker **Albumin**	Albumin is a good measure of liver function. Decreased levels can indicate an injured or diseased liver or kidney disease.
Liver biomarker **Total protein test**	A total protein test is used to measure albumin and all other proteins in the blood. Total protein levels are used in the evaluation of nutritional status and many diseases.
Liver biomarker **Globulins**	Globulins play an important role in helping to fight infection.

Other Important Biomarker	Why Is It Important?
Liver biomarker **Albumin-globulin ratio**	The ratio of albumin to globulin helps identify the presence of liver and kidney diseases.

How Biomarker Results Are Applied to Your Treatment Plan

You've completed the comprehensive initial biomarker testing, so what happens next?

Your physician will point out associations in the biomarker results to identify actual or potential disease processes–the upstream view of your health status. For example, you might have some elevated inflammation and increased liver enzymes, suggesting the presence of a liver disorder. Additionally, if your weight-related biomarkers indicate a large degree of fat versus lean tissue, you could have fatty liver disease, which may account for the liver inflammation.

Your health care team will customize a treatment plan for you based, in part, on their assessment of these initial biomarker results. Your health will be assessed continuously, and what's important is the rate of change over time–not on any single measurement.

Your physician and health coach will continue to evaluate key biomarkers to reassess your response to treatments. With each successive test, the information becomes more powerful, enabling your health care team to identify which types of treatment are improving your health and steering your away from prediabetes and diabetes.

If your initial lab testing reveals out-of-range results in your liver biomarkers, your physician might order testing for hepatitis. If you are on testosterone therapy, additional sex hormone biomarkers will be measured in order to assess the effectiveness of this supplementation. Lastly, the physician may order testing on any number of additional biomarkers based on your test results.

Improving Your Biomarker Numbers

Comprehensive treatment, hard work, commitment and improved education will help you reverse the onset of diabetes. Throughout the 12-month program, you will feel better, have more energy and achieve significant overall health improvement. Your biomarkers will start to improve, indicating less visceral fat cells producing less pro-inflammatory markers, which, in turn, allows for improved insulin sensitivity. This leads to improvement of your insulin dynamics, moving you further away from diabetes.

The long-term affects are profound. Moving from prediabetes to a healthy state minimizes the natural aging process. Since the conditions associated with prediabetes are recognized early and treated effectively, the additional risk of associated diseases, such as early atherosclerosis, is minimized. Your quality of life will grow dramatically, and you will know how to protect yourself from the devastating consequences of diabetes.

Defeating prediabetes and living a long, healthy life is your reward.

Concierge Nutrition

Concierge
Nutrition

Chapter 7

Total Nutrition

Most Americans are overfed and undernourished, which has contributed to an epidemic of obesity and type 2 diabetes. It turns out, you really are what you eat: Food can make you sick or help keep you healthy.

Healthy and balanced nutrition means eating the right type of foods to help the body function optimally. Good nutrition provides energy, promotes good sleep, prevents disease, and gives the body what it needs to stay healthy.

Here's a rundown of key nutrients, what they do for the body and the best food sources for each nutrient.

The Skinny on Fat

Fats are an important part of any diet. They support several functions in the body, acting as essential nutrients that provide energy to your body. Fats also produce hormones that are vital to regulate cell and organ activity, and help vitamins like vitamins A, D, E, and K function effectively.

The two most important good fats are the omega-3 fats eicosapentaenoic acid (EPA) and docosahexaenoic acid (DHA). Omega-3 fats are used to build healthy cells and make hormones and substances that affect nearly every body system. Studies show that supplementing with these fats helps boost heart health, lower triglycerides and decrease blood pressure. Omega-3 fats can be found in oily fish such as salmon, mackerel, anchovies, sardines, tuna and trout, and in plant oils such as flaxseed oil.

Choosing the Right Fats

There are several kinds of fat. Some are healthy, some aren't, and some are toxic.

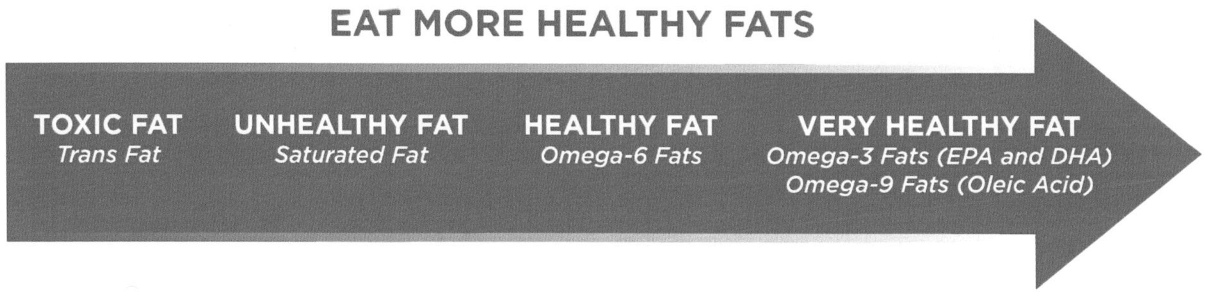

EAT MORE HEALTHY FATS

TOXIC FAT	UNHEALTHY FAT	HEALTHY FAT	VERY HEALTHY FAT
Trans Fat	*Saturated Fat*	*Omega-6 Fats*	*Omega-3 Fats (EPA and DHA)* *Omega-9 Fats (Oleic Acid)*

Oleic acid, an omega-9 fatty acid, helps enable the passage of nutrients and waste in and out of cells. A good source of this fatty acid is olive oil, which contains about 80% oleic acid. Olive oil helps lower blood sugar and blood pressure and reduces blood clotting. It also helps raise protective HDL cholesterol and lower harmful LDL cholesterol.

Omega-6 fats compete with omega-3 fats to perform many of the same functions, although the omega-6 fats produce more inflammation. It's important to eat a small amount of omega-6 fats, but to not eat so much as to render the healthy omega-3s ineffective or to cause unwanted inflammatory effects. It's recommended that you eat no more than four parts of omega-6 fatty acids for every one part of omega-3 fatty acids. Most Americans eat 25 parts of omega-6s for every one part of omega-3–far more than the recommended amount! Omega-6 fats can be found in most vegetable oils (such as corn and sunflower oil), poultry, eggs, avocados, and nuts.

Saturated fats should be limited to 7% of all calories, or about 10 grams a day. These fats can harden cell walls and slow the passage of nutrients and waste products in and out of cells. Diets high in saturated fats are associated with many diseases, including cardiovascular disease and cancer.

Trans fats have been chemically modified to prolong their shelf life. They increase LDL cholesterol and decrease HDL cholesterol. Anything labeled "partially hydrogenated" on food labels contains unhealthy trans fat and should be avoided.

Other Nutrients to Know

Cholesterol is made by the body and ingested in the foods we eat. "Good" HDL cholesterol protects against heart disease and strokes, while "bad" LDL cholesterol is unhealthy and promotes heart disease. You can avoid unhealthy cholesterol by limiting your intake of saturated fat from animal-based foods, found in meat, poultry, milk, cheese, and eggs or products made from them.

Sodium (salt) can contribute to high blood pressure, a condition that often occurs with prediabetes. Avoiding processed foods is a good way to limit sodium.

Fiber comes in two forms, both of which are good! Soluble fiber slows the passage of food through the digestive system, helps keep blood sugar and insulin levels steady, and prevents spikes in blood sugar. Soluble fiber is found in oatmeal, nuts, seeds, lentils, blackberries, broccoli, Brussels sprouts and sweet potatoes. Insoluble fiber promotes the passage of food through the digestive system. People who suffer from irregular digestion, including constipation, can benefit from insoluble fiber as it softens and adds bulk to stool. Foods rich in insoluble fiber include whole grain foods, green beans, cauliflower, and potatoes with the skin on.

Whole grains are a powerhouse of nutrition for your body. They contain the germ, endosperm and bran parts of the grain. (Refined grains are stripped of the germ and bran, which removes most nutrients and fiber.) Whole grains can lower fasting insulin levels, improve insulin sensitivity, decrease blood pressure,

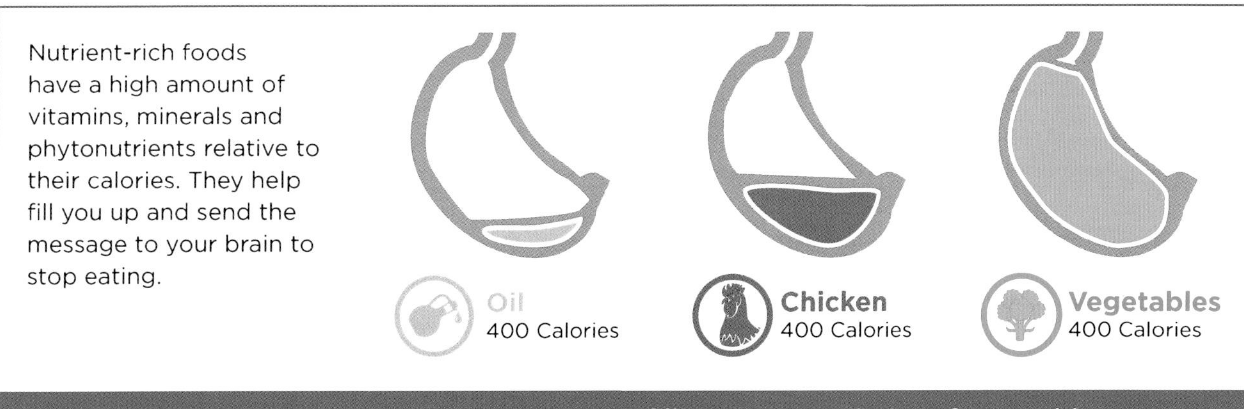

Nutrient-rich foods have a high amount of vitamins, minerals and phytonutrients relative to their calories. They help fill you up and send the message to your brain to stop eating.

As you can see, 400 calories of chicken isn't as filling as 400 calories of vegetables.

and decrease LDL cholesterol and triglycerides. Whole grain foods include whole wheat flour, whole wheat pasta, popcorn, quinoa, brown rice, oats, and spelt. Try to limit consumption of refined grains such as white bread, enriched pasta, white rice, white flour, and products made with white flour.

Phytonutrients are chemicals that protect plants from a wide variety of diseases, and they offer disease protection for people too. Plants contain thousands of phytonutrients—which give plants their color and odor—so try to eat a variety of colorful, flavorful plant-based foods to ensure you get the widest array of phytonutrients. Phytonutrients can decrease inflammation, raise HDL cholesterol, lower LDL cholesterol, and help with insulin resistance.

Organic or Non-Organic?

You may wonder if you should buy organic foods. Nutrition-wise, organic and non-organic foods have the same amount of nutrients. Organic foods usually cost more but may have more flavor. If you're concerned about harmful health effects from pesticides, chemicals and genetically modified foods, you may want to buy organic, especially for fruits and vegetables where you eat the skin, such as apples and peaches. It may also be a good idea to buy organic soy, wheat and corn products. (Non-organic soy, wheat and corn are the grains that are most commonly altered and most likely to cause allergies or sensitivities. Buying organic may eliminate these sensitivities.) When buying non-organic produce, be sure to wash pesticides and chemicals from fruits and vegetables before you eat them.

How Much Should I Eat?	
Fiber	30-40g a day
Saturated Fat	<7% of total calories, or no more than 13mg a day for a 2,000-calorie diet
Sodium	<2,300mg a day or <1,500mg a day if you have high blood pressure
Cholesterol	None on PURE eating days, up to 200mg a day on VITALITY eating days

FOOD CONTINUUM CHART

Unhealthy Choice (Least Nutritious) to Healthier Choice (Nutrient-Rich)

	LEAST NUTRITIOUS					NUTRIENT-RICH
MEAT	Hot dogs Deli meat Organ and muscle-based meats	Dark poultry meat Rack of lamb Pork chops	Prime cuts of beef Trimmed lamb Pork Loin	Egg whites Extra lean beef (eye round, top round, sirloin tip, top sirloin) Choice or select beef	Wild game White poultry meat Vegetarian meat substitute	
SEAFOOD	Puffer fish Carp Perch Shark	Catfish Tilapia Orange roughy	Shrimp Shellfish Crab	Black cod Sole Red snapper	Mahi-mahi Ahi tuna Halibut	Salmon Trout Sardines
DAIRY PRODUCTS	Heavy cream Non-dairy creamers (Coffee-mate) Half and half	Whole milk products (ice cream) Flavored yogurt	2% milk products Sour cream Coconut milk ice cream	Skim milk products Plain nonfat Greek yogurt Soy ice cream	Soy, almond or rice milk Cream cheese substitute Sour cream substitute Sorbet	
CHEESE	Velveeta Processed cheese slices Laughing Cow	Ricotta Cream cheese Brie	Parmesan Gruyere/Swiss Manchago	Nonfat mozzarella Goat cheese Nonfat cottage cheese	Soy, almond or rice cheese	
SALAD GREENS			Iceberg lettuce	Boston (butter) lettuce Red leaf lettuce	Romaine lettuce Cabbage Oak leaf lettuce	Kale Spinach
SWEETENERS	Artificial sweeteners High-fructose corn syrup Corn sugar	Sugar in the Raw Evaporated cane juice Brown sugar	Maple syrup Molasses Coconut syrup	Agave nectar Honey	Date sugar Puréed dried dates Dried figs	
OILS AND FATS	Palm oil Margarine Lard	Peanut oil Soybean oil Butter	Coconut oil Sesame oil Canola oil	Butter substitute PAM Original and olive oil spray Omega-3 fortified oils	Walnut oil Avocado oil	Olive oil

FOOD CONTINUUM CHART

Unhealthy Choice (Least Nutritious) to Healthier Choice (Nutrient-Rich)

	LEAST NUTRITIOUS					NUTRIENT-RICH
STARCHY VEGETABLES	Hash brown patties Instant potatoes Potato chips	Packaged or canned potatoes White potatoes	Canned or frozen pumpkin Zucchini Peas	Light-colored beans Sweet potatoes Squash	Lentils Red potatoes Edamame	Dark-colored beans Purple potatoes
NOODLES AND PASTA	Fried chow mein noodles Ramen noodles	Egg noodles Couscous Semolina pasta	Spinach and artichoke pasta Rice noodles Gluten-free pasta	Whole wheat couscous Whole wheat orzo Spelt pasta	Whole wheat pasta Quinoa pasta Brown rice pasta	
BAKED GOODS	Donuts Cake Cinnamon rolls	Cookies Biscuits Crescent rolls	Fortified white bread Pancakes Muffins	Whole wheat bread products Whole wheat crackers	Multigrain products	Sprouted multigrain products
GRAINS	Enriched grain cereals	White rice Bleached white flour Masa	Wild rice Cornmeal	Whole grains (wheat, brown rice, buckwheat, teff, quinoa, farro, wheatberry, oats, barley, spelt) Whole grain products (flour, bread, pasta, oatmeal, popcorn)		Sprouted whole grains Sprouted multigrain products Sprouted grain cereal
FRUITS				Grapes Citrus fruits Melons	Kiwi Strawberries Apples	Berries Pomegranates Cherries
NUTS				Macadamia nuts Pine nuts Brazil nuts	Cashews Pistachios Hazelnuts	Walnuts Pecans Almonds
SEEDS					Sunflower seeds Hemp seeds Sesame seeds	Chia seeds Flaxseeds Pumpkin seeds

Chapter 8

Concierge Nutrition

The PURE Plan

The PURE Plan jumpstarts the healing process. For 10 days you'll eat completely plant-based foods that have no cholesterol, added sugar, chemicals, preservatives, food coloring or texturizers. You will abstain from eating meat while on the PURE Plan; instead, you will get protein from other food sources during this time. PURE foods are low in sodium and rich in vitamins, minerals and protective phytonutrients. You'll get a diverse array of nutrients by eating a wide variety of foods from the list, so don't be afraid to try foods you haven't eaten before!

Eat your first meal after you wake up, and be sure not to skip meals or starve yourself during the day. Eat a snack to stave off hunger between meals, but limit snacking to once daily–it's ideal to allow your stomach to rest for several hours between meals. Try to avoid or limit caffeine and alcohol.

Follow the PURE Plan for the first 10 days. After that, you'll start the VITALITY Plan, which is the plan you'll follow for life. At each visit your physician will evaluate your diet and may recommend that you repeat the PURE Plan.

PURE Plan Daily Food Requirements

While on the PURE Plan, you will eat these foods daily:

 3-10 servings of whole grains. One serving equals:

- 1/2 cup cooked brown rice, cooked grain, 100% whole grain pasta or hot cereal (such as oatmeal)
- 1 ounce uncooked whole grain pasta, brown rice or other grain
- 1 slice 100% whole grain bread
- 1 small (1 ounce) 100% whole grain muffin
- 1 cup 100% whole grain ready-to-eat cereal
- 1 1/2 tablespoons (16 grams) whole grain ingredients, such as whole grain flour, for cooking

 5 servings of vegetables, half raw. One serving equals:

- 1/2 cup cooked or 1 cup raw vegetables

 3 servings of fruit, with at least one serving of berries. One serving equals:

- One piece of fruit or 1/2 cup fruit (fresh or frozen) or 8 ounces fruit juice

 1/2-2 servings of beans/legumes. One serving equals:

- 1/2 cup

 1/2-1 serving of nuts and seeds. One serving equals:

- 1/4 cup

 1-2 servings of olive oil. One serving equals:

- 1 tablespoon

PURE Foods to Eat

Here is a complete list of what you can eat for 10 days:

VEGETABLES

Acorn squash
Amaranth
Artichoke
Arugula
Asparagus
Avocado
Baby greens (any kind)
Bamboo shoot
Beet greens
Beetroot
Beets
Bell pepper
Bitter melon/bitter gourd
Bok choy
Broadleaf arrowhead
Broccoli
Broccoli rabe
Broccolini
Brussels sprout
Butternut squash
Cabbage
Caper
Carrot
Cassava
Cauliflower
Celeriac
Celery
Chayote
Chickweed
Chicory
Chinese artichoke
Chinese mallow
Collard greens
Cucumber
Daikon
Dandelion
Eggplant/aubergine/brinjal
Endive
Fiddlehead
Garden rocket
Garlic
Ginger
Greater plantain
Green bean
Hamburg parsley
Horseradish
Ivy gourd
Jalapeno
Jerusalem artichoke
Jícama
Kai-lan
Kale
Kohlrabi
Leek
Lettuce
Lotus root
Miner's lettuce
Mizuna greens
Mushroom
Mustard
Napa cabbage
New Zealand spinach
Onion
Parsnip
Pea sprouts/leaves
Pearl onion, spring onion/scallion
Peas
Poblano pepper
Poke
Pumpkin
Radicchio
Radish
Red potato
Rutabaga
Salsify
Shallot
Snap peas
Snow peas
Sorrel
Spinach or baby spinach
Sprouts (any kind)
Squash
Squash blossoms
Summer purslane
Sweet pepper
Sweet potato
Swiss chard
Taro
Tatsoi
Tomatillo
Tomato
Turnip
Turnip greens
Water chestnut
Watercress
West Indian gherkin
Wild leek
Winter melon
Winter purslane
Yacón
Yam
Yarrow
Zucchini

LEGUMES

Azuki bean
Black-eyed pea
Chickpea
Fava bean
Garbanzo
Green bean
Guar
Lentil
Lima bean
Mung bean
Okra
Pea
Pigeon pea
Snap pea
Snow pea
Soybean

SEA VEGETABLES

Dulse or dillisk
Hijiki
Kombu
Mozuku
Nori
Ogonori
Sea grape
Sea kale
Sea lettuce
Wakame

FRUITS

Acai
Apples
Apricots
Bananas
Blackberries
Blueberres
Cherries
Cranberries
Grapefruit
Grapes
Jackfruit
Kiwis
Lemons
Limes
Longan fruit
Lychee
Mangoes
Nectarines
Oranges
Peaches
Pears
Plums
Pomegranates
Pomelo
Star fruit
Strawberries

NUTS

Almonds
Brazil nuts
Cashews
Chestnuts
Filberts or hazelnuts
Peanuts
Pecans
Pine nuts
Pistachios
Walnuts

SEEDS

Chia seeds
Flaxseeds
Hemp seeds
Poppy seeds
Pumpkin seeds
Safflower seeds
Sesame seeds
Sunflower seeds

WHOLE/SPROUTED GRAINS

Amaranth
Barley maize
Brown rice
Buckwheat
Farro
Kamut
Millet
Oat
Quinoa
Rye
Spelt
Teff
Triticale
Wheat

OILS, SAUCES & SUBSTITUTIONS

Apple cider vinegar
Bragg Liquid Aminos
Brewer's yeast
Hot sauce (sriracha, Cholula or your favorite brand)
Low-sodium soy sauce
Olive oil, including cooking spray (PAM)
Plum vinegar
Red or white cooking wine
Red wine vinegar
Sherry or champagne vinegar
Whole grain mustard

BEVERAGES

Green tea
Herbal tea
Hibiscus tea
Sparkling water
Unsweetened seltzer
White tea

PURE Foods to Avoid

Avoid these foods while on the PURE Plan:

Alcohol

Canned fruit

Chocolate

Coffee

Corn products

Crackers

Dairy products (sour cream, cottage cheese, yogurt, cream cheese, cheese, ice cream)

Deep-fried food

Eggs

Energy bars

Jams and jellies

Lunch meats

Margarine and butter

Mayonnaise

Meat, poultry, fish, seafood (including canned products and lunch meats)

Packaged cereals (unless they are sprouted whole grain)

Packaged chips

Pancakes

Pasta

Prepared salad dressings

Refined oils (soybean, peanut)

Soda

Sugar (brown sugar, molasses, agave, honey) (Note: If you MUST use table sugar, try to limit use to 2-5 teaspoons per day.)

Sugar substitutes (Stevia, Equal)

Syrups

White bread

White flour

White rice

10 Tips for PURE Plan Success

1. **Start juicing!** Having trouble getting your daily recommended amount of fruits and vegetables? Put your fruits and vegetables into a juicer and drink them down! Two 8-ounce glasses of juice can give you 4-5 servings of fruits and vegetables.

2. **Snack on veggies.** Fill a one-gallon plastic bag halfway with raw vegetables and fruit. Commit to eating all of it throughout the day. Fruits and vegetables that are easily portable include cherry tomatoes, celery, carrots, sliced bell peppers, sliced cucumber, broccoli florets, cauliflower florets, zucchini, green beans, blueberries, strawberries, raspberries, blackberries, cherries, and grapes.

3. **Buy whole grains, nuts and seeds in bulk.** Select flavors that you know you like and don't be afraid to try something new.

4. **Purchase several kinds of whole grains.** Buy whole grains that require preparation, such as whole grain pasta, brown rice, farro or quinoa. Cook enough whole grains for five days and store in your fridge. When you need to make a quick dish, your whole grains will already be cooked and ready to go–just add vegetables and sauce.

5. **Freeze sauce in an ice-cube tray.** Make sauce ahead of time so that when you need it, you can punch out a few cubes and you're ready to go.

6. **Shop the perimeter of the grocery store.** Most processed, unhealthy foods are on shelves in the middle of the store. Avoid or minimize time in the aisles and focus on the perimeter, with emphasis on the produce section. This will increase your odds of making healthy purchases. Or, visit your local health food store or organic market for an even greater selection of nutritious food. If a food has a label on it, you might want to consider whether you want to purchase it or not.

7. **Get colorful.** Fruits and vegetables come in a variety of colors. Typically the darker the color, the more nutrients. Try to get as many colors as possible on your plate–it'll help you get the daily recommended amount of nutrients. Remember, nutrients work together, not alone. Eating a limited variety of foods, even healthy foods, will not give you all the nutrients you need. Eating a wide variety of colorful foods is the best way to deliver the most nutrients to your body.

8. **Take control of your eating.** Use these 10 days to become aware of when you're eating, how you're eating and what you're eating. Try to become aware of how often you eat processed foods. You may notice that it can be difficult to find whole foods when you're not at home. Start thinking about your strategies to overcome this inconvenience (see Tip No. 2).

9. **Eat at least one new food a day.** You won't like everything you eat, but your inventory of healthy food choices won't grow unless you experiment with new foods. Once you discover a food you like, add it to your weekly menu. Variety is a key part of your new healthy diet.

10. **Aim for a steady intake of calories throughout the day.** Don't skip breakfast or starve yourself. Your blood sugar will be more balanced over the course of the day if your caloric intake is steady.

What to Expect When Eating PURE Foods

Withdrawing from your old foods and adopting new, nutritious foods may have a few side effects. You may experience:

Fatigue. If this happens, increase your whole grain intake. Make sure you're well hydrated and you're taking in enough calories. Don't starve yourself during the day.

Headaches and moodiness. Many people experience headaches and moodiness when withdrawing from caffeine. You may want to wean yourself off rather than going cold turkey. Unless contraindicated, an over-the-counter pain medication can help alleviate a headache.

Hunger and cravings. If you feel hungry, then you need to eat. Choose a low-calorie, high-fiber snack, such as a handful of almonds with a banana, an apple or cherry tomatoes. If you have a craving, try to identify what it is you want (sweet, salty, chewy, crunchy) and replace it with a healthier substitution.

Bloating and gas. If your diet is currently low in fiber, increasing fiber too quickly may cause cramping, gas and bloating. To avoid these side effects, add fiber to your diet slowly, increasing the amount each week until you reach your goal. Increase your activity and make sure you drink enough fluids. Water and tea are good choices to help process fiber.

Dizziness or mental fog. A quick walk outside may help alleviate these symptoms. A nutrient-dense snack may also help. Make sure you're well hydrated. If symptoms continue, you may want to take a short nap.

Constipation. While most people experience improved digestion with a high-fiber diet, some people may experience constipation. Try cutting back on your total fiber but increase your insoluble fiber intake by eating more whole grain foods (bread, pasta, cereal), brown rice, nuts, seeds, carrots, cucumbers, zucchini, celery, tomatoes, green beans, cauliflower and red potatoes with the skin on. Make sure you're well hydrated and are getting enough exercise. If constipation continues, discuss it with your physician.

Frustration. It may seem difficult to know what to eat or how to put a delicious meal together. Use the

Concierge Nutrition recipes as often as you can. Your coach is there to help you with any problems you may have with meal preparation. If you plan on dining out, visit the restaurant's website first. Many fast-food restaurants have online nutrition calculators you can use to put together a meal. Plan nutritious and tasty meals before you arrive so that your meals are satisfying and you're not lured into choosing less healthy options.

Bad breath, increased body odor and acne. Some people may experience an increase in these symptoms which are related to the detoxification process. Symptoms should clear up as the body detoxifies.

Increased cost. Once you are proficient in shopping for healthy foods, you'll find that you're actually saving money. That's because our recipes and menus are designed to be more cost-effective than you're probably used to. You may find initially that getting started costs a little more compared to the cost of foods which have little to no nutrition and are loaded with salt, unhealthy fat and sugar, giving them a long shelf life at low cost for the manufacturer. Whole foods, prepared at home, will produce healthier meals at reduced cost to you in the long run.

Enhanced taste sensation. Most people find they experience an increased taste sensation. This, in turn, leads to greater enjoyment of meals and the ability to cut back on salt and sugar.

Weight loss. If you're overweight, you'll probably experience significant weight loss. Enjoy it!

Increased energy. Most people with prediabetes experience fatigue. Increased energy may be one of the first positive effects that you notice. Use this new energy to further your activity goals, adding in some additional steps or using your energy towards activities you previously didn't have the energy for.

Better digestive health. Your digestive system will be healing along with the rest of your body. Processed foods are hard on the digestive system, and when you remove them your system will start to heal. You may experience a decrease in bloating, constipation, diarrhea, gas and other symptoms. You may also have more bowel movements than you're used to.

The VITALITY Plan

The purpose of the VITALITY plan is to get the maximum amount of nutrients in your body in the minimum amount of calories. VITALITY foods are loaded with protein, fiber, healthy fats, vitamins, minerals and phytonutrients. Some VITALITY foods are exceptionally nutrient-rich, making them superfoods. These foods are the building blocks of good nutrition and healthy bodily function. Loaded with antioxidants, anti-inflammatory properties and other disease-fighting agents, VITALITY foods are the key to getting and staying well-nourished.

The VITALITY Plan is a lifelong eating plan. To get the vitamins and nutrients you need for good health, you should follow the plan after completing the PATHFinder Program.

VITALITY Plan Daily Food Requirements

While on the VITALITY Plan, you will eat these foods daily:

 3-10 servings of whole grains. One serving equals:

- ½ cup cooked brown rice, cooked grain, 100% whole grain pasta or hot cereal (such as oatmeal)
- 1 ounce uncooked whole grain pasta, brown rice or other grain
- 1 slice 100% whole grain bread
- 1 small (1 ounce) 100% whole grain muffin
- 1 cup 100% whole grain ready-to-eat cereal
- 1 ½ tablespoons (16 grams) whole grain ingredients, such as whole grain flour, for cooking

 5 servings of vegetables, half raw. One serving equals:

- ½ cup cooked or 1 cup raw vegetables

 3 servings of fruit, with at least one serving of berries. One serving equals:

- One piece of fruit or ½ cup fruit or 8 ounces fruit juice

 ½-2 servings of beans/legumes. One serving equals:

- ½ cup

✓ ½-1 serving of nuts and seeds. One serving equals:

- ¼ cup

 1-2 servings of olive oil. One serving equals:

- 1 tablespoon

 2-4 ounces of lean meat, poultry, fish or seafood

 1 glass of red wine (optional)

What to Expect When Eating VITALITY Foods

By following the plan, you will feel satiated after every meal, lose weight, get better sleep and have higher energy levels. Your biomarkers will show improvement, including your prediabetes, cardiovascular and inflammatory biomarkers. You will likely see a reduction in uric acid levels, if you have high levels. You may also experience better gastrointestinal health—including regular bowel movements and a decrease in symptoms associated with irritable bowel syndrome—and improvement in existing diseases such as arthritis, painful joints, acne, headaches, and high blood pressure.

> **TIP**
>
> Not all foods in health food stores are healthy. Read nutrition labels and avoid foods with trans fats, added sugars, food coloring and texturizing agents. Better yet—avoid foods with labels!

Some people also notice an improvement in their complexion. The skin may take on an orange hue, which is due to increased carotenes in the diet (from vegetables). If you experience this, don't be alarmed. It's a sign of good nutrition!

Your body will experience improved health in a short time, compared to how long it took to get here, but you shouldn't expect immediate results or rapid weight loss. It took time for your body to develop prediabetes, and it will take some time for you to reverse the decline in your health. Be as diligent as possible with your eating plan and you'll see changes over the months.

VITALITY Foods to Eat

Continue to eat all the foods on the PURE list, plus add:

- Agave nectar or honey (1-2 teaspoons per day)
- All nuts
- Almond milk
- Cheese substitutes (almond, soy, rice)
- Coconut milk, creamer and water
- Cornstarch
- Cough drops (as needed)
- Dried fruits (such as apples, apricots, blueberries, cherries, cranberries, currants, dates, figs, goji berries, pineapple, plums, prunes, raisins, strawberries)
- Earth Balance or Smart Balance butter substitute
- Egg whites
- Freeze-dried fruit or vegetables
- High-quality baking powder
- High-quality baking soda
- Hominy
- Lean meats, fish or seafood, 2-4 ounces per day
- Mints (a maximum of 3 per day)
- Pomegranate, blueberry or acai juice
- Popcorn (plain)
- Rice milk
- Rolled oats or oat groats
- Seitan
- Soy creamer
- Soy milk
- Soy protein powder
- Sprouted and seeded crackers
- Sugar-free gum
- Tahini
- Teff flour
- Tempeh
- Tofu
- Tofutti cream cheese substitute
- Tofutti sour cream substitute
- V8 vegetable juice
- Vegenaise mayonnaise substitute
- Vegetarian meat substitutes
- Whole grain breads, tortillas, English muffins, flat bread, naan bread
- Whole grain pasta (whole wheat, brown rice or quinoa pasta)
- Red wine (optional)

VITALITY Foods to Avoid

Continue to avoid all prohibited foods on the PURE list.

TIP

Soy binds to estrogen receptor sites in the body, producing the same effects as estrogen without actually increasing the level of estrogen. For this reason, soy products are often thought of as "natural estrogen." Many studies show that soy can help relieve the symptoms of menopause. Soy also decreases cholesterol, blood pressure and osteoporosis. Some researchers believe that soy products may stimulate breast cancer growth, though many experts disagree, as Asian women consume large quantities of soy without experiencing higher rates of breast cancer. If you're taking hormone replacement medication, talk to your physician about the use of soy products and risk for breast cancer. Some women increase their soy intake and are able to discontinue hormone replacement therapy.

Experiment with Concierge Nutrition Recipes

Cooking at home will allow you to build your healthy meal preparation skills and become familiar with the foods you're feeding your body. We encourage you to try as many recipes as possible. You may not like every dish, but sampling a wide variety will allow you to discover a handful of favorites to incorporate into your life. By the program's end, you should have at least 25 new meals that you enjoy.

To enhance the flavor of any meal, simply add one of our tasty sauces. When you find a food substitute you love, add it to a new meal!

Remember, it's important to stick to the PURE Plan for the first 10 days. Afterward, feel free to turn a PURE recipe into a VITALITY recipe by adding 2-4 ounces of lean meat.

Getting There Faster

The closer you stay to whole foods, or PURE Plan food, the faster your body will respond to good nutrition. To quicken your efforts, we recommend that you adopt dietary principles practiced in "Blue Zones," areas of the world where people are known to live longer, higher-quality lives. There are a few key nutritional habits scientists have learned from these regions. Blue Zone populations:

- Get most dietary protein from plant-based foods, primarily vegetables and beans
- Eat meat infrequently–usually once a week
- Consume complex carbohydrates, such as whole grains
- Eat a low-fat diet with a focus on foods high in omega-3 and omega-9 fatty acids

- Load up on antioxidants and phytonutrients, found in nuts, seeds and plants
- Consume foods that protect against diabetes, heart disease and cancer, found in green tea, dark and leafy vegetables, cruciferous vegetables, berries, nuts, and seeds

Make the Nutrition Plan Work for You

As the year progresses you'll become more skilled at shopping and preparing healthier foods. Experiment as often as possible with new foods and recipes, and visit a local health food store—or the health foods section of a grocery store—to get more familiar with healthy foods. Above all, keep your diet packed with as many natural foods as possible.

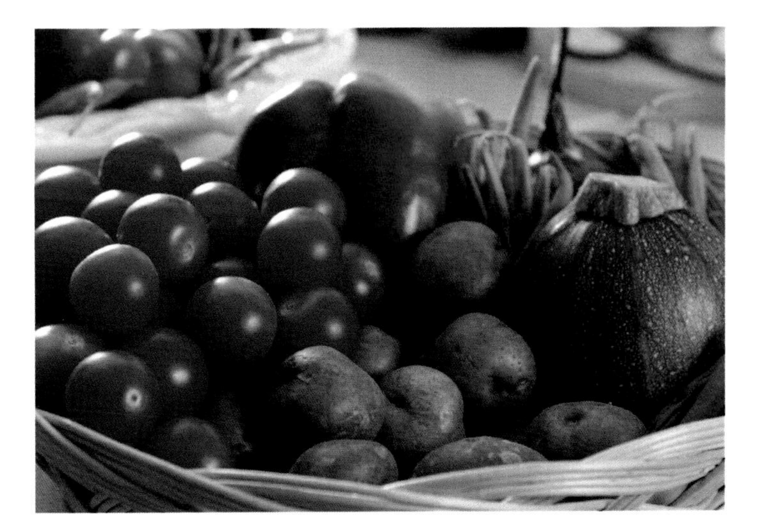

Food Basics

What Is Sour Cream?

Sour cream is cream (a milk product) that has been soured by adding bacteria or acids to it. Many forms also have a thickening agent added. Tofutti sour cream substitute is made primarily from soybean oil and protein. It tastes similar to sour cream but has fewer calories and no cholesterol.

What Is Cream Cheese?

Cream cheese is a white cheese made from whole milk and added cream. It's high in calories and unhealthy fats and contains cholesterol. Vegetarian cream cheeses are made from oils such as coconut, sunflower and soybean oil. They're creamy, tasty and have no cholesterol.

What Is Mayonnaise?

Mayonnaise is traditionally made by adding oil to an egg yolk. Oil and egg yolk don't normally mix, so the combination has to be emulsified. The protein in the egg yolk serves to stabilize the mixture. Vegenaise is made with healthy canola oil and soy protein rather than egg. It tastes great, has healthier fats and no cholesterol.

Transition Foods That Can Help

These foods mimic the flavors of their unhealthy counterparts and make your meals more healthful. Reading nutrition labels will enable you to make healthier choices as well. We're confident that you and your family will love the taste of healthy substitutions!

INSTEAD OF THIS...	TRY THIS...
Bacon and sausage	Veggie bacon and sausage
Beef	Veggie beef
Boxed cereal	Whole grain cereal
Butter	Earth Balance, Smart Balance or Benecol butter substitute
Cheeseburger	Veggie burger
Chicken	Veggie chicken
Chips	Freeze-dried vegetable chips, baked corn chips
Chocolate	Cacao nibs, 80% dark chocolate
Coffee and tea	Pero, decaf coffee or herbal tea
Corn dog	Veggie corn dog
Cream cheese	Tofutti cream cheese substitute
Creamer	Soy, almond, coconut, or rice creamer
Eggs	Egg Beaters or egg whites
Hot dog	Veggie hot dog
Ice cream	Soy, coconut, almond, or rice ice cream
Mayonnaise	Vegenaise
Meat chili	Veggie chili
Milk	Soy, almond or coconut milk
Soda	Sparkling water or seltzer
Sour cream	Tofutti sour cream substitute
Sugar	Dried fruit, honey, agave, puréed dates, coconut nectar
White bread, muffins and tortillas	Sprouted grain breads, English muffins and tortillas

Getting Started: Stocking the Pantry for the VITALITY Plan and Lifelong Healthy Eating

Preparing your pantry is your first priority. Here's how to do it:

Step 1: Eliminate unhealthy foods!

Throw out all foods with "partially hydrogenated" on the label. Discard all oils except olive, canola or sesame. Also, check the oils you're keeping to make sure they haven't gone rancid. Get rid of white flour foods (bread, pasta, crackers, pancakes, waffles, cookies, cake, breakfast breads, muffins), white rice, lunch meats, mayonnaise, butter, margarine, all dairy products (milk, cheese), yogurt (unless it's plain or Greek), jams and jellies, soda, syrup, salad dressing, breaded foods, chips, pretzels, cereal (unless it's whole grain), energy bars and any food that has added sugars, salt and saturated fat, or is high in cholesterol, low in fiber or non-whole grain.

Step 2: Stock your pantry, fridge and freezer with healthy staples.

Oils

- Extra virgin olive oil
- Canola oil
- Sesame oil
- *PAM* cooking spray

Sauces and Condiments

- *Vegenaise* mayonnaise substitute
- Hot sauce such as *Cholula* or sriracha
- Agave syrup (maple-flavored or regular) or honey
- Reduced-sodium soy sauce or *Bragg Liquid Aminos*
- Specialty vinegars, such as red wine and champagne vinegar
- Mustards, such as whole grain, honey, Dijon and yellow mustard

Herbs and spices

- Allspice, basil, bay leaves, ground pepper, cayenne and chili powder, cinnamon, cloves, coriander, cumin, curry powder, dill, garlic powder, ground ginger, mint, nutmeg, onion powder, oregano, paprika, crushed red pepper, rosemary
- Low-sodium *Spike* seasoning
- Spice blends: Southwestern spice blend, Moroccan ras el hanout, Indian garam masala, curry, pumpkin spice, French herbes de Provence, Italian herb seasoning, Chinese five-spice, *Mrs. Dash* seasonings

Nuts and seeds (raw, unroasted and salt-free)

- Almonds, walnuts, pecans, hazelnuts, Brazil nuts, pine nuts, cashews, peanuts, pistachio nuts
- Sesame, pumpkin, sunflower, chia, hemp, ground flaxseeds
- Tahini, almond butter, peanut butter, cashew butter

Dried or dehydrated foods

- Mushrooms (shiitake, porcini)
- Beans: lentils (red, green, brown, and French), kidney, pinto, black beans, cannellini, adzuki and chickpeas (garbanzo)
- Fruit: currants, goji berries, raisins, dates, prunes, apricots, apples, cranberries, blueberries, cherries, strawberries, apricots
- Dehydrated fruits and vegetables: apples, strawberries, bananas, mangoes, peas, mixed veggies
- Seaweed: nori, kombu, wakame or hijiki

Whole grains

- Farro, quinoa, wheatberry, polenta, bulgur wheat, barley, millet, brown rice, amaranth, buckwheat groats
- Whole wheat bread/tortilla/flat bread, naan, English muffins, pasta, oatmeal, couscous, brown rice pasta
- Whole grain, trans fat-free crackers such as *Health Valley* whole wheat crackers, *Kashi TLC* crackers, *Reduced Fat Triscuits*, *Wasa Lite Rye Crispbread*, baked and trans fat-free whole grain tortilla chips, whole grain pretzels, *Dr. Kracker* whole grain crackers, whole wheat pita bread, whole wheat pita crisps

- Whole-grain cold cereals (Note: Choose cereals that contain 5 grams or more of dietary fiber and fewer than 8 grams of sugar per serving.)
- Brown rice cakes, popcorn cakes such as *Snyder's* oat bran or honey wheat
- Plain popcorn or light (98% fat-free) microwave popcorn
- Whole-wheat flour and whole-wheat pastry flour

Canned foods

- Tuna, salmon, diced tomatoes, crushed tomatoes, tomato sauce, tomato paste, low-sodium and sugar-free marinara sauce
- Canned beans, chickpeas, pinto, navy, black, adzuki, cannellini, red beans
- 98% fat-free cream of mushroom or chicken soups (such as *Campbell's Healthy Request*)
- Reduced-sodium chicken, beef and vegetable broths
- Coconut milk
- Boxed soy or almond milk

Freezer foods

- Frozen vegetables and vegetable blends without added sauces, gravies and sodium (such as corn, broccoli, cauliflower, green beans, peas, spinach, asparagus, squash, carrots, sweet potato, diced red potato)
- Frozen fruits without added sugar (such as blueberries, strawberries, raspberries, cherries, mango, pineapple, acai, cranberries)
- Frozen soybeans (edamame)
- Frozen veggie burgers, veggie bacon, veggie chicken patties, veggie chicken nuggets, veggie chicken strips (such as *Boca*, *Yves*, *Morningstar Farms*, or *Gardenburger*)
- Frozen brown rice
- Sprouted whole grain breads, English muffins, tortillas, and pitas
- Ground chicken or turkey
- Skinless white breast chicken or turkey meat
- Turkey or chicken sausage
- Pork tenderloin, trimmed of fat

- Bison
- Lean ground beef such as ground round or ground sirloin (When buying beef, look for words like "round" or "loin" and choose lean cuts—the less marbling, the lower the fat content.)
- Assorted fish: wild salmon, halibut, flounder, red snapper, mackerel, wild trout, herring, and tuna

Fridge foods

- Tofu: silken (for sauces), firm or extra firm (for stir-fry)
- *Vegenaise* mayonnaise substitute
- *Tofutti* sour cream substitute
- *Tofutti* cream cheese substitute
- *Earth Balance* butter substitute
- Cheese substitute (almond, soy or rice)
- Soy, almond or coconut milk
- Egg whites
- Soy creamer or coconut milk creamer
- Coconut water

Step 3: Prepare nutritious meals!

Use the recipes as a guide. Again, stick to the plan as much as possible for the fastest results. Be sure to include plenty of variety and to experiment with new foods. Some recipes are spiced fairly lightly, so if you're a person who likes spice and heat in food, feel free to add more.

Helpful Cooking Techniques

How to Steam-Sauté

This quick and easy technique of cooking vegetables uses the least amount of oil and prevents the nutrient loss that commonly occurs with boiling. The water evaporates during cooking and the oil caramelizes vegetables and brings out their delicious, sweet flavors.

Every 1 pound of vegetables is cooked with:

- ⅓ cup water and 2 teaspoons olive oil

Preparation: Heat a skillet over medium-high heat with water and olive oil until boiling. Add vegetables, cover and let cook for 5 minutes. Stir and cook uncovered for 2 minutes until water evaporates completely and vegetables are bright in color, indicating doneness. Most vegetables take 7 minutes to cook thoroughly. Potatoes take 15 minutes to steam if cut uniformly and added to boiling water.

How to Quick Roast

Roasting allows the sugars in vegetables to caramelize without making them mushy. This method allows you to pop the vegetables in the oven, walk away and return to perfectly roasted vegetables ideal for any meal.

Every 1 pound of vegetables is cooked with:

- 1 tablespoon olive oil and pinch of salt
- Olive oil spray (PAM)

Preparation: Preheat oven to 425 degrees. Toss washed vegetables with olive oil. (It's okay if the vegetables are a little damp.) Spread vegetables over foil-lined, lightly sprayed baking sheet, making sure vegetables do not touch. Sprinkle pinch of salt over the vegetables and roast for 20 minutes.

How to Quick Grill

This speedy method allows you to toss the ingredients on the grill and return to perfectly cooked vegetables that are crispy, tender and ready to serve or store in the fridge for later use. Cut vegetables long and lengthwise so they don't fall between the grill and are easy to handle with tongs. Potatoes and sweet potatoes take longer to grill; cook those first then add the other vegetables 10 minutes later so that all vegetables are ready to eat at the same time.

Every 1 pound of vegetables is cooked with:

- 1 tablespoon olive oil and pinch of salt
- Olive oil spray (PAM)

Preparation: Preheat grill to 425 degrees. Toss washed vegetables with olive oil. Lightly spray a grill basket with PAM and spread vegetables inside, making sure vegetables do not touch. Sprinkle pinch of salt over the vegetables and close the grill to cook for 7 minutes. Turn vegetables over and cook for 5-10 minutes more.

Some vegetables will require modified cooking times. Asparagus and kale are usually done in 7-10 minutes total. Potatoes take 20 minutes to cook through, depending on the size and thickness of the sliced potatoes. If grilling potatoes, put them on the grill first for 10 minutes covered, then add the other vegetables.

Cooking Whole Grains

This easy method allows you to quickly mix the ingredients over the stove, walk away and return to cooked grains that are fluffy, tender and delicious every time. We recommend that you cook 2 whole grains each week.

Preparation: Put whole grain and water in a saucepan and cover. Cook on high heat until boiling. Reduce to lowest heat setting and cook for the time listed in the chart below. DO NOT lift lid or stir before cooking time has ended. Stirring can disrupt the cooking process and cause the grains on the bottom to overcook while leaving the top grains raw. Note: Bulgur wheat is not brought to a boil; instead, pour boiling water over bulgur and let soak for 10-15 minutes.

Cooking time can vary. To check for doneness, remove lid and taste with a fork. If the grain is not done, add a little more water, cover and cook for an additional 5 minutes.

1 CUP	WATER	COOKING TIME	YIELDS
Amaranth*	2 cups	20-25 min	3 1/2 cups
Barley, pearl	2 1/2 cups	40 min	2 1/2-3 cups
Buckwheat	2 cups	20-25 min	4 cups
Bulgur wheat	1 cup	10-15 min	2 cups
Cornmeal (polenta)*	4 cups	25-30 min	2 1/2 cups
Farro	3 cups	25 min	2 cups
Kamut	3 cups	60 min	2 cups
Millet*	2 1/2 cups	25-35 min	4 cups
Oats, rolled	1 cup	5 min	1 1/2 cups
Oats, steel-cut	4 cups	20-25 min	4 cups
Quinoa*	2 cups	15 min	3 cups
Rice, black*	2 cups	35 min	2 cups
Rice, brown*	2 cups	40 min	2 cups
Rice, red*	2 cups	45 min	2 cups
Wheatberry	3 cups	45 min	2 cups

*Gluten-free *Note: Some people with gluten intolerance may be able to tolerate rolled or steel-cut oats.*

Cooking Legumes

Dried beans and legumes, except for black-eyed peas and lentils, require soaking in room-temperature water, a step that rehydrates them for even cooking and a tender, silky texture. Before soaking, pick through the beans, discarding any discolored or shriveled ones or any foreign matter. Depending on how much time you have, choose one of the following soaking methods:

- **Slow soak.** In a stockpot, cover 1 pound dried beans with 16 cups water and 3 tablespoons salt. Cover and refrigerate 6-8 hours or overnight. This method, called "brining," will break down oligosaccharides, or carbohydrates that cause gas. Be sure not to soak the beans for more than 24 hours; it will cause the beans to lose flavor and develop a mealy texture.

- **Hot soak.** In a stockpot, bring 16 cups water and 3 tablespoons salt to a boil. Add 1 pound dried beans and return to a boil. Remove from the heat, cover tightly and set aside at room temperature for 2-3 hours.

- **Quick soak.** In a stockpot, bring 16 cups water and 3 tablespoons salt to a boil. Add 1 pound dried beans and return to a boil. Boil 2-3 minutes. Cover and set aside at room temperature for 1 hour.

To prepare legumes: After soaking, rinse beans, dispose of water, and add beans to stockpot. Cover the beans with three times their volume of water. Add herbs or spices as desired. Bring to a boil. Reduce the heat and simmer gently, uncovered and stirring occasionally, until tender. The cooking time depends on the type of bean, but start checking after 45 minutes. Add more water if the beans become uncovered. Beans are done when they can be easily mashed between two fingers or with a fork. To freeze cooked beans for later use, immerse them in cold water until cool, drain well and freeze.

Fast, Convenient and Nutritious VITALITY Plan Meals

Many people avoid cooking because they think it's time-consuming and troublesome. The following meal plans are designed to give you maximum nutrition with minimum effort. Each meal has a low-fat source of protein, whole grains and plenty of vegetables.

What's for Lunch?

It's important that you have a nutritious midday meal. To ensure you're getting a varied, healthy meal, we recommend that you make a Bento box, which is a traditional home-packed meal common in Japan. You don't have to pack Japanese food in the Bento box; we just think the arrangement of a Bento box will help ensure you're getting an adequate variety of food. You can buy a Bento lunch box online, or just use a few plastic containers to hold the different types of food to keep in your regular lunch bag.

To make your own Bento box, use this formula for every lunch:

- Pack 1-2 servings of each:
  - ✓ Whole grains (such as bread, crackers, pasta, rice, or quinoa)
  - ✓ Veggies
  - ✓ Fruit
  - ✓ Legumes (such as garbanzo, black or cannellini beans, or peas)

- Optional items:
  - ✓ Nuts and seeds
  - ✓ Lean meats and seafood

A Weekly Lunch Menu

Not sure which foods to pack in your lunch box? Try any of these combinations.

American Lunch Box

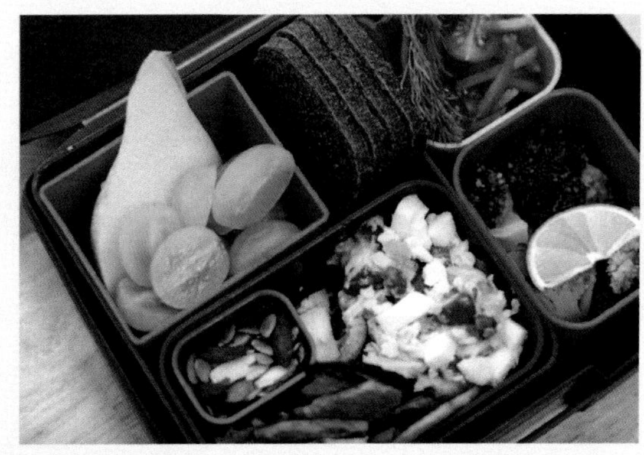

- Whole grain toast triangles, Lemony Chicken Salad, sliced cucumbers, carrots, cherry tomatoes, cantaloupe, blackberries, dried apricots, and walnuts.
- Grilled Pesto Chicken Sandwich, veggie chips, Creamy Tomato-Basil Soup, apples and grapes, dried blueberries, and almonds.
- Tuna Pasta Salad, sliced cucumbers, cherry tomatoes, spinach, melon balls and grapes, dried cranberries, and pumpkin seeds.
- Egg salad with rye toast triangles, root veggie chips, cherry tomatoes, carrots, steamed broccoli, pears and grapes, dried goji berries, and pumpkin seeds.

Mediterranean Lunch Box

- Whole grain pita triangles, hummus, sliced cucumbers, carrots, cherry tomatoes, olives, almonds, grapes and apple slices, and Fig Bar.
- Romesco Sauce, Savory Italian Meatloaf balls, whole grain toast, steamed green beans and carrots, raspberries and grapefruit, pistachios, and currants.
- Hot Artichoke-Spinach Dip, whole grain crackers, cherry tomatoes, cucumber slices, carrots, grapes, apples, dried figs, and walnuts.
- Walnut Pesto, whole grain rigatoni, cherry tomatoes, steamed broccoli and cauliflower, kiwi, strawberry, dried blueberries, and sunflower seeds.

Mexican Lunch Box

- Baked sprouted corn tortilla triangles, Zesty Mexican Bean Dip, 1/2 avocado and lime wedge, fresh corn and cherry tomatoes, Green Poblano Sauce, mango and pineapple, and Five-Star Brownie.
- Veggie cheese and black bean quesadillas, Salsa Caliente, 1/4 avocado, bell peppers, carrots, apples, bananas, pecans, and cacao nibs.
- Southwestern Salad Bowl, 1/4 avocado, bell peppers, Cool Garden Vegetable Gazpacho, oranges, blueberries, kiwi, and pumpkin seeds.
- BLT Breakfast Burrito, 1/4 avocado, cherry tomatoes, carrots, green beans, peach, blueberries, dried apricots, and almonds.

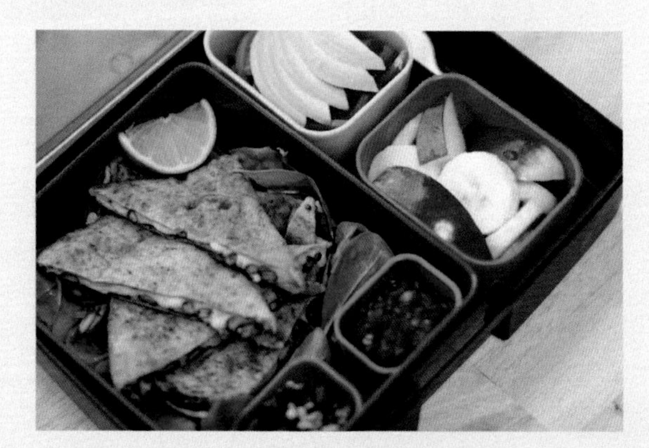

Asian Lunch Box

- Cooked short-grain brown rice, cooked extra-firm tofu cut into triangles with Sesame-Ginger Sauce, steamed snap peas and edamame, orange wedges and raspberries, and Coconut-Chia Seed Pudding.
- Creamy Asian Sesame Noodle Salad, raw spinach, cherry tomatoes, sliced jicama, pears and plums, and Fig Bar.
- Oven-Roasted Sweet Potatoes with Curry Dip, steamed cauliflower, carrots, tomatoes, papaya and mango, pistachios, and dried goji berries.
- Sesame Ahi Salad, 1/4 avocado, steamed broccoli, edamame, plum, nectarine, wasabi peas, and almonds.

What's for Dinner?

Making dinner is a snap! Just follow these simple instructions.

1. Steam, grill, broil, roast or poach 1 serving (2-4 ounces) of lean, meat, fish, or poultry. You can use 1-2 teaspoons olive oil, coconut oil, safflower oil, or butter substitute to grill, broil, roast or sauté.

2. Cook 1-2 cups whole grain quinoa, brown rice, whole grain pasta, brown rice pasta, grits, or oatmeal. Or, serve 1 slice sprouted grain bread or flatbread with your meal.

3. Prepare 1-3 cups raw leafy vegetables or 1-3 cups cooked vegetables. Variety is key to getting the most nutrients, flavors, textures and satisfaction from your meal. Prepare at least 2-5 different vegetables, raw or cooked.

4. Add 1 serving (1/2 cup) legumes.

5. Add a sauce ($^1/_2$ cup) to your meal:

    - Alfredo Sauce - Great with chicken, halibut or shrimp, scallops, or bass.
    - Romesco Sauce - Delicious with cod, halibut, mahi mahi, salmon, chicken or beef, scallops, tuna, or red snapper.
    - Chinese Black Bean Sauce - Ideal for chicken, tofu, mahi mahi, cod, or salmon.
    - Walnut Pesto - Serve with cod, salmon, chicken or turkey, shrimp, trout, or tuna.
    - Green Poblano Sauce - Pair with cod, salmon, halibut, trout, tuna, red snapper, bass, chicken, beef, or turkey.

6. Top with 1 tablespoon nuts or seeds.

7. Include 1-2 servings fresh fruit or berries for dessert.

A Weekly Dinner Menu

Try these tasty dinner combinations. Each makes 1 serving.

Italian Dinner #1

- 4 ounces sliced chicken
- 1 cup whole grain linguine
- 1-3 cups mixed spinach, mushrooms, bell pepper, onion and asparagus
- $^1/_2$ cup green beans
- $^1/_2$ cup Alfredo Sauce
- 1 tablespoon pine nuts
- Chives for garnish
- Melon or nectarines for dessert

Italian Dinner #2

- 4 ounces salmon
- 1 cup farro
- 1-3 cups mixed broccolini, mushrooms, tomatoes, asparagus and onion
- ½ cup cannellini beans
- ½ cup Walnut Pesto
- 1 tablespoon chopped walnuts
- Basil for garnish
- Oranges or strawberries for dessert

Middle Eastern Dinner

- 4 ounces shrimp
- 1 cup whole wheat couscous or quinoa
- 1-3 cups mixed broccolini, mushrooms, shallots, carrots
- ½ cup chickpeas
- ½ cup Romesco Sauce
- 1 tablespoon sliced almonds
- Parsley for garnish
- Nectarines or figs for dessert

Asian Dinner

- 4 ounces sliced lean beef
- 1 cup brown rice
- 1-3 cups mixed broccoli, carrots, bell peppers, shitake mushrooms
- ½ cup green beans
- ½ cup Chinese Black Bean Sauce
- 1 tablespoon sesame seeds
- Green onions for garnish
- Pears or kiwi for dessert

Mexican Dinner

- 4 ounces red snapper
- 1-2 corn tortillas
- 1-3 cups mixed zucchini squash, carrots, corn, spinach
- ½ cup pinto beans
- ½ cup Green Poblano Sauce
- 1 tablespoon chia seeds
- Garnish with green onions
- Pineapple or mango for dessert

Chapter 9

Healthy Menus

We've put together two weeks of delicious meals for you. Use these menus as a guide to plan your meals for the week. To help you prepare, we've included shopping lists that can help keep you organized at the grocery store. For the first week, you will eat a combination of Mexican and Mediterranean foods. The second week is packed with American- and Asian-inspired fare.

To minimize cooking, we recommend buying several sauces and pairing them with certain dishes. However, if you want to prepare all of your own food, you can substitute the following store-bought sauces with the corresponding recipe (found in the Prediabetes Recipes chapter):

- Buy red salsa or make our Salsa Caliente
- Buy green (tomatillo) salsa or make our Green Poblano Sauce
- Buy pesto or make our Walnut Pesto
- Buy hummus or make our Fresh Garlic-Lemon Hummus
- Buy marinara sauce or make our Garden Marinara Sauce
- Buy black beans or make our Zesty Mexican Bean Dip

Week 1:

Start the week by preparing the Creamy Herb Dressing and Alfredo Sauce. Double both recipes and freeze half of each to use in recipes for week 2.

MONDAY: MEXICAN

Breakfast	Lunch	Snack	Dinner
Southwestern Breakfast Burrito Vegetable juice or V8	Rice and vegetable bowl with brown rice, zucchini, avocado, mushrooms, and spinach, topped with Salsa Caliente Mango and strawberries	Banana or apple with almond butter	2-3 burritos with black beans, tortilla, brown rice, spinach, alfalfa sprouts, tomato, avocado, Southwestern spice, 1 tablespoon rice or almond cheese, and diced beef or steak Kiwi and blackberries

TUESDAY: MEDITERRANEAN

Breakfast	Lunch	Snack	Dinner
Scrambled egg white with spinach and hummus on toast Green Gourmet Smoothie	Mixed baby greens salad with julienned carrots, tomatoes, avocado, zucchini, Creamy Herb Dressing and sprouted grain toast (hummus or avocado, optional) Cherries and strawberries	Breakfast Berry Parfait	Quinoa or brown rice noodles and vegetables (spinach, mushrooms, bell pepper, onion, asparagus), salmon or trout, topped with Alfredo Sauce Nectarines and blackberries

WEDNESDAY: MEXICAN

Breakfast	Lunch	Snack	Dinner
Southwestern Breakfast Burrito Vegetable juice	Mexican salad (mixed baby greens with zucchini, carrots, corn, spinach, cilantro, avocado, brown rice, and 1 tablespoon rice or almond cheese) with lime juice Mango and blackberries	Banana or apple with almond butter	1-2 tortillas with chicken and cooked vegetables (zucchini, carrots, corn, spinach, cilantro) with green salsa, 1 tablespoon rice or almond cheese, and brown rice Nectarines and raspberries

THURSDAY: MEDITERRANEAN			
Breakfast Breakfast Berry Parfait and almond butter on toast Vegetable juice	**Lunch** Pesto with whole grain pasta and vegetables (brocollini, mushrooms, tomatoes, asparagus, onion) Oranges and cherries	**Snack** Hummus and vegetables with whole grain pita crisps	**Dinner** Whole grain pasta and vegetables (brocollini, mushrooms, tomatoes, asparagus, onion) with ground beef or ground turkey, Garden Marinara Sauce, and 1 tablespoon rice or almond cheese Strawberries and blueberries

FRIDAY: MEDITERRANEAN			
Breakfast Scrambled egg white with spinach and hummus on toast Green Gourmet Smoothie	**Lunch** Whole grain pasta and vegetables (brocollini, mushrooms, tomatoes, asparagus, onion), Garden Marinara Sauce and 1 tablespoon rice or almond cheese Oranges and blackberries	**Snack** Breakfast Berry Parfait	**Dinner** Mixed baby greens salad with julienned carrots, tomatoes, avocado, zucchini with Creamy Herb dressing and sprouted grain toast (hummus or avocado, optional), shredded chicken Cherries and strawberries

SATURDAY: MEXICAN			
Breakfast Southwestern Breakfast Burrito Vegetable juice	**Lunch** Rice and vegetable bowl with brown rice, zucchini, avocado, mushrooms, spinach, red salsa, and 1 tablespoon rice or almond cheese Mango and strawberries	**Snack** Banana or apple with almond butter	**Dinner** Mexican salad (mixed baby greens with zucchini, carrots, corn, spinach, cilantro, avocado brown rice, 1 tablespoon rice or almond cheese) with lime juice, diced steak Mango and blackberries

SUNDAY: MEXICAN			
Breakfast Breakfast Berry Parfait Almond butter on toast Vegetable juice	**Lunch** 2 burritos with black beans, tortilla, brown rice, spinach, alfalfa sprouts, tomato, avocado, and 1 tablespoon rice or almond cheese Kiwi and blackberries	**Snack** Hummus, vegetables and whole grain pita crisps	**Dinner** 1-2 tortillas with chicken and cooked vegetables (zucchini, carrots, corn, spinach, cilantro), green salsa, 1 tablespoon rice or almond cheese, and brown rice Nectarines and raspberries

Grocery List for Week 1 (Serves 2)

The grocery list assumes that you have none of the food items in your pantry.

4 avocados

1 bunch asparagus

1 bunch broccolini

1 bag julienned carrots

2 packages sliced mushrooms

5 poblano peppers (omit if buying pre-made green salsa)

2 zucchini

4 tomatoes

3 onions

2 red bell peppers

1 green bell pepper

1 package alfalfa sprouts

6-8 ounces bagged baby greens

6-8 ounces bagged spinach

2 pounds red potatoes

8-10 ounces frozen spinach

8-10 ounces frozen corn

1 bunch cilantro

1 large bulb garlic (or minced in a jar)

4 apples

8 bananas

4 limes

4 lemons

3 mangos

2 pounds strawberries

3 kiwi

2 packages blackberries

2 pounds cherries

4 nectarines/peaches

2 packages raspberries

4 oranges

1 package blueberries

2 packages frozen cherries

2 packages frozen mixed berries

1 package frozen pineapple or mangoes, dried blueberries or currants

1 pound brown rice

½ pound quinoa

1 package corn or multigrain tortillas

1 box sprouted grain cereal or granola

1 loaf sprouted grain bread

2 boxes quinoa or brown rice pasta

1 box multigrain or whole wheat pita crisps

8 ounces rice cheese

8 ounces almond butter

2 pounds raw cashew pieces

1 ½ pounds almond slivers, pecans and walnuts

15 ounces cold-milled flaxseed meal

1 carton egg whites

24 ounces plain nonfat Greek yogurt

64 ounces pomegranate-blueberry juice

1 six-pack V8 vegetable juice

1 package silken tofu

2 cans low-sodium black beans

8 ounces hummus

1 ½ pounds lean beef steak

½ pounds ground beef, bison or turkey

½ pound shrimp

3 pounds chicken breasts

1 ½ pounds salmon, trout, halibut or cod

25 ½ ounces low-sodium marinara sauce (if you don't prepare Garden Marinara Sauce)

25 ½ ounces red salsa (if you don't prepare Salsa Caliente)

25 ½ ounces green salsa (if you don't prepare Green Poblano Sauce)

25 ½ ounces pesto (if you don't prepare Walnut Pesto)

Additional items: vinegar, salt, pepper, olive oil, agave nectar or honey, cumin, Southwestern chili powder blend, Italian seasoning, hot sauce (Cholula or Tabasco), crushed red pepper (optional), vanilla extract, brewer's yeast (optional), Vegenaise, Earth Balance or Smart Balance butter substitute

Week 2:

Start the week by preparing the Hot Artichoke-Spinach Dip, Coconut Curry Sauce, and Sesame-Ginger Sauce, which will be used as a salad dressing. Double the recipe for the Coconut Curry Sauce.

MONDAY: AMERICAN

Breakfast	Lunch	Snack	Dinner
Cereal with fruit, nuts and almond or soy milk Green Gourmet Smoothie	2 slices bread topped with Hot Artichoke-Spinach Dip and tomato Apples and blackberries	6 almonds with 2 cups air-popped popcorn, 1 tablespoon pumpkin seeds	White fish (cod, halibut, trout) and vegetables (green beans, carrots, broccoli, peas) and brown rice with Alfredo Sauce Blueberries and strawberries

TUESDAY: ASIAN

Breakfast	Lunch	Snack	Dinner
Sausage and Egg English Breakfast Muffin Vegetable juice	Baby greens, bell peppers, snap peas, carrots, radish with Sesame-Ginger Sauce and brown rice topped with 1/2 tablespoon almonds, cashews or peanuts Mango and strawberries	Hot Artichoke-Spinach Dip with sprouted grain toast	Coconut Curry Sauce with chicken over brown rice or quinoa and vegetables (broccoli, carrots, bell peppers, shitake mushrooms, snap peas or edamame) Cantaloupe and blueberries

WEDNESDAY: AMERICAN

Breakfast	Lunch	Snack	Dinner
Cereal with fruit, nuts and almond or soy milk Green Gourmet Smoothie	Baby greens with green beans, carrots, broccoli, peas, Creamy Herb Dressing and sprouted grain toast Cantaloupe and blueberries	6 almonds with 2 cups air-popped popcorn 1 tablespoon pumpkin seeds	Shrimp with whole grain orzo and green beans, carrots, broccoli, peas, cherry tomatoes, and Alfredo Sauce Mango and kiwi

THURSDAY: ASIAN

Breakfast	Lunch	Snack	Dinner
Fresh fruit and 2 slices toast with almond butter sprinkled with cacao nibs Vegetable juice	Coconut Curry Sauce with chicken over brown rice or quinoa and vegetables (broccoli, carrots, bell peppers, shitake mushrooms, snap peas, edamame) Cantaloupe and blueberries	Hot Artichoke-Spinach Dip with vegetables (carrots, celery, peppers, broccoli) and nuts	Baby greens, bell peppers, snap peas, carrots, radish with Sesame-Ginger Sauce, brown rice and shredded chicken Blueberries and strawberries

FRIDAY: AMERICAN

Breakfast	Lunch	Snack	Dinner
Sausage and Egg English Breakfast Muffin Vegetable juice	2 slices bread topped with Hot Artichoke-Spinach Dip and tomato Apples and blackberries	6 almonds with 2 cups air-popped popcorn, 1 tablespoon pumpkin seeds	Roasted vegetables (broccoli, green beans, bell peppers) over greens, salmon or trout, rotini pasta, and Creamy Herb Dressing Cantaloupe and raspberries

SATURDAY: ASIAN

Breakfast	Lunch	Snack	Dinner
Cereal with fruit and nuts and almond and soy milk Green Gourmet Smoothie	Baby greens salad with bell peppers, snap peas or edamame, carrots, radish and tomatoes topped with olive oil and lemon juice, garnished with walnuts and served with sprouted grain toast Mango and strawberries	Coconut Curry Sauce with raw or steamed vegetables (carrots, celery, peppers, broccoli)	Beef and vegetable stir-fry with 2 cloves garlic, 1 tablespoon sesame oil, $^{1}/_{2}$ diced onion, 2 tablespoons soy sauce and 1 teaspoon agave nectar, over brown rice or quinoa and vegetables (bok choy, snap peas or edamame, julienned carrots, red bell peppers) Apples and blackberries

SUNDAY: AMERICAN

Breakfast	Lunch	Snack	Dinner
Fresh fruit and 2 slices toast with almond butter sprinkled with cacao nibs Vegetable juice	Steamed broccoli, green beans, and bell peppers over greens and rotini pasta with Creamy Herb Dressing Cantaloupe and raspberries	Hot Artichoke-Spinach Dip with sprouted grain toast	Chicken and peas, carrots, onions, red potatoes, mushrooms over quinoa with Alfredo Sauce Blueberries and strawberries

Grocery List for Week 2 (Serves 2)

2 bunches broccoli

1 bunch celery

1 bag julienned carrots

1 package sliced mushrooms or dried shiitake mushrooms

1 bunch bok choy

2 red bell peppers

4 shallots

1 bunch fresh lemongrass

1 bunch green onions

1 bunch cilantro

1 large bulb garlic (or minced in a jar)

1 package cherry tomatoes or 4 tomatoes

1 bunch celery

1 pound green beans

16 ounces bagged baby greens

1 bunch radishes

8-10 ounces frozen spinach

8-10 ounces frozen peas

8-10 ounces frozen snap peas or edamame

4 apples

8 bananas

4 limes

4 lemons

3 mangoes

2 pounds strawberries

3 kiwi

2 packages blackberries

1 cantaloupe

2 packages blueberries

2 packages frozen cherries

2 packages frozen mixed berries

1 package frozen pineapple or mangoes

1 package dried cranberries or blueberries

14 ounces artichokes

2 cans coconut milk

19 ounces cannellini beans

1 package cooked egg white patties or 1 box egg whites

1 package veggie sausage patties

1 pound brown rice or quinoa

1 package sprouted grain English muffins

1 loaf sprouted grain bread

1 box whole grain or whole wheat orzo

1 package brown rice or quinoa rotini pasta

1 box whole grain cereal

1 package roasted sesame seeds

½ pound almonds or pecans

1 pound walnuts

8 ounces almond butter

1 jar tahini

1 carton almond or soy milk (unsweetened)

15 ounces cold-milled flaxseed meal (omit if leftover from last week)

8 ounces grated parmesan cheese

8 ounces package rice cheese

8 ounces pumpkin seeds

1 bottle low-sodium soy sauce or Bragg Liquid Aminos

64 ounces pomegranate-blueberry juice

1 six-pack V8 vegetable juice

1 pound lean beef steak

½ pound shrimp

2 pounds chicken breasts or tenders

1 pound wild salmon, trout, halibut or cod

1 package silken tofu

Additional items:
Curry powder blend, sherry wine vinegar, Dijon mustard, cacao nibs, Vegenaise, Tofutti sour cream substitute or plain nonfat Greek yogurt, Tofutti cream cheese substitute, brewer's yeast, sesame oil, Earth Balance or Smart Balance butter substitute

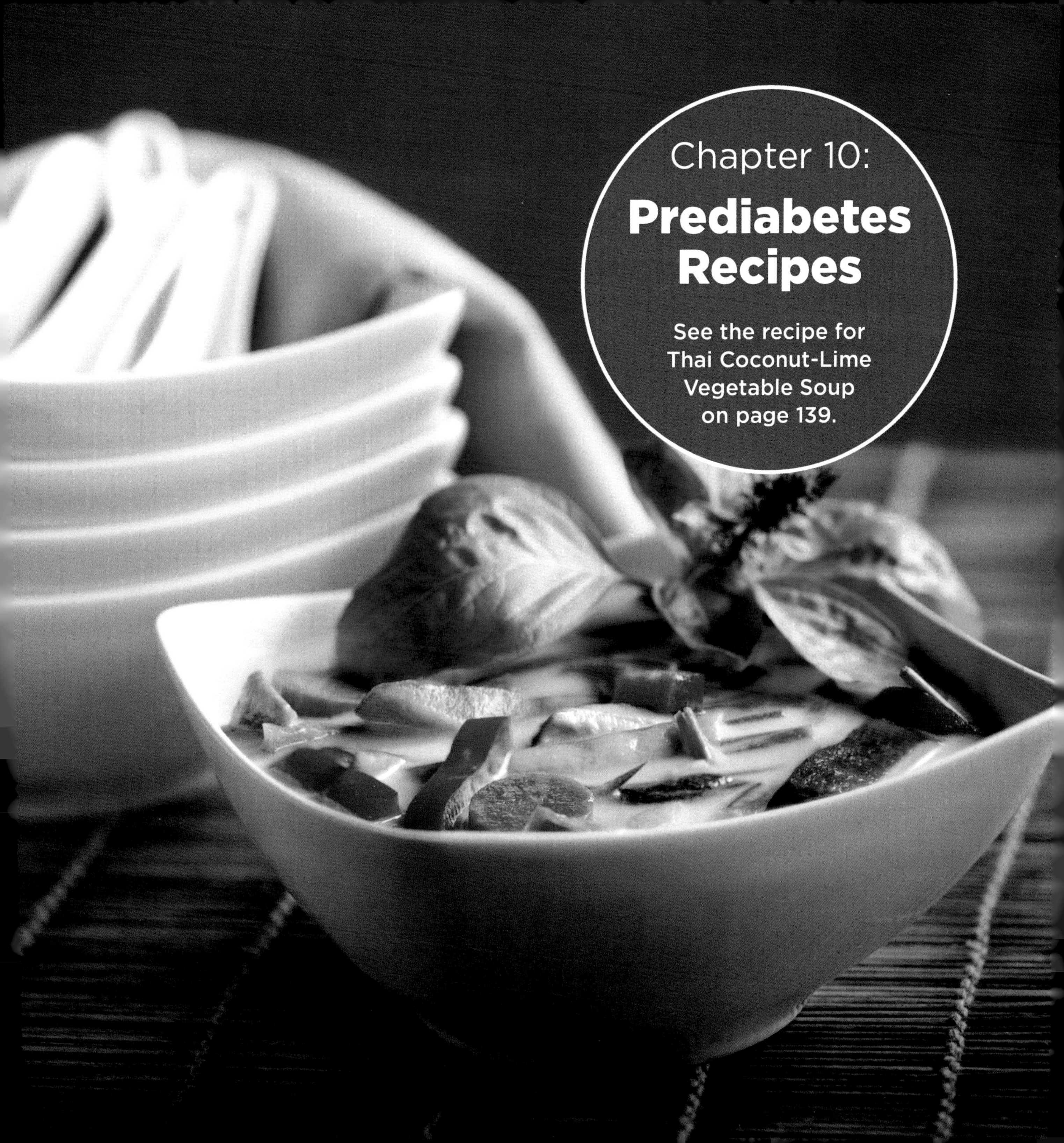

Chapter 10: Prediabetes Recipes

See the recipe for Thai Coconut-Lime Vegetable Soup on page 139.

Introduction

Concierge Nutrition includes more than 100 delicious recipes designed to meet your nutritional needs. Try as many new recipes as you can: Discovering new meals that you enjoy is critical to your long-term success.

When cooking new meals, it might take more time at first, which may be frustrating. Try easier recipes initially or work on a healthier version of your favorite dish. Find recipes for different situations: dinner at home with the family during a busy workweek, a potluck luncheon, backyard barbecue, or an elegant holiday dinner. Use the recipes often and be proactive about eating nutritious, delicious foods!

Each recipe features icons that indicate how many servings of nutrients are in one meal serving. Here are the nutrient categories:

RECIPE KEY

Nuts and Seeds

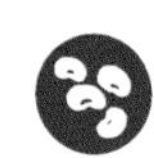
Beans and Legumes

Vegetables

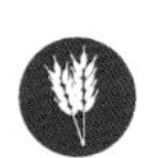
Whole Grains

Fruits

Oils

Lean Meats, Eggs & Cheese

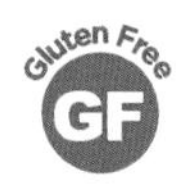

Gluten-Free

Many recipes contain gluten, but they can be made gluten-free by changing the whole grain in the recipe for a gluten-free whole grain.

Some recipes are higher in calories than others. If you're working on weight loss, choose a different recipe or decrease your portion size.

And, yes, there is a dessert section! These recipes are healthier than their traditional versions, but they're still desserts, which means they should be savored only once in a while.

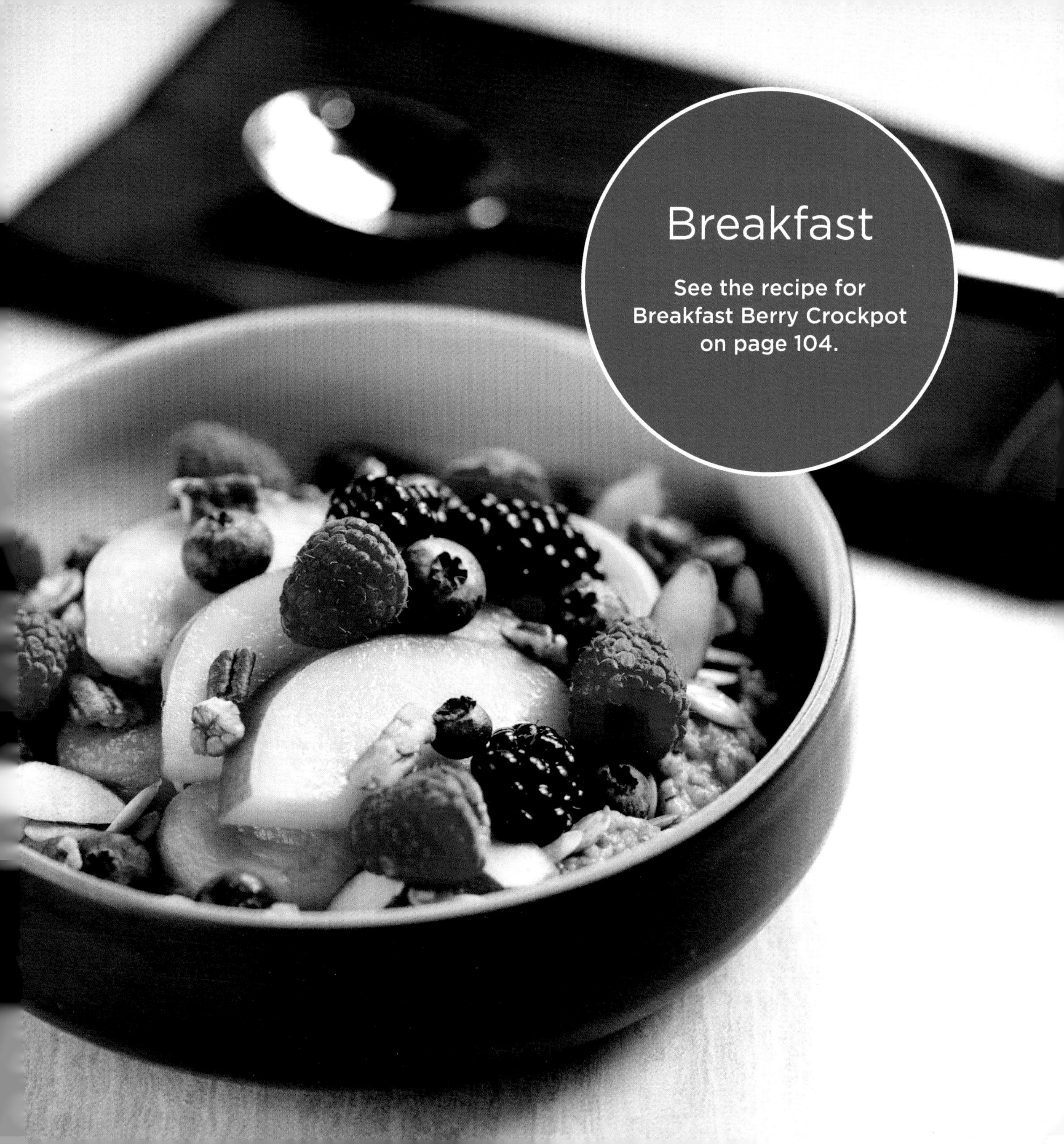

Breakfast

See the recipe for Breakfast Berry Crockpot on page 104.

Recipe Index

0 0 1 0 0 1 0

Gluten Free GF

Serves 2

Asian Breakfast Rice Bowl

Start your day with a tasty, nutritious meal that's both heart-healthy and anti-inflammatory. Dark, leafy greens packed with folic acid can help reduce risk for heart disease, while the dish's star spice, turmeric, fights inflammation and cancer-causing free radicals.

½ onion, chopped
8 ounces mushrooms, sliced or diced
2 cloves minced garlic
2 cups spinach or kale, chopped
1 pound firm tofu, drained and mashed
1 teaspoon turmeric
2 teaspoons Bragg Liquid Aminos or low-sodium soy sauce
2 cups cooked short-grained brown rice

Preparation

1. Steam-sauté onions, garlic and mushrooms until tender, approximately 5-7 minutes. Add tofu, turmeric and soy sauce and warm until heated through.

2. Toss in spinach or kale until wilted. Serve on top of rice.

Per Serving: 418 calories, 11g total fat, 0g saturated fat, 0mg cholesterol, 395mg sodium, 292mg potassium, 56g total carbohydrate, 5g dietary fiber, 26g protein

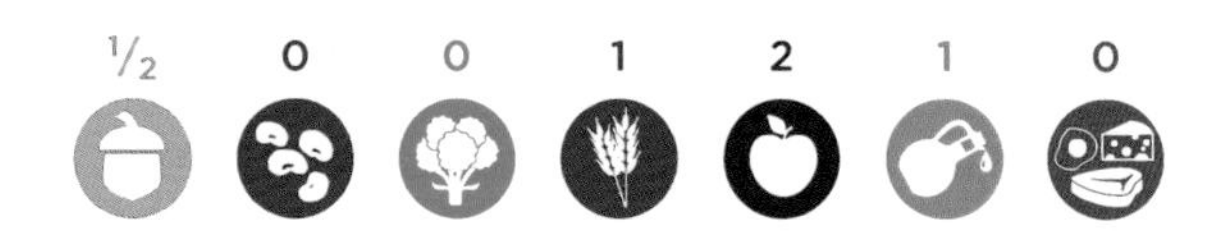

Serves 4

Berry Breakfast Crockpot

Fiber-rich 10-grain cereal teams with inflammation-fighting flaxseeds, heart-healthy nuts and dried fruit to create a delicious hot breakfast cereal. Berries are considered a superfood because they're very low in calories and high in nutrients, antioxidants and anti-inflammatory phytonutrients.

1 cup 10-grain hot cereal
1 1/4 cup soy, almond or coconut milk
2 cups water
1/4 cup diced nuts, such as almonds, raw cashews, walnuts, or pecans
1/4 cup dried fruit, such as dried cherries, blueberries, goji berries, cranberries, or diced apricots
4 pitted dates or 1/4 cup date pieces
1/4 teaspoon salt
1 cinnamon stick
2 sliced bananas
1 cup fresh berries, washed and diced
2 tablespoons flaxseed meal

Preparation

1. Pour all ingredients, except flaxseed meal, bananas and fresh berries, into a crockpot and cook on low overnight, or cook in a saucepan for 10 minutes.

2. Add flaxseed meal, bananas and fresh berries. Drizzle with more soy milk if desired.

Per Serving: 368 calories, 6g total fat, 1g saturated fat, 0mg cholesterol, 196mg sodium, 605mg potassium, 68g total carbohydrate, 11g dietary fiber, 11g protein

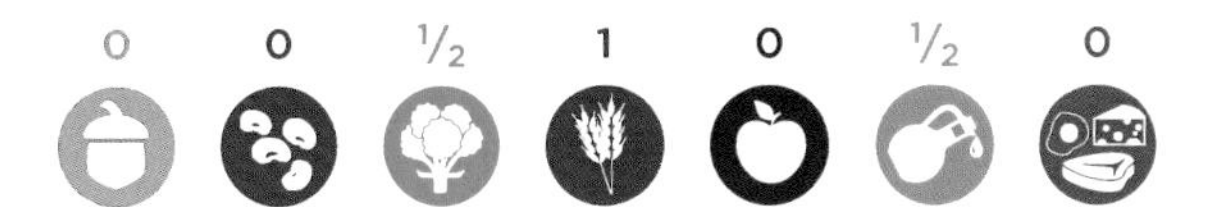

Serves 1

BREAKFAST

BLT Breakfast Burrito

Prepare several of these tasty burritos at the beginning of the week to have on hand for a quick, satisfying breakfast. Dark, leafy greens containing folic acid promote heart health, and avocado adds a dose of healthy monounsaturated fats. Can be refrigerated for up to seven days or individually wrapped and frozen for up to three months.

1 sprouted whole grain tortilla
2 slices Morningstar Stripples
1/2 teaspoon Dijon mustard
1 egg white patty or 1 egg white, scrambled
1/2 tablespoon shredded non-dairy rice cheese
1 cup baby greens, spinach, arugula, or baby kale
Sliced tomato or avocado, optional

Preparation

1. Prepare several at a time. Lay each tortilla flat and spread with mustard. Top with Stripples, egg white and optional tomato or avocado. Sprinkle with rice cheese.

2. Roll up and wrap in plastic wrap or parchment paper, twisting the ends. Stack in gallon-size plastic freezer bag and store in the refrigerator or freezer.

3. Before eating, warm in microwave for 1-2 minutes. Serve warm.

Per Serving: 360 calories, 14g total fat, 1g saturated fat, 46mg cholesterol, 724mg sodium, 441mg potassium, 39g total carbohydrate, 11g dietary fiber, 21g protein

0 0 0 1/3 1/4 0 0

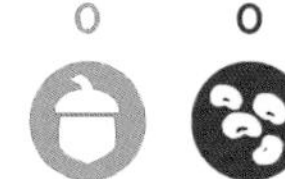 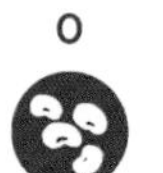  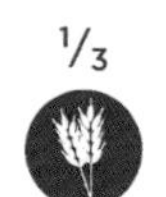  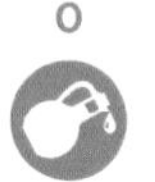 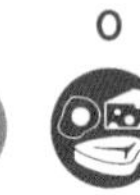

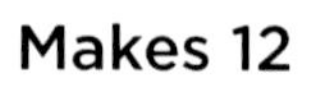

Makes 12

Blueberry Breakfast Muffins

Bite into one of these muffins right out of the oven, when it's hot and fresh! An excellent source of B vitamins and high in magnesium and manganese, flaxseed helps fight inflammation. Fresh blueberries are a powerful antioxidant, aiding your body in combating cancer-causing free radicals. These muffins aren't only delicious, they're good for you too!

1 cup whole wheat flour
3/4 cup plus 2 tablespoons all-purpose flour
1 1/2 teaspoons baking powder
1 teaspoon ground cinnamon
1/2 teaspoon baking soda
1/4 teaspoon salt
2 large eggs
1/2 cup pure maple syrup
1 cup nonfat buttermilk
1/4 cup canola oil
2 teaspoons freshly grated orange zest
1 tablespoon orange juice
1 teaspoon vanilla extract
1 1/2 cups fresh blueberries
1 tablespoon sugar
3 tablespoons flaxseed meal

Preparation

1 Preheat oven to 400 degrees. Coat 12 muffin cups with cooking spray.

2 Add whole-wheat flour, all-purpose flour, baking powder, cinnamon, baking soda and salt; whisk to blend. Whisk eggs and maple syrup in a medium bowl until smooth. Add buttermilk, oil, orange zest, orange juice and vanilla; whisk until blended.

3 Make a well in the dry ingredients and stir in the wet ingredients with a rubber spatula just until moistened. Fold in blueberries. Scoop the batter into the prepared muffin cups. Sprinkle the tops with sugar.

4 Bake the muffins until the tops are golden brown and spring back when touched lightly, 15 to 25 minutes. Sprinkle the tops with flaxseed meal. Let cool in the pan for 5 minutes. Loosen edges and transfer from pan to a wire cooling rack.

Per Serving: 192 calories, 7g total fat, 1g saturated fat, 36mg cholesterol, 191mg sodium, 12mg potassium, 29g total carbohydrate, 2g dietary fiber, 4g protein

0 0 1 0 0 1 0

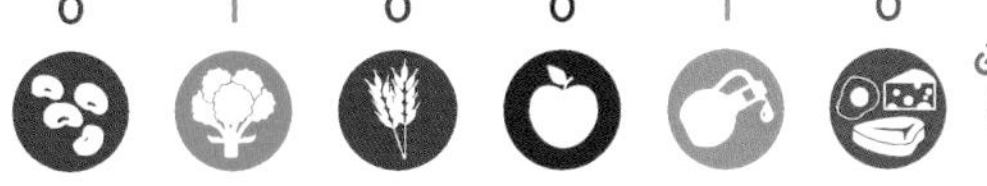

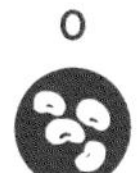
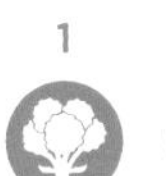
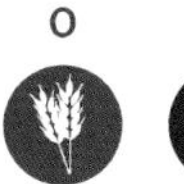
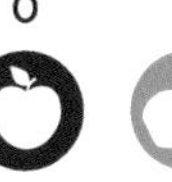
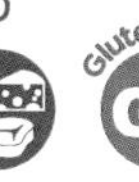
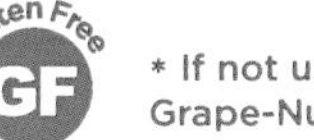

* If not using Grape-Nuts or granola

Serves 4

Breakfast Berry Parfait

This delicious parfait is a snap to make! Top with fresh fruit and flaxseed for a high-calcium, fiber-rich breakfast. Keep the parfait fresh in the refrigerator for up to seven days.

4 cups mixed fresh or frozen fruit

3 tablespoons agave nectar

1/4 cup dried fruit, blueberries, goji berries, cranberries, diced apricots or pitted dates

1 pound plain nonfat Greek yogurt

1 pound silken (soft) tofu

2 teaspoons vanilla extract

1 sliced banana, for garnish

1 tablespoon flaxseed meal

1/2 tablespoon granola or Grape-Nuts cereal

Preparation

1. Mix fresh fruit, agave nectar and dried fruit in a bowl.
2. In a blender, add Greek yogurt, silken tofu and vanilla extract, and blend until creamy and smooth.
3. In a tall glass layer 1/4 cup fruit, 1/4 cup yogurt, 1/4 cup fruit, then 1/4 cup yogurt. Cover and store in the refrigerator until ready to serve.
4. Top with sliced banana, flaxseed meal and granola or Grape-Nuts cereal.

Per Serving: 150 calories, 2g total fat, 0g saturated fat, 4mg cholesterol, 30mg sodium, 313mg potassium, 25g total carbohydrate, 2g dietary fiber, 9g protein

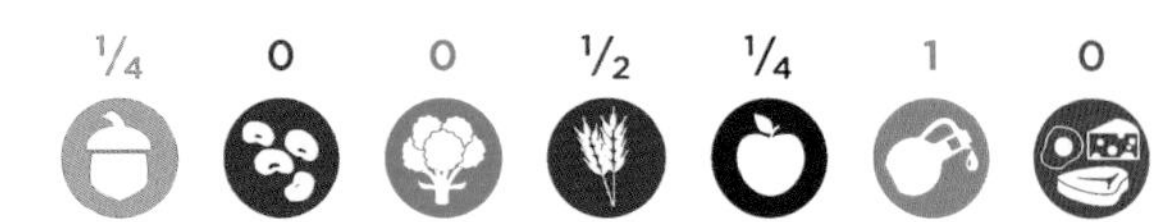

Makes 12

Chocolate-Pecan Oat Cakes

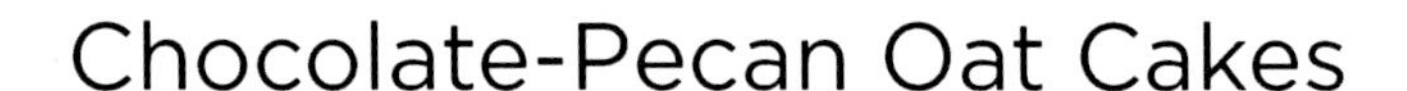

These hearty, whole grain cookies are based on the traditional oat cakes carried by Scottish shepherds. Oats are full of fiber, making these oat cakes an ideal breakfast or midday snack for people with prediabetes. These breakfast cakes get an extra nutritional boost from pecans which contain sterols, a substance that helps decrease levels of harmful LDL cholesterol.

1 cup unbleached flour

½ cup whole wheat or spelt flour

¾ cup Earth Balance butter substitute

1 cup bulgur wheat soaked in warm water for 15 minutes and drained

3 cups old-fashioned rolled oats (not instant)

1 cup dried dates puréed with 1 cup water

2 tablespoons honey or agave nectar

1 pinch salt

¼ cup chocolate chips

¼ cup pecans

Preparation

1 Preheat oven to 400 degrees.

2 Mix dry ingredients. Add butter substitute and blend with pastry tool or fork into pea-sized pieces, then add dates and honey.

3 Spoon into 2-inch balls; place on cookie sheet and bake for 15 minutes. Remove from oven and mash each ball with spatula until about ⅓-inch thick. Bake for 5 more minutes. Remove and cool on a wire rack for 10 minutes.

4 Serve warm. Top with fruit compote if desired.

Per Serving: 314 calories, 15g total fat, 5g saturated fat, 0mg cholesterol, 124mg sodium, 99mg potassium, 43g total carbohydrate, 6g dietary fiber, 8g protein

<1/3 0 0 <1/2 Trace Trace 0

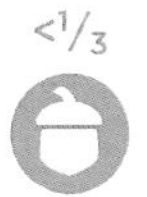 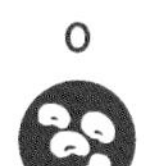 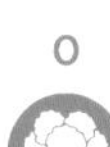 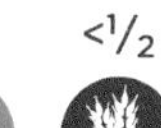   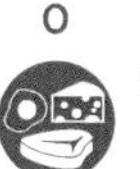 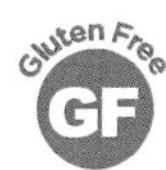

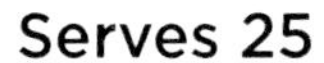

High-Protein Granola

This filling breakfast cereal is loaded with complex carbs and protein. Flaxseed, one of the most nutrient-dense foods on the planet, teams up with antioxidant-packed nuts and berries for a tasty, healthful breakfast option. Flaxseed meal loses its omega-3 properties when heated, so add it to cold foods or use as a topping.

6 cups old-fashioned rolled oats (not instant)

3 cups Ezekiel high-protein sprouted grain cereal

1 cup soy protein powder

1 1/4 cup flaxseed meal

3/4 cup Smart Balance cooking oil

1 cup honey, agave nectar or maple syrup

1 pinch salt

1 cup raw nuts

1 cup dried berries

1/2 cup seeds, such as pumpkin, sunflower, hemp or sesame

Preparation

1. Preheat oven to 325 degrees. Mix oats, cereal and soy protein powder.

2. Warm cooking oil and honey in a saucepan over medium heat until hot and viscous, about 2-3 minutes.

3. Combine dry cereal mixture with warm oil and honey mixture. Toss to combine and pour onto foil- or parchment-lined baking sheet. Sprinkle with salt. Bake for 12 minutes, stir and bake for another 5 minutes, or until it's golden. Check frequently to avoid burning.

4. Combine raw nuts, seeds, berries and flaxseed meal with hot golden granola. Cool and store in airtight container in refrigerator for up to three months. Serve 1/2 cup granola with soy milk.

Per Serving: 293 calories, 16g total fat, 2g saturated fat, 0mg cholesterol, 83mg sodium, 69mg potassium, 34g total carbohydrate, 3g dietary fiber, 6g protein

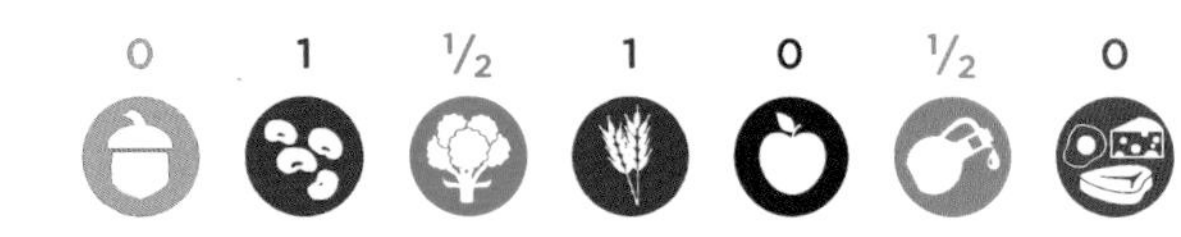

Serves 2

Mexican Migas

This classic Mexican breakfast gets a healthy makeover with inflammation-fighting spinach and iron-rich cumin. This satisfying breakfast also doubles as a healthful quick dinner.

1 tablespoon olive oil
1 corn tortilla, diced
2 pinches cumin, Southwestern spice mix or taco seasoning
2 pinches salt
1 serving Egg Beaters
1 cup baby spinach
1 tablespoon shredded non-dairy rice cheese or 1 diced avocado
1/4 cup salsa
Chopped cilantro or sliced green onions for garnish, optional

Preparation

1. Heat olive oil in a skillet. Add spices and corn tortillas and cook over medium heat until crispy.

2. Pour in Egg Beaters and scramble until cooked, about 3 minutes. Add spinach and heat until thoroughly warmed.

3. Divide onto two plates and top with rice cheese and salsa. Top with cilantro or green onions for added flavor. Serve with whole grain toast or vegetarian refried beans.

Per Serving: 241 calories, 8g total fat, 1g saturated fat, 0mg cholesterol, 707mg sodium, 245mg potassium, 28g total carbohydrate, 5g dietary fiber, 10g protein

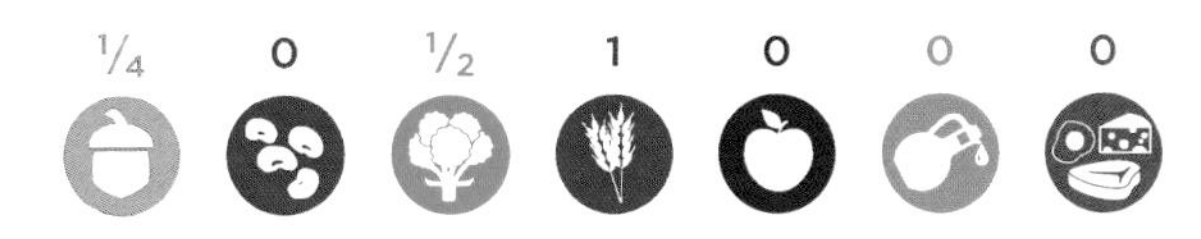

Makes 1

Sausage and Egg English Breakfast Muffin

Build a week's worth of these sandwiches for a delicious, on-the-go breakfast! Just zap in the microwave and stuff with a handful of veggies before you head out the door. Dark, leafy greens give you a shot of folic acid while avocado nourishes the body with healthy monounsaturated fats. Wrap them individually and warm in the microwave before serving.

1 sprouted grain English muffin, split
1/2 tablespoon Walnut Pesto or store-bought pesto
1/2 teaspoon favorite hot sauce
1 egg white patty
1 veggie sausage patty
1/2 tablespoon shredded non-dairy rice cheese
1 handful baby greens, spinach, arugula, or kale
Sliced tomato
Sliced avocado

Preparation

1. Split muffins and spread pesto on one muffin half, then sprinkle hot sauce on the other half.

2. Lay veggie sausage and egg white patty on one half, sprinkle with rice cheese and top with other half of muffin. Make several and put in freezer-safe plastic sandwich bags. Can refrigerate for up to five days, or freeze for up to three months.

3. Before eating, cook in microwave for 1-2 minutes or toast in oven for 10 minutes at 375 degrees. Add greens, tomato and avocado.

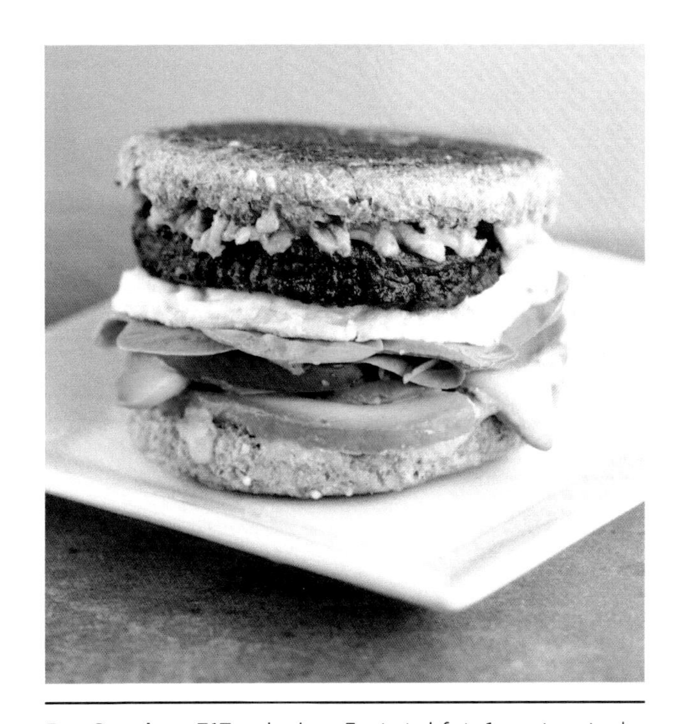

Per Serving: 317 calories, 5g total fat, 1g saturated fat, 0mg cholesterol, 711mg sodium, 563mg potassium, 42g total carbohydrate, 9g dietary fiber, 26g protein

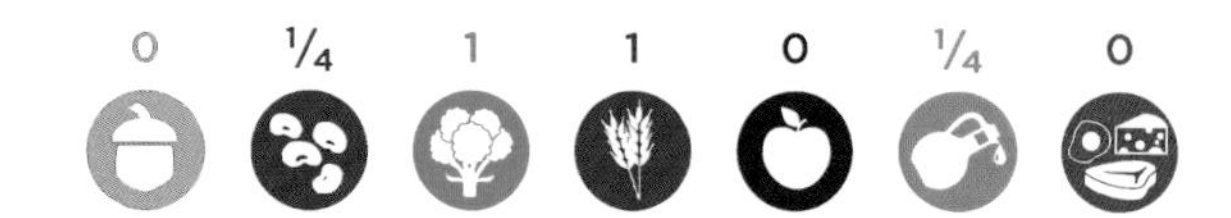

Serves 8

Southwestern Breakfast Burritos

Start your day with a high-protein meal that will boost your energy and keep you feeling fuller longer. Spinach promotes heart health and fights inflammation, and beans are an excellent source of fiber.

2 tablespoons olive oil, divided

2 cups diced or shredded frozen potatoes, white or red

1 cup Egg Beaters

1 teaspoon salt

2 pinches Southwestern seasoning or taco seasoning

1/2 cup shredded non-dairy rice cheese

Favorite hot sauce to taste

1 cup baby spinach

1 cup vegetarian refried beans

1 cup salsa

8 whole wheat, sprouted grain or brown rice tortillas

Sliced avocado

Preparation

1. Heat 1 tablespoon of olive oil in a 10-inch skillet and cook potatoes until lightly browned. Season with salt, transfer potatoes to a plate and set aside.

2. In same skillet, heat 1 tablespoon oil and scramble Egg Beaters and top with Southwestern seasoning. Fold in spinach if you prefer or add it fresh before serving.

3. Warm tortillas in microwave for 1 minute until pliable. Lay out 8 tortillas and spread with 2 tablespoons of vegetarian refried beans, top with rice cheese, potatoes and Egg Beaters. Top with hot sauce.

4. Roll burritos individually in parchment paper or Saran Wrap, twisting the ends. Pack them in a freezer-safe plastic bag and refrigerate until ready to eat. Warm in microwave for 40 seconds to 1 minute. After warming, open burrito and add baby greens and salsa, and serve.

Per Serving: 295 calories, 7g total fat, 1g saturated fat, 0mg cholesterol, 516mg sodium, 236mg potassium, 41g total carbohydrate, 6g dietary fiber, 13g protein

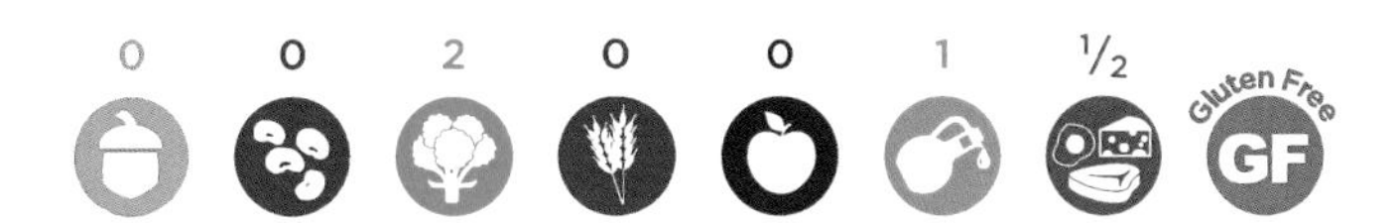

Serves 2

Spanish Torta

A healthy take on the classic Spanish omelet, this dish uses less cooking oil and healthy Egg Beaters for a low-fat, low-cholesterol version. Red bell peppers are packed with beta-carotene and free radical-fighting antioxidants. Serve warm or at room temperature for breakfast, lunch or a light dinner with a mixed baby green salad.

2 tablespoons olive oil, divided

1 small onion, diced

2 cups diced frozen potatoes, white or red

1 cup baby spinach

1/2 cup peas, red bell peppers, diced, or roasted green chilies

1 teaspoon salt

1/4 teaspoon ground pepper

1/2 cup silken tofu, puréed

1/2 cup Egg Beaters

2 tablespoons cornstarch

1/8 teaspoon turmeric and 1/8 teaspoon paprika, or 1/4 teaspoon thyme, optional

Preparation

1. Heat 1 tablespoon of olive oil in 10-inch nonstick skillet. Add onions and cook until tender, about 2-3 minutes. Add potatoes with 2 tablespoons of water, cover and cook on medium-low for 5 minutes.

2. Add spinach and red bell peppers. Cook until spinach is wilted and add optional spices if desired. Pour contents into a bowl.

3. In blender, purée silken tofu, Egg Beaters, cornstarch, salt and pepper until smooth. Pour contents in bowl and fold to combine. Add peas.

4. Heat 1 tablespoon oil in skillet over high heat and pour bowl contents into the hot pan and reduce heat to medium. Cover and cook for 5 minutes. Uncover and loosen edges with a spatula.

5. Slide torta onto a plate, cover with pan and flip torta back into the skillet. Cook for another 5 minutes. Let cool for 15 minutes. Serve as an appetizer with fresh aioli or over baby greens.

Per Serving: 342 calories, 15g total fat, 2g saturated fat, 0mg cholesterol, 175mg sodium, 619mg potassium, 40g total carbohydrate, 5g dietary fiber, 14g protein

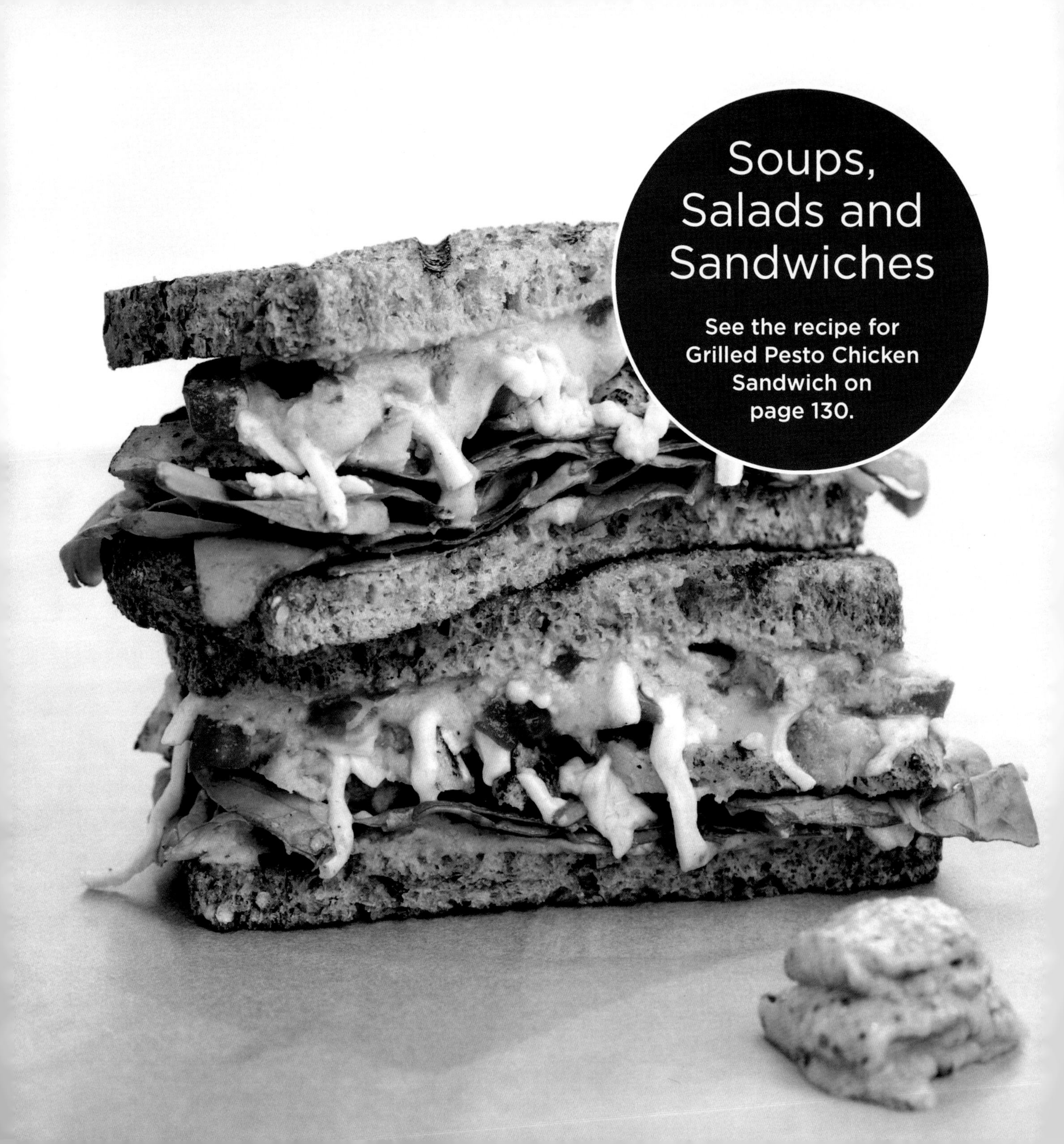

Soups, Salads and Sandwiches

See the recipe for Grilled Pesto Chicken Sandwich on page 130.

Recipe Index

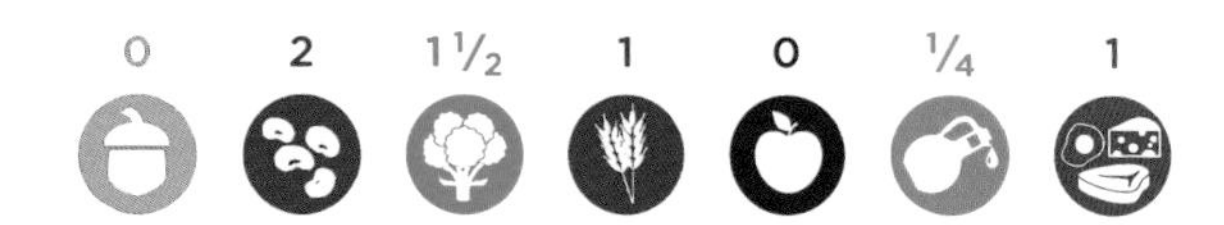

Serves 1

Black-Eyed Pea Salad with Grilled Meat

An ideal lunch or light supper, this hearty salad features black-eyed peas that provide slow, steady energy to fuel you through the day. Lean beef is an excellent source of vitamin B12, which aids in nervous system function and regulation of homocysteine levels.

1 celery rib, diced
1/2 green onion, sliced
1/2 can black-eyed peas, rinsed, white beans or edamame
1/2 cup cherry tomatoes, halved, or diced red bell pepper
1/4 teaspoon Italian seasoning
1/8 teaspoon ground pepper
Lemon juice from half a lemon
1/2 teaspoon olive oil
1 pinch allspice
1/2 cup sliced grilled beef, chicken, fish or veggie meat
1 cup baby greens
1 slice sprouted whole grain bread

Preparation

1. Toss all ingredients except beef, baby greens and bread. Spoon salad mixture over baby greens and top with sliced grilled meat and extra lemon wedges. Serve with bread on the side.

Per Serving: 378 calories, 6g total fat, 0g saturated fat, 57mg cholesterol, 384mg sodium, 696mg potassium, 42g total carbohydrate, 9g dietary fiber, 36g protein

1/2  1/4 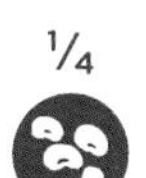 1 1/4  0 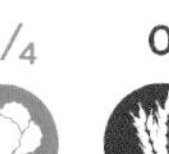 0 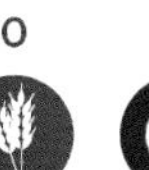 1/16 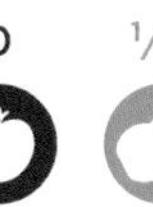 0 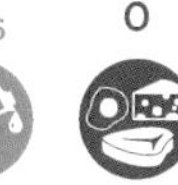 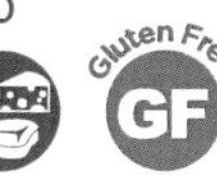

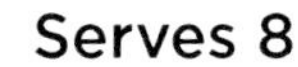

Serves 8

Caesar Salad with Garlicky Walnuts

This classic salad is pumped up with extra phytonutrients from raw greens and tossed with a healthy version of Caesar dressing. Top the garlicky walnuts with brewer's yeast, which tastes similar to grated parmesan cheese and helps with blood sugar regulation and fat metabolism.

6 cups baby mixed greens, such as spinach, romaine lettuce, arugula and red lettuce

2 large tomatoes, diced, or 1 cup halved cherry tomatoes

1 can low-sodium garbanzo beans, rinsed and drained

2 cups diced kale

1/4 cup raw cashews or Vegenaise mayonnaise substitute

1/4 cup water

2 lemons juiced, 1 zested

1 teaspoon hot sauce or 1/8 teaspoon crushed red pepper, cayenne or ground pepper

1/2 teaspoon plus 1/4 teaspoon salt

4 cloves garlic, mince 2 and leave 2 whole

1/2 tablespoon olive oil or Earth Balance butter substitute

1 cup crushed walnuts

1/2 tablespoon brewer's yeast, optional

Preparation

1 In blender, add raw cashews or mayonnaise substitute, lemon juice, lemon zest, hot sauce, whole garlic cloves, and 1/2 teaspoon salt. Purée ingredients until smooth and creamy. Add more water if the mixture is too thick.

2 In a large bowl, toss dressing with kale and let set until slightly wilted, about 5 minutes.

3 In a small skillet, heat olive oil and add garlic when pan is shimmering. Add walnuts and roast slightly until fragrant, about 4-7 minutes. Remove from heat and toss with 1/4 teaspoon salt and brewer's yeast. Set aside to cool.

4 Add mixed greens, tomatoes and garbanzo beans to the kale. Toss to coat and serve salad with garlicky walnuts on top.

Per Serving: 182 calories, 13g total fat, 1.5g saturated fat, 0mg cholesterol, 424mg sodium, 228mg potassium, 13.5g total carbohydrate, 4.5g dietary fiber, 6g protein

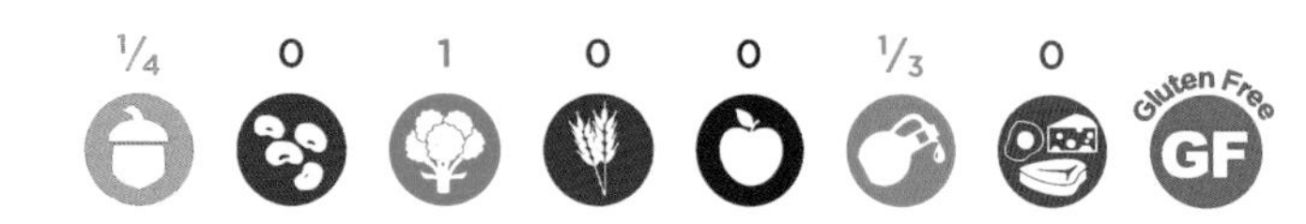

Serves 6

Chilled Cucumber-Avocado Soup

Cool cucumber and heart-healthy avocados make a delicious combination in this recipe. The good fats in avocados can help reduce total cholesterol, elevate "good" cholesterol, and control blood glucose levels. If you use fresh herbs, double the amount recommended in the recipe, as dried herbs have a more concentrated flavor. Serve the soup chilled.

2 English cucumbers

1 avocado, pitted and peeled

1/2 cup plain nonfat Greek yogurt or Tofutti sour cream substitute, or 1/4 cup raw cashews or blanched almonds

2 handfuls of baby spinach

1/2 tablespoon dried tarragon, basil or cilantro

4 cups water

1/2 teaspoon lemon zest and 1 lemon, juiced

Salt and ground pepper or hot sauce

Tarragon or parsley sprigs for garnish

Preparation

1. Add all the ingredients in a large pot and purée using an immersion blender. Adjust the consistency with more water if desired. Chill.

2. Divide soup evenly into four bowls, garnish with tarragon and serve.

Per Serving: 73 calories, 3g total fat, 1g saturated fat, 2mg cholesterol, 73mg sodium, 143mg potassium, 7g total carbohydrate, 2g dietary fiber, 3g protein

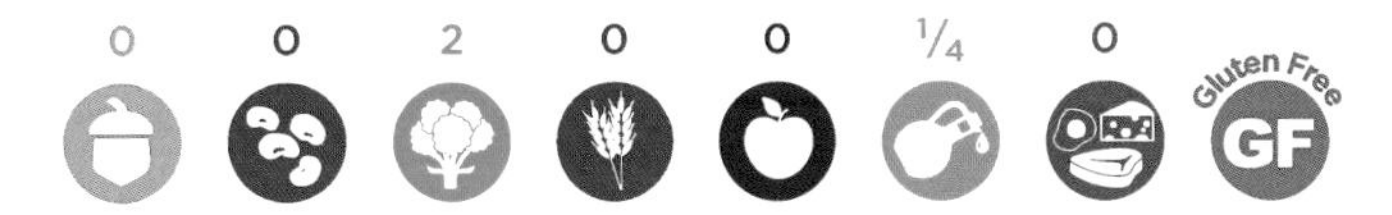

Serves 6

Cool Garden Vegetable Gazpacho

This soup is best made with fresh summer vegetables and should be served chilled on a warm day. Carrot juice will nourish your body with carotenoids, powerful antioxidants that help to reduce disease-causing free radicals.

1 tablespoon olive oil

1/2 onion, diced

4 cloves garlic, diced

1/2 teaspoon ground cumin

2 tablespoons sherry or red wine vinegar, or 1 lime, juiced

1 English hothouse cucumber or regular cucumber, peeled and seeded

1 red bell pepper, diced

1 poblano or jalapeno pepper, or bell pepper

6 plum tomatoes (2 pounds)

1 1/2 cups tomato juice

1 1/2 cup carrot juice

1 teaspoon hot sauce to taste or black pepper

1 1/2 teaspoon salt to taste

Fresh cilantro or basil for garnish

Preparation

1 In a small skillet, heat olive oil and sauté onion and garlic until cooked through; add 1 teaspoon water to prevent browning. Once water is evaporated, add cumin and toast for 30 seconds. If using red wine vinegar or sherry, pour in pan and scrape the pan. Add contents to blender.

2 In blender, combine cucumbers, red bell pepper, poblano, tomatoes, tomato juice, carrot juice, hot sauce and salt. Pulse to blend; don't let the mixture get too smooth. Garnish and serve chilled.

Per Serving: 88 calories, 3g total fat, 0g saturated fat, 0mg cholesterol, 129mg sodium, 510mg potassium, 16g total carbohydrate, 3g dietary fiber, 2g protein

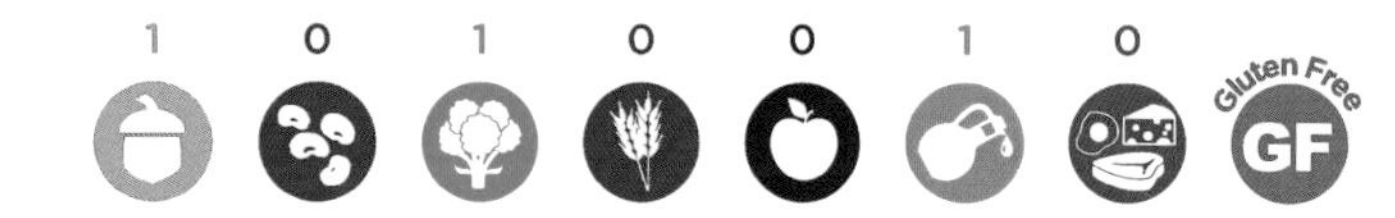

Serves 6

Corn and Summer Vegetable Chowder

Fresh summer produce is showcased in this delicious corn chowder! Chowder is traditionally made with heavy cream, which is high in saturated fat, calories and cholesterol. Using non-dairy substitutes allows you to avoid the harmful effects of bad fats and reap the nutritious benefits of soy, almonds or cashews.

3 tablespoons Earth Balance or Benecol butter substitute

1 large onion, diced (1/2 cup)

2 medium zucchini, diced, or 2 diced celery ribs

2 diced carrots

1 can roasted green chilies or 1 roasted poblano chili

3 medium red potatoes (about 1 1/2 pounds), diced into 1/4-inch cubes

1 1/2 cup diced green beans, fresh or frozen

1/2 teaspoon dried thyme

4 ears corn, kernels removed (about 4 cups), or 2 cans corn, drained

2 cups water or 2 14.5-ounce cans of low-sodium vegetable broth

1 cup soy milk, almond milk or soy creamer, or 1 cup cashew cream (3/4 cup cashews puréed with 3/4 cup water)

3 tablespoons cornstarch

1/3 cup plain nonfat Greek yogurt or Tofutti sour cream substitute

Coarse salt and ground pepper

1/4 teaspoon cayenne pepper

Preparation

1. In a large saucepan over medium heat, melt butter substitute and cook onions and zucchini for 3 minutes. Add carrots, potatoes, thyme and green chilies.

2. Pour in water and simmer for 20 minutes. Stir in corn and green beans and cook for 8-10 minutes.

3. Meanwhile, whisk corn starch with soy milk and slowly whisk into soup pot and continue to cook until boiling. After soup begins to thicken, stir in Greek yogurt.

4. Add salt and pepper to taste. Simmer on low for another 10 minutes or check potatoes for tenderness before serving.

Per Serving: 239 calories, 7g total fat, 2g saturated fat, 1mg cholesterol, 153mg sodium, 743mg potassium, 37g total carbohydrate, 5g dietary fiber, 9g protein

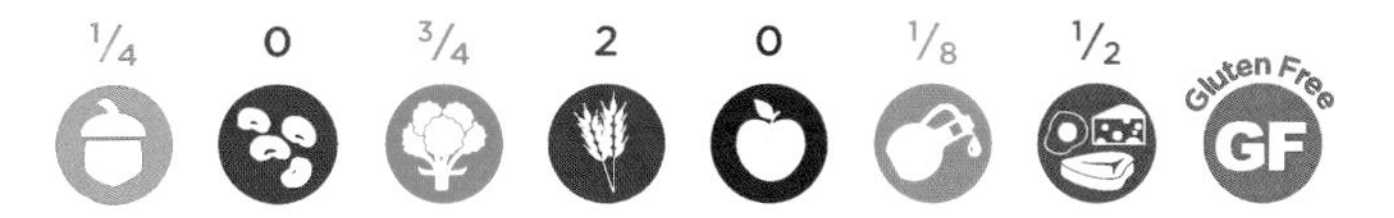

Serves 8

Creamy Asian Sesame Noodle Salad

This protein-packed dish is delicious served warm, and tastes just as good served cold the next day. Sesame and sesame oil should only be used in low heating conditions, such as in soups or salad dressing. Loaded with calcium and iron, sesame can be a powerful supplement to your diet.

1 pound whole grain linguine pasta or gluten-free brown rice pasta

1 tablespoon sesame oil

1/4 cup tahini (sesame paste) or peanut butter

1/4 cup plus 3 tablespoons water

2 teaspoons sriracha or hot sauce, or 1/2 teaspoon crushed red pepper or cayenne pepper

3 tablespoons Bragg Liquid Aminos or low-sodium soy sauce

2 tablespoons red wine vinegar or apple cider vinegar

2 tablespoons minced garlic, divided

1 cup julienned carrots

4 cups sliced kale or bok choy

1 package chopped veggie chicken, or 1 pound cooked chicken breasts, shredded

1/2 tablespoon sesame seeds for garnish

2 tablespoons crushed peanuts for garnish

1/2 bunch scallions, diced, for garnish

Mixed baby greens or shredded romaine lettuce

Preparation

1. Cook pasta until al dente and then drain and rinse under cold water until cool. Add the pasta back to the cooking pot, toss with 1/4 teaspoon of sesame oil, and set aside.

2. In a small saucepan, heat the remaining sesame oil until the pan shimmers. Add 1 tablespoon garlic and cook about 30 seconds; don't let the garlic brown. Add 1/4 cup water to the pan. When the water begins to boil, add carrots and kale. Steam the vegetables for 7-10 minutes until tender.

3. In a medium bowl, stir 3 tablespoons water, tahini, hot sauce, soy sauce, vinegar and 1 tablespoon garlic and whisk until creamy. Add water to thin the mixture if necessary.

4. Toss tahini dressing with noodles, steamed vegetables and chicken. Pour noodle salad over mixed baby greens and top with scallions, sesame seeds and peanuts.

Per Serving: 402 calories, 14g total fat, 2g saturated fat, 0mg cholesterol, 378mg sodium, 306mg potassium, 52g total carbohydrate, 10g dietary fiber, 21g protein

¼ ½ 1 ½ 0 1 0

  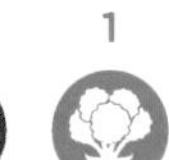 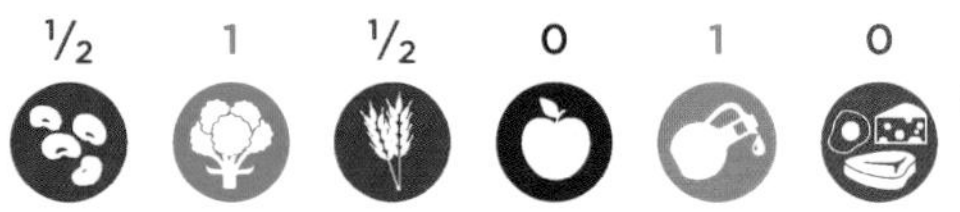 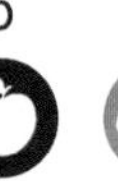 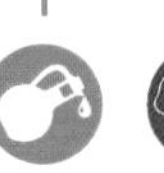 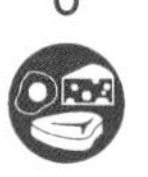

* Can be gluten free if you use brown rice noodles to replace whole grain pasta

Serves 6

Creamy Macaroni-Potato Salad

When you want a creamy salad, this one will satisfy! Red potatoes are a better choice than russet potatoes because of its deeper hue, which makes it a more nutrient-dense vegetable. One medium red potato has 5 grams of protein and less starch than a russet potato. The skin is packed with nutrients, so keep the skin on potatoes for extra nutrition.

½ box whole grain pasta (fusili, elbows, bowtie, or penne)

3 pounds diced red potatoes

1 pound or package fresh green beans or snap peas, steamed and blanched

1 cup frozen edamame or green peas, blanched

1 can drained cannellini beans

4 celery ribs, diced

1 bell pepper, diced

2 cups carrots, julienned

1 cup parsley or kale, diced

½ cup Vegenaise mayonnaise substitute

½ cup Tofutti sour cream substitute or plain nonfat Greek yogurt

2 lemons juiced, 1 zested

¼ teaspoon ground pepper

1 teaspoon hot sauce or sriracha

1 teaspoon salt

1 tablespoon flaxseed meal for garnish

½ bunch green onions, diced, for garnish

6 cups fresh baby greens, optional

Preparation

1. In a large saucepan, boil water and salt. Add the potatoes and cook for 10 minutes. Then add pasta to the potatoes and cook for an additional 12 minutes. Drain in a colander.

2. In a separate large bowl, mix mayonnaise substitute, sour cream substitute, lemon juice, lemon zest, black pepper, hot sauce and salt. Add vegetables to the bowl and reserve the baby greens.

3. Add pasta and potatoes to the bowl and combine. Spoon 1 cup of macaroni-potato salad on top of 1 cup baby greens. Garnish with flaxseed and green onions. Serve chilled.

Per Serving: 512 calories, 15g total fat, 1g saturated fat, 1mg cholesterol, 626mg sodium, 1064mg potassium, 74g total carbohydrate, 16g dietary fiber, 21g protein

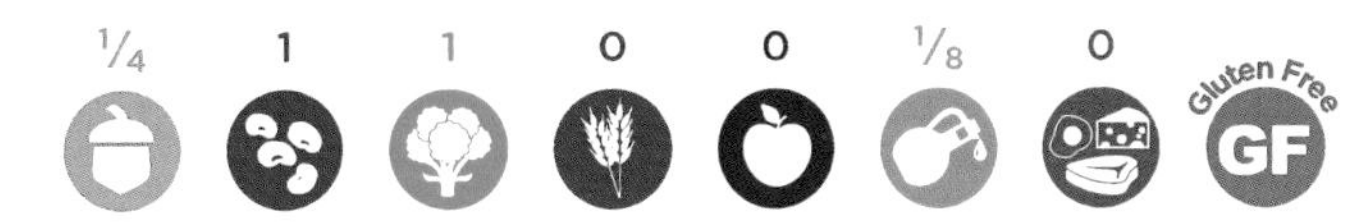

Serves 8

Creamy Tomato-Basil Soup

Tomato soup gets a healthy makeover in this nutrient-rich, high-protein version. Tomatoes have lycopene, a potent antioxidant that becomes more abundant when cooked. Studies show that lycopene has heart-healthy benefits and can reduce inflammation.

4 tablespoons Earth Balance butter substitute or olive oil

4 cups fresh tomatoes, cored, peeled and chopped, or 4 cups canned whole tomatoes, crushed

2 15-ounce cans diced tomatoes with juice and 2 cans water

1 8-ounce can low-sodium tomato sauce and 1 can water

2 diced carrots

2 diced red potato or 2 diced zucchini squash

1 large shallot or ¼ cup diced onion

1 cup low-sodium cannellini, navy or cooked lentils

1 cup soy creamer, or ½ cup raw cashews puréed with ¾ cup water

¼ teaspoon cracked black pepper or 1/8 teaspoon crushed red pepper

Salt to taste

1 handful baby spinach, optional

Lemon juice, optional

⅔ cup chopped fresh basil leaves or 5 tablespoons dried basil for garnish

Preparation

1. Combine tomatoes, tomato sauce, water, diced carrots, potato, shallot, and beans in a large stock pot. Simmer for 30 minutes.

2. Purée in small batches in blender or with an immersion blender. Blend in basil, soy creamer and butter substitute, and season with salt and pepper.

3. Add spinach if desired. Allow to wilt before serving. Finish with lemon juice and serve with basil as garnish.

Per Serving: 203 calories, 8g total fat, 2g saturated fat, 0mg cholesterol, 184mg sodium, 617mg potassium, 28g total carbohydrate, 8g dietary fiber, 7g protein

¼ 0 1 1 ¼ ½ 1

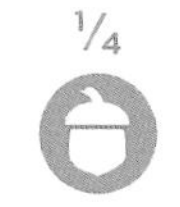 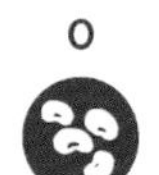     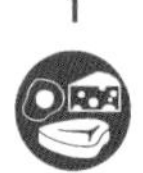

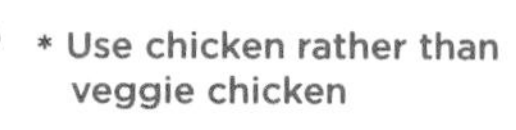
* Use chicken rather than veggie chicken

Serves 4

Curried Apple Chicken Salad

This healthy chicken salad option blends fruits, vegetables and meat for a salad rich in nutrients and protein. The tasty salad gets an extra boost with the addition of turmeric, a spice found in curry powder blends that has been used for thousands of years to strengthen the immune system, relieve inflammation and improve digestion.

1 package veggie chicken strips, diced, or 1 pound cooked chicken breasts, diced

½ cup raw cashews or walnuts, diced

½ cup grapes, halved

2 celery ribs, diced, or 1 stalk bok choy, finely diced

1 apple, diced

2 tablespoons dried currants or cranberries

4 cups baby greens

4 slices sprouted whole grain bread, toasted, or 2 cups whole grain flatbread crackers, divided

Dressing:

1 green onion, sliced

1 teaspoon curry powder

2 tablespoons Vegenaise mayonnaise substitute

Juice from half a lemon

½ teaspoon agave nectar

1 tablespoon water

Preparation

1 In large bowl, mix onion, curry powder, mayonnaise substitute, lemon juice, agave nectar and water. Add chicken, cashews, grapes, celery, apple and dried currants.

2 Divide baby greens into 4 servings and top with chicken salad. Serve with toast.

Per Serving: 378 calories, 12g total fat, 2g saturated fat, 68mg cholesterol, 233mg sodium, 606mg potassium, 36g total carbohydrate, 7g dietary fiber, 35g protein

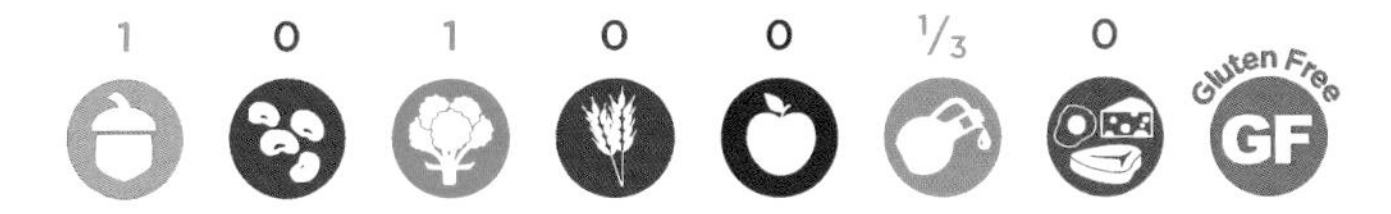

Serves 6

Curried Parsnip and Carrot Soup

Parsnips are a cold-weather vegetable that pair nicely with carrots in this British soup. These two closely related taproots are rich in antioxidant compounds that are anti-inflammatory and anti-fungal. This gluten- and dairy-free soup is perfect for a chilly night, and can be eaten the next day as a filling lunch.

- 2 tablespoons Earth Balance butter substitute
- 2 large onions, diced
- 4 parsnips, peeled and diced
- 4 large carrots, diced
- 3 red potatoes, diced
- 1/4 cup sherry
- 1 1/2 cup raw cashews puréed with 1 cup water, or 1 cup soy creamer
- 1 tablespoon curry powder
- 1 teaspoon salt
- teaspoon pepper
- 2 tablespoons fresh parsley for garnish
- 4 cups water

Preparation

1. Melt the butter substitute in a pan and sauté onions until tender. Add curry powder and stir. Add 1/2 cup water and steam-sauté parsnips, carrots and potatoes for 15 minutes. Add sherry and 3 1/2 cups water. Simmer for 15 minutes.

2. In a blender, purée soup with puréed cashews. Season with salt and pepper and garnish with parsley.

Per Serving: 218 calories, 4g total fat, 1g saturated fat, 0mg cholesterol, 473mg sodium, 718mg potassium, 39g total carbohydrate, 7g dietary fiber, 4g protein

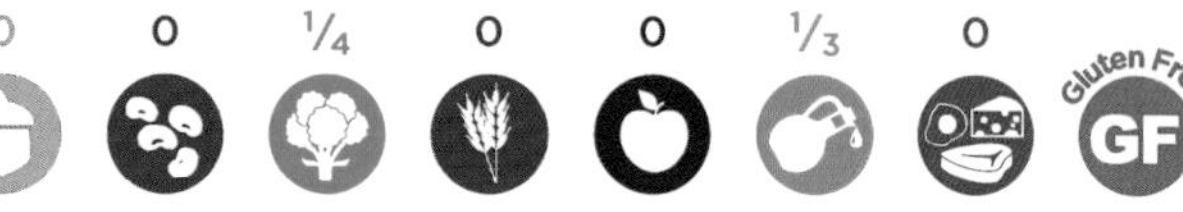

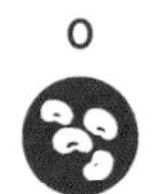
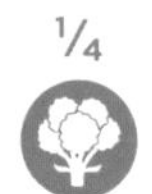
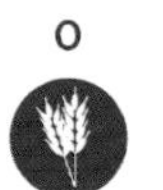
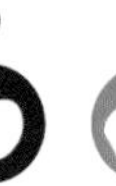

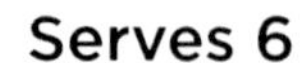

Serves 6

Ginger-Miso Soup

Miso paste and tofu are soy products that play an important role in improving bone health and reducing risk for cancer and heart disease. The addition of ginger makes this soup elegant and flavorful.

6 cups water

1 diced carrot

2 tablespoons fresh ginger, sliced or minced

2 cups diced cabbage, bok choy, wakame seaweed, or a combination

1 package firm tofu, diced

1/4 cup miso paste (barley or rice miso)

1 sliced green onion

1 teaspoon sesame oil

1/2 teaspoon low-sodium soy sauce or Bragg Liquid Aminos

1/4 teaspoon dried chili peppers, optional

Preparation

1 In a large stock pot, bring the water, carrot and ginger to a medium boil for 7 minutes.

2 Add vegetable greens and cook for 4 minutes. Lower heat and stir in miso paste until completely dissolved.

3 Stir in tofu, onion and sesame oil. Season with soy sauce and serve. Make a large batch and freeze for up three months.

Per Serving: 66 calories, 3g total fat, 1g saturated fat, 0mg cholesterol, 183mg sodium, 203mg potassium, 5g total carbohydrate, 2g dietary fiber, 5g protein

0 1/2 2 1 1/2 0 1/6 1/4

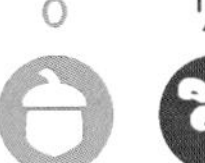 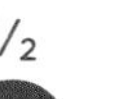 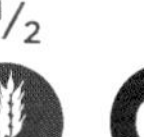 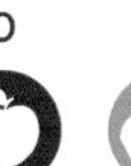 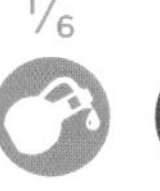 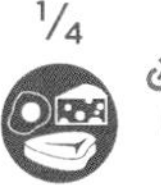

Gluten Free GF 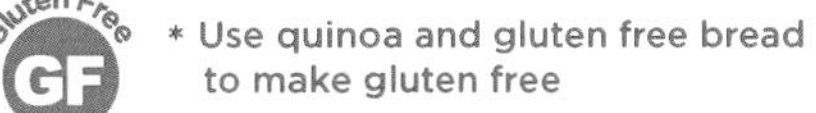

* Use quinoa and gluten free bread to make gluten free

Serves 1

Greek Salad with Sardines and Wheat Berries

This classic salad gets a nutritional overhaul with omega-3-rich sardines and vitamin-packed whole grains. Providing anti-inflammatory effects, this salad works well for lunch or a light dinner.

1 1/2 cups mixed baby greens, or spinach and romaine lettuce

1/2 green onion or 1 tablespoon diced red onion

1/4 cup white beans, butter beans or cannellini beans

1/4 cup cherry tomatoes, halved, or 1 sliced tomato

1/4 cup diced red bell pepper

1/4 cup sliced cucumber

1 celery rib or 1 carrot, diced

1/4 teaspoon dried oregano or Italian seasoning

1/8 teaspoon pepper

1/2 cup cooked wheat berries, farro or quinoa

1/2 slice toasted sprouted grain bread or 1/4 cup whole grain flatbread crackers

Dressing:

Lemon juice from half a lemon

1/2 teaspoon olive oil

1/2 tablespoon water

2 sardines, chopped, or 1 ounce tuna

1 tablespoon feta cheese

1 tablespoon olives

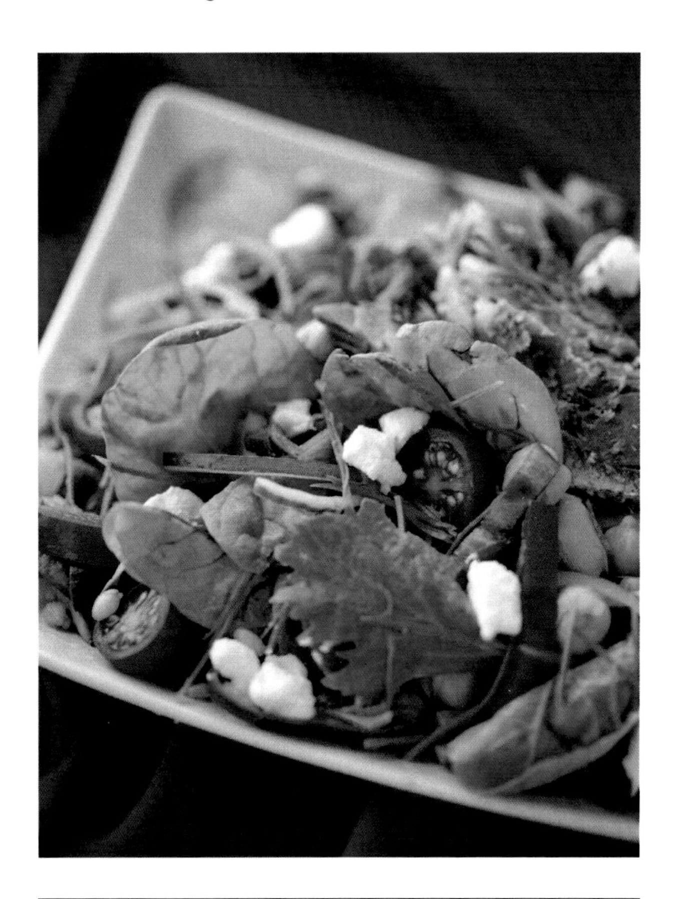

Preparation

1 In large bowl, mix lemon juice, olive oil, water, and sardines. Toss with feta cheese and olives.

2 Add salad ingredients and toss. Before serving, top with wheat berries or quinoa. Serve with toast.

Per Serving: 486 calories, 9g total fat, 2g saturated fat, 27mg cholesterol, 259mg sodium, 230mg potassium, 85g total carbohydrate, 17g dietary fiber, 26g protein

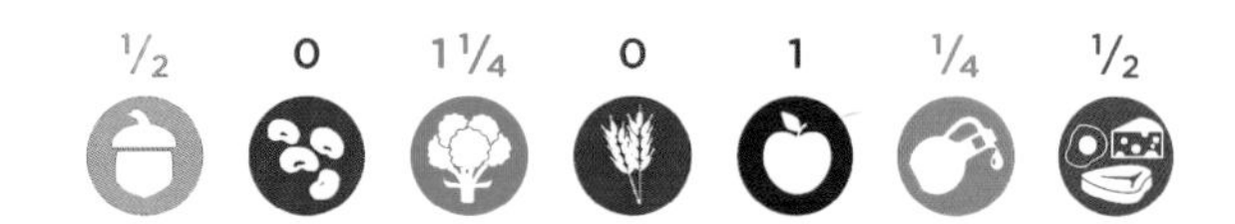

Serves 2

Green Salad with Apples, Berries and Goat Cheese

Goat cheese contains selenium, an antioxidant that promotes a healthy heart and immune system. Selenium also plays an important role in healthy thyroid function. Leafy greens make this refreshing salad a good source of fiber, iron and calcium.

2 1/2 cups mixed baby greens or romaine lettuce, spinach and kale

1/4 cup diced goat cheese

1/8 cup diced walnuts or pecans

1 celery rib, diced

1 diced apple

1 tablespoon dried currants or cranberries

1 cup diced strawberries

1/2 cup blueberries, raspberries or blackberries

Dressing:

1 lemon, juiced

1 teaspoon agave nectar

2 tablespoon water

1/2 tablespoon coconut oil or olive oil

1/4 teaspoon salt

1/8 teaspoon black pepper

1 tablespoon shallots, green onion or red onion

Preparation

1 Toss greens, cheese, walnuts, celery, fruit and berries in a bowl.

2 In a blender, purée lemon juice, agave, water, coconut oil, salt, pepper and shallots.

3 Pour over salad ingredients and toss. Serve with whole grain toast.

Per Serving: 232 calories, 12g total fat, 6g saturated fat, 18mg cholesterol, 398mg sodium, 197mg potassium, 30g total carbohydrate, 5g dietary fiber, 6g protein

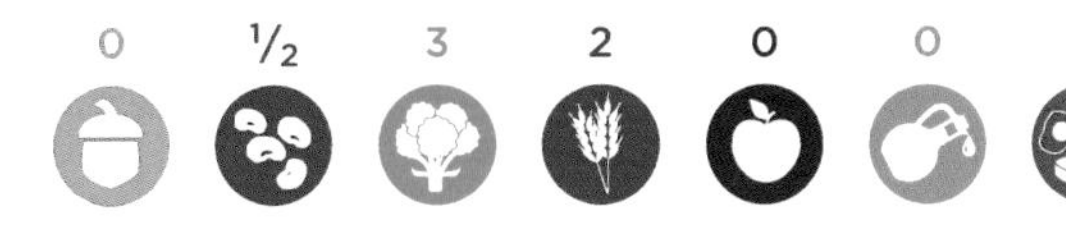

Serves 1

Grilled Garden Panini

Leftover vegetables can be used to make a delicious grilled panini sandwich for picnics, a weekend lunch or light dinner. This dish features mushrooms, which contain large amounts of selenium, riboflavin, vitamin B, potassium and vitamin D.

1 cup (8 ounces) sliced mushrooms
1/2 cup sliced onions
2 tablespoons hummus
1/4 cup chopped cilantro
1 roasted red bell pepper (or use from a jar, drained)
1/4 cup sliced cucumbers, pickles or pepperoncini
1 handful spinach or arugula
2 slices sprouted whole grain bread

Preparation

1. Sauté mushrooms on high heat with a little water for two minutes, then add onions until soft.
2. Heat skillet to medium heat. Spread 1 tablespoon hummus on each slice of bread and place one slice onto the skillet with hummus side up.
3. Pile mushrooms, onions, cilantro, cucumbers, and spinach on top of hummus and top with the other slice of bread. Use a saucepan or plate and press down on the sandwich.
4. Cook until bottom slice is golden, about 3 minutes. Flip sandwich over and brown the opposite side. Slice and serve.

Per Serving: 337 calories, 7g total fat, 1g saturated fat, 0mg cholesterol, 309mg sodium, 500mg potassium, 55g total carbohydrate, 13g dietary fiber, 15g protein

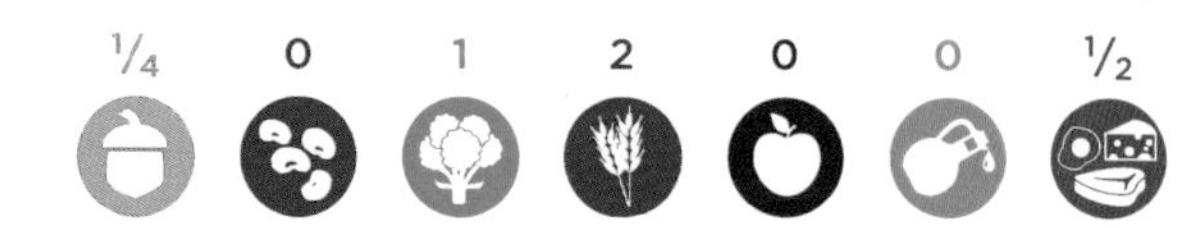

Serves 1

Grilled Pesto Chicken Sandwich

Loaded with big flavors, this grilled cheese is a rib sticker! Our recipe uses non-dairy cheese, which has zero cholesterol, trans fat or lactose. Layered with chicken, tomato, spinach and walnut pesto, it's nutritious and tummy-filling.

2 ounces diced or sliced chicken breast or veggie chicken, cooked

2 slices sprouted grain bread or English muffin

2 slices tomato

1 tablespoon Walnut Pesto (recipe in Sauces section)

1/2 cup baby greens

1 tablespoon shredded non-dairy rice, almond or soy cheese, or low-fat mozzarella

1/4 teaspoon hot sauce

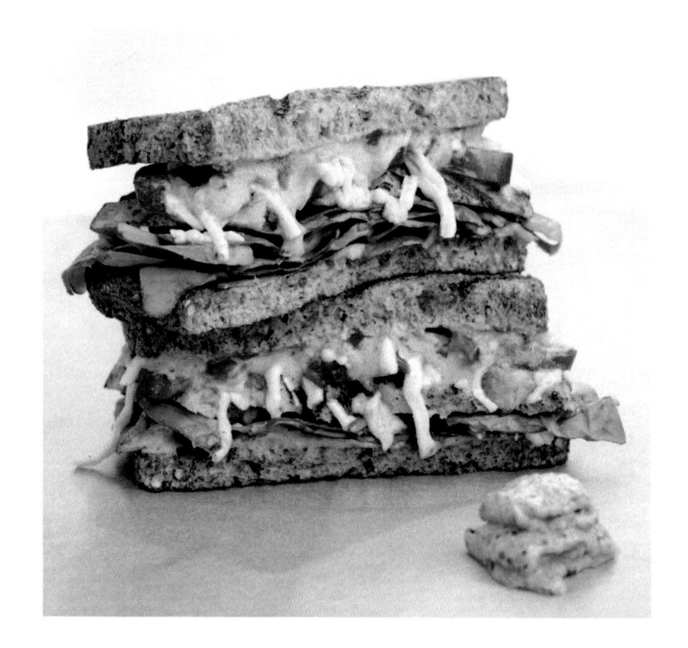

Preparation

1. Spread 1/2 tablespoon Walnut Pesto on each slice of bread and add tomato and baby greens.
2. Sprinkle hot sauce on chicken and top with rice cheese and bread.
3. Grill in a pan, or cook in panini press or toaster oven for 3 minutes. If cooking in a pan, spray with PAM cooking oil spray and grill on medium-low heat for 3 minutes on each side.

Per Serving: 303 calories, 9g total fat, 2g saturated fat, 35mg cholesterol, 324mg sodium, 371mg potassium, 35g total carbohydrate, 7g dietary fiber, 25g protein

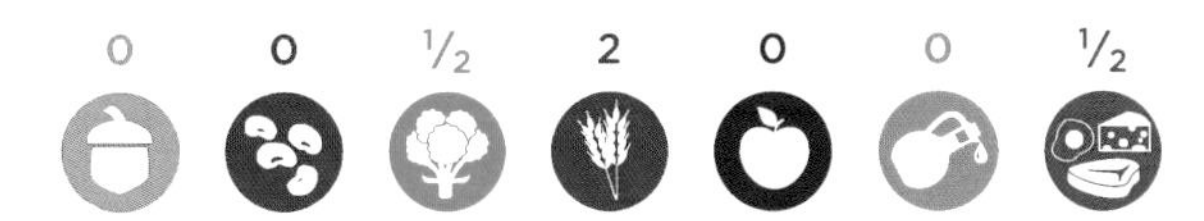

Serves 1

Hot Salmon Sandwich

Salmon comes in many varieties and forms (frozen, fresh, wild and canned). All forms of salmon are loaded with healthy fats, vitamins and minerals. Select your favorite form of salmon for this tasty sandwich.

2 ounces salmon
1 splash low-sodium soy sauce or Bragg Liquid Aminos
2 slices sprouted grain bread or 1 sprouted grain bun
¼ avocado, mashed or sliced
¼ teaspoon hot sauce
1 teaspoon Dijon mustard
½ cup baby greens
2 slices tomato
2 tablespoons sprouts or shredded carrots
Sliced onions or pickled onions

Preparation

1. Poach or boil salmon on the stove with ¼ cup water and soy sauce. Cover the pan and cook for 3-4 minutes.

2. Toast bread and spread one side with avocado. Sprinkle hot sauce on avocado. Spread Dijon mustard on other side.

3. Stack the salmon, baby greens, tomato, sprouts, and onions in the sandwich, and serve.

Per Serving: 353 calories, 9g total fat, 1g saturated fat, 32mg cholesterol, 311mg sodium, 633mg potassium, 38g total carbohydrate, 10g dietary fiber, 26g protein

SOUPS, SALADS AND SANDWICHES

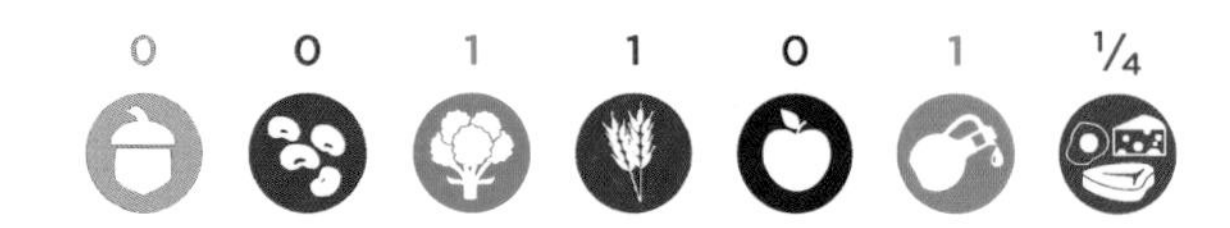

Serves 4

Lemony Chicken Salad

This zesty, refreshing chicken salad is packed with diced red bell peppers, fresh lemon and leafy greens. Rich in vitamins A and C, this nutritious dish makes a scrumptious lunch.

4 celery ribs, diced

1 bell pepper, diced

1/4 cup parsley, chopped

2 green onions, sliced

1 package (8 ounces) chicken-flavored seitan (wheat gluten) or non-breaded veggie chicken strips, cooked and diced, or 1/2 pound cooked chicken breasts, diced

4 whole sprouted grain rolls or bread

2 cups shredded kale or spinach

1 large tomato, sliced

1 tablespoon grainy mustard, optional

Dressing:

1/4 cup Vegenaise mayonnaise substitute

2 tablespoons Tofutti sour cream substitute or plain nonfat Greek yogurt

1 teaspoon lemon juice

1/2 teaspoon hot sauce or ground pepper to taste

1/4 teaspoon salt

Preparation

1 In a large bowl, whisk mayonnaise substitute, sour cream substitute, lemon juice, hot sauce and salt.

2 Combine celery, bell pepper, parsley, green onions and chicken with dressing. Toast rolls and spread with mustard if desired. Line rolls with greens and tomatoes. Fill with chicken mixture.

Per Serving: 273 calories, 12g total fat, 1g saturated fat, 0mg cholesterol, 552mg sodium, 286mg potassium, 28g total carbohydrate, 5g dietary fiber, 12g protein

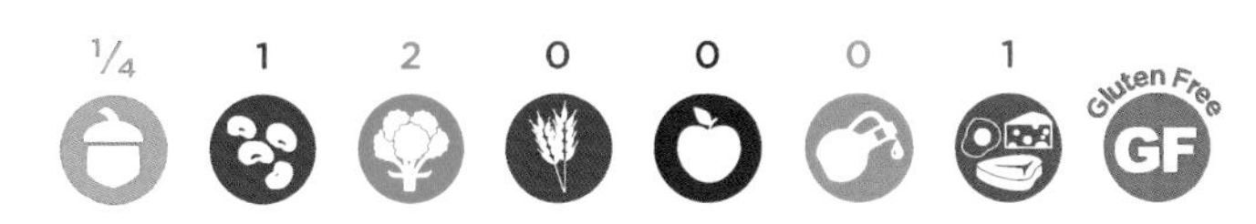

Serves 1

Mexican Taco Salad

Our taco salad recipe is full of bold flavors, nutritious veggies and heart-smart cheese. Using non-dairy cheese eliminates lactose and large amounts of saturated fat and cholesterol, while black beans add essential protein and fiber. We like ours with baked corn tortillas for added crunch and authentic flavors.

1/2 cup cooked ground beef, vegetarian beef crumbles or diced chicken

1/4 cup black beans

1/2 teaspoon taco seasoning

1 1/2 cup mixed baby greens

1/4 red bell pepper, diced

1/4 cup diced tomato

1/8 cup frozen corn, thawed

1 carrot, diced

1 celery, diced

1/2 avocado, diced

1 tablespoon shredded non-dairy rice, almond or soy cheese

1 corn tortilla, baked and sliced, or 1/2 cup baked corn tortilla chips

1 green onion, sliced

Fresh lime wedges

1 tablespoon cilantro, optional

1/2 tablespoon flaxseed meal

Preparation

1 In a bowl, mix the ground beef with beans and taco seasoning. Combine and toss the mixed baby greens, red bell pepper, tomatoes, corn, carrot, celery, avocado, rice cheese, and corn tortilla.

2 Add green onion, cilantro and lime wedges. Sprinkle with flaxseed before serving.

Per Serving: 449 calories, 13g total fat, 2g saturated fat, 60mg cholesterol, 337mg sodium, 1065mg potassium, 45g total carbohydrate, 17g dietary fiber, 34g protein

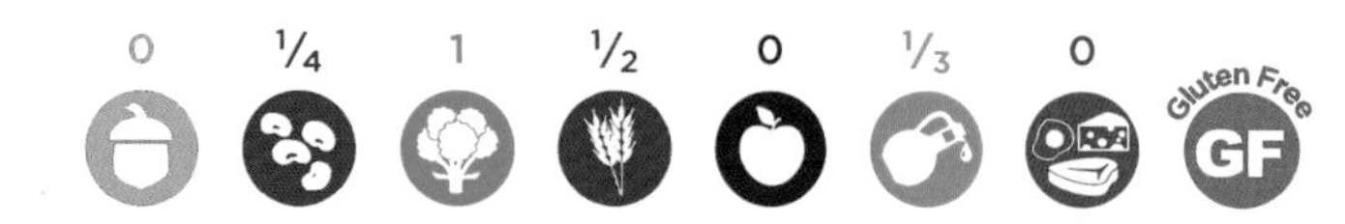

Serves 6

Quinoa Tabbouleh

Fresh herbs, lemon zest and quinoa make this side dish aromatic and outstanding! Quinoa is rich in magnesium, a mineral that, when packed into a diet, may reduce risk for type 2 diabetes and high blood pressure, studies say. High in protein, quinoa tends to be well tolerated by people with gluten sensitivity. Serve this dish as a light meal with hummus and whole grain flatbread.

2 cups cooked quinoa
1/3 cup lemon juice
2 tablespoons lemon zest
1 bunch chopped green onions
2 bunches chopped parsley
1 bunch chopped mint
1 cup diced celery
1 hothouse cucumber, peeled, seeded and chopped
1 cup cooked lentils or chickpeas
1 package cherry tomatoes, diced
2 tablespoons olive oil
1 tablespoon garlic
3 teaspoons ground coriander seed
2 teaspoons cumin
1 teaspoon allspice
1/2 teaspoon cinnamon
1 teaspoon salt
1 teaspoon ground pepper

Preparation

1. Combine cooked quinoa, lemon juice, lemon zest, green onion, parsley, mint, celery, cucumbers and chickpeas.

2. Heat oil in pan and add garlic, coriander seed, cumin, allspice and cinnamon. Stir until garlic is lightly browned and spices are fragrant.

3. Fold into quinoa mixture. Season with salt and pepper. Cover and chill.

4. Add tomatoes before serving and garnish with parsley. Serve with flatbread, falafel, tahini sauce, and pickled beets for a traditional Lebanese meal.

Per Serving: 293 calories, 8g total fat, 1g saturated fat, 0mg cholesterol, 439mg sodium, 724mg potassium, 43g total carbohydrate, 10g dietary fiber, 11g protein

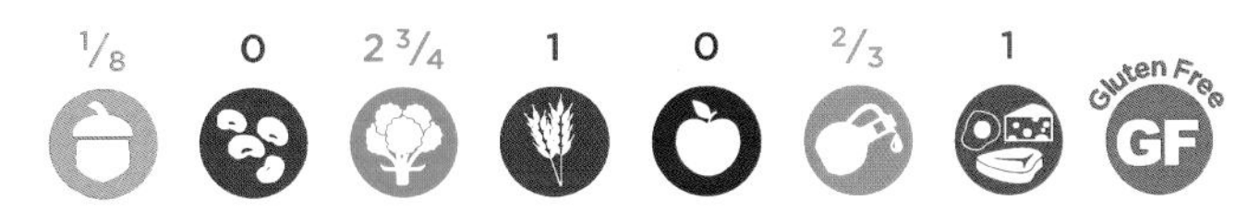

Serves 1

Sesame Ahi Salad

Tuna, as well as salmon and sardines, are high in omega-3 fatty acids, which help raise protective HDL cholesterol levels. You'll love the taste of this crisp, satisfying salad!

1 teaspoon sesame oil

4 ounces ahi tuna

1 1/2 cups mixed baby greens (or romaine lettuce, spinach and kale)

1/2 cup shelled edamame

1/4 red bell pepper, diced

1/4 cup snap peas diced, or green beans

1 carrot or celery rib, diced

1 sheet of toasted nori seaweed, folded and sliced or cut in pieces with scissors

1/2 cup brown rice, cooked

Dressing:

1/2 tablespoon rice vinegar

1/2 teaspoon agave nectar

1 tablespoon water

1 teaspoon sesame oil

1 teaspoon low-sodium soy sauce or Bragg Liquid Aminos

1 teaspoon raw sesame seeds

1/8 teaspoon crushed red pepper or 1/4 teaspoon sriracha

1 tablespoon shallots, green or red onion

Preparation

1 Heat sesame oil in a pan over high heat. Sear fish for 30 seconds on both sides.

2 In a large bowl, toss baby greens, edamame, red bell pepper, snap peas, carrot, and nori.

3 In a blender, purée vinegar, agave, water, sesame oil, soy sauce, sesame seeds, crushed red pepper and shallots. Pour dressing over salad ingredients, toss and serve with sliced ahi on top. Serve with cooked brown rice.

Per Serving: 498 calories, 19g total fat, 1g saturated fat, 43mg cholesterol, 303mg sodium, 630mg potassium, 49g total carbohydrate, 15g dietary fiber, 44g protein

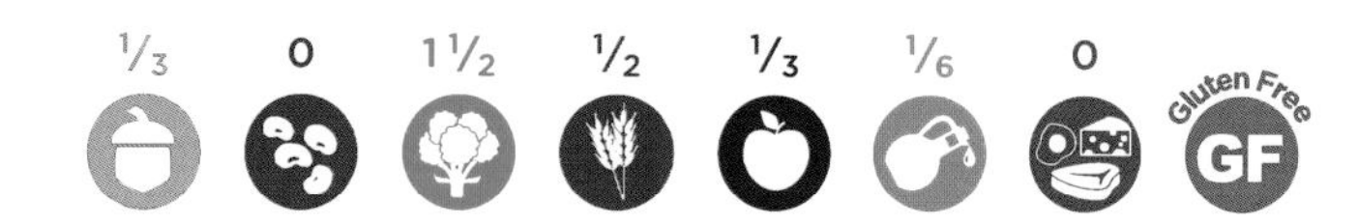

Serves 6

Sesame-Lime Rice Salad Bowl

Tofu, a staple of Asian diets, absorbs flavors well, making it ideal for savory marinades. This flavorful and filling rice salad bowl balances traditional Asian flavors for a perfect, delicious light meal. Serve chilled.

3/4 cup Sesame-Lime Sauce (recipe in Sauces section)

2 pouches Uncle Ben's Brown Rice, steamed according to package instructions

1 package diced veggie chicken strips, diced seiten (wheat gluten), or diced firm tofu, cooked

6 cups romaine lettuce

1 cup shredded carrots

2 celery ribs, diced

1 red bell pepper, diced

1 cup defrosted frozen peas, diced sugar peas, snap peas or green beans

1 cup cherry tomatoes, halved

2 tablespoons dried cranberries or 1 diced apple

1/2 cup cilantro

1 tablespoon flaxseed meal

1 tablespoon peanuts or almonds

Preparation

1. Prepare Sesame-Lime Sauce.

2. In a large bowl, toss lettuce, carrots, celery, red bell pepper, peas, cherry tomatoes, dried cranberry, and cilantro with Sesame-Lime Sauce. Chill.

3. Right before serving, add brown rice and veggie chicken, and toss salad well. Top with flaxseed meal and peanuts.

Per Serving: 286 calories, 7g total fat, 1g saturated fat, 0mg cholesterol, 217mg sodium, 364mg potassium, 41g total carbohydrate, 6g dietary fiber, 15g protein

1/2 0 1 0 0 1/2 1

 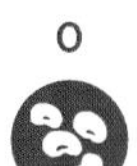  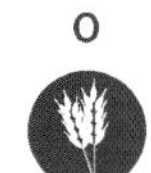 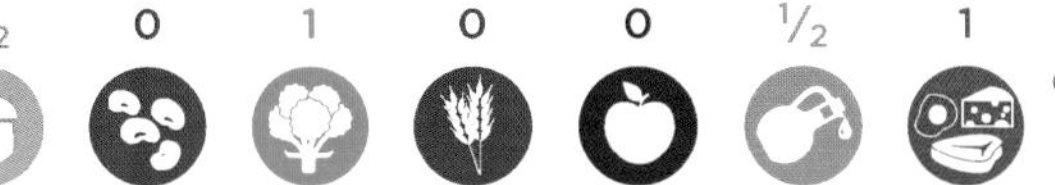  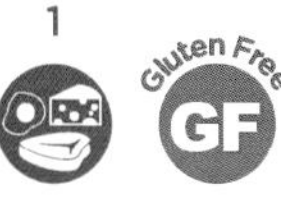

Serves 6

Southern Sweet Potato and Pumpkin Soup

This sweet, creamy soup will satisfy your hunger and tickle your taste buds! Sweet potatoes contain vitamin A, a fat-soluble vitamin required for vision. It can also boost immune function and bone development. People with prediabetes are at risk for vision problems, which makes supplementing with this vitamin all-important.

1/4 cup Earth Balance butter substitute
2 large onions, diced
1 15-ounce can pumpkin purée
5 1/2 cups water
4 carrots, washed and diced (leave skin on)
2 sweet potatoes, peeled and diced
1/4 cup sherry
1 cup raw cashews or 1 cup soy creamer
1 tablespoon thyme
4 tablespoons fresh parsley or chives
Salt and pepper

Preparation

1. In a saucepan, melt butter substitute over medium heat. Sauté onions until tender, add 1/2 cup water and steam-sauté carrots and sweet potatoes covered for 15 minutes.
2. Add sherry, thyme, pumpkin purée and 5 cups water. Simmer for 15 minutes.
3. Purée soup in blender or with an immersion blender. Add cashews and purée again.
4. If soup is too thick, add more water. Season with salt and pepper. Garnish with parsley.

Per Serving: 288 calories, 16g total fat, 3g saturated fat, 0mg cholesterol, 187mg sodium, 227mg potassium, 31g total carbohydrate, 6g dietary fiber, 6g protein

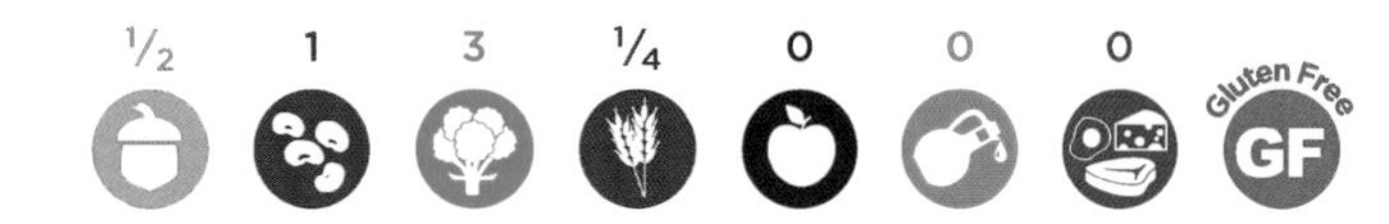

Serves 4

Southwestern Salad Bowl

Most green leafy vegetables contain iron. Pairing them with vitamin C-rich foods such as lime juice enhances the iron absorption. Chock-full of protein and fiber, this salad bursts with flavors and textures.

2 cups frozen green beans, thawed and cut

1 can low-sodium black beans or pinto beans

1 can petite diced low-sodium tomatoes

1 can corn

½ package of high-quality taco seasoning

4 cups baby spinach or greens

1 pouch Uncle Ben's Brown Rice, prepared according to package instructions

1 avocado, diced

1 tablespoon shredded non-dairy rice, almond or soy cheese

2 tablespoons cilantro, chopped

2 tablespoons chopped walnuts or pumpkin seeds for garnish

4 lime wedges for garnish

Preparation

1. Drain the black beans, tomatoes and corn and combine them with taco seasoning in a medium bowl. Add green beans to the mixture.

2. Divide the spinach into four bowls, sprinkle with brown rice and top with black bean salad mixture. Top with diced avocado, rice cheese, cilantro, walnuts and garnish with limes. Serve warm or cold.

Per Serving: 384 calories, 12g total fat, 1g saturated fat, 0mg cholesterol, 254mg sodium, 1082mg potassium, 23g total carbohydrate, 17g dietary fiber, 14g protein

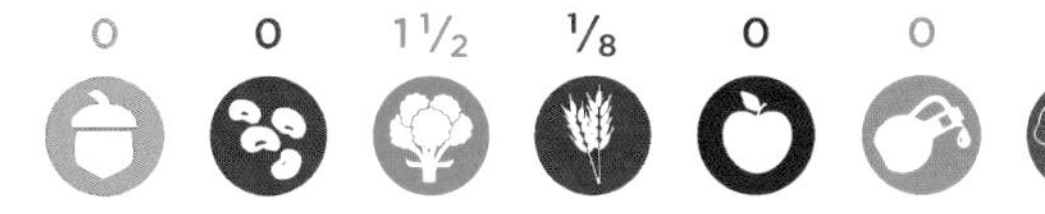

Serves 8

Thai Coconut-Lime Vegetable Soup

This savory recipe is adapted from a classic comfort soup in Thailand. The creamy broth is enriched with coconut milk and loaded with good fats. Coconut milk is rich with manganese, an essential mineral that helps with carbohydrate and fat breakdown. Serve this to your family for a fast, deep-flavored weekday meal.

1 tablespoon olive oil
3 shallots, peeled and diced
2 celery ribs, small dice
4 carrots, small dice
2 cloves garlic, minced
1/2 jalapeno, poblano chili (less spicy) or green bell pepper, diced
1 tablespoon ginger, minced
1 cup chopped mushrooms (preferably dried shiitake mushrooms soaked in hot water for 10 minutes)
1 can coconut milk
3 cups vegetable stock or water
1 teaspoon honey or agave nectar
1/2 bunch chopped kale leaves, de-stemmed
1 cup diced snap peas
4 tablespoons vegan fish sauce or low-sodium soy sauce
1 cup firm tofu, diced, or 1 cup diced veggie chicken
1 lime, juiced
1/4 cup cilantro, chopped

Preparation

1. In large pot, sauté shallots on low heat with olive oil for 3 minutes. Add celery and carrots. Cook for 8 minutes or until tender.

2. Add jalapenos, ginger, garlic and mushrooms. Cook for 2 minutes. Add coconut milk, vegetable stock and honey. Bring to a simmer and cook for 15 minutes.

3. Add kale, snap peas, fish sauce and tofu. Cook for 4 minutes.

4. Remove from heat. Add cilantro and lime juice and serve.

Per Serving: 150 calories, 12g total fat, 9g saturated fat, 0mg cholesterol, 57mg sodium, 211mg potassium, 11g total carbohydrate, 3g dietary fiber, 5g protein

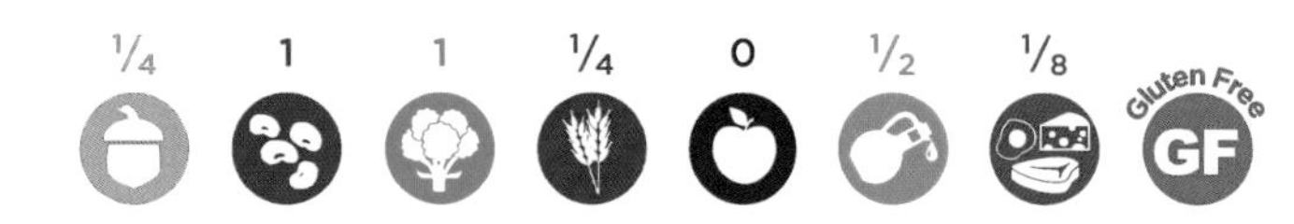

Serves 4

Three-Bean Salad with Almond and Lemon

Oleic acid is the healthy omega-9 fat found in olive oil. This healthy fat works with the omega-3 fat DHA to make cells more responsive to insulin. Serve with grilled shrimp or salmon for a hearty, satisfying meal.

2 tablespoons olive oil

1 lemon, juiced and zested

1 small shallot or 2 cloves garlic

2 medium zucchini, thinly sliced

1 cup frozen peas, thawed, or 2 cups steamed green beans

1 can low-sodium kidney beans

1 can navy or cannellini beans

1/4 cup chopped almonds, roasted

1 tablespoon dried dill or 1/4 cup fresh dill

1 cup soaked bulgur wheat, cooked quinoa or cooked brown rice

2 ounces crumbled goat cheese, or chopped parsley, mint, basil, or cilantro

Salt and pepper

Preparation

1. Combine the first four ingredients in a blender, adding 2 tablespoons of water until the lemon zest is finely minced.

2. Place bulgur wheat in a large heat-proof bowl and add 2 cups of boiling water and let it stand until tender, about 10-15 minutes. Season with salt and pepper.

3. In a large bowl, add zucchini, peas, beans, almonds, and dill and toss with the dressing. Let set for 10-15 minutes until the zucchini softens slightly. Top with goat cheese. Serve salad over bulgur wheat. Can be kept refrigerated for up to five days.

Per Serving: 429 calories, 16g total fat, 3g saturated fat, 5mg cholesterol, 90mg sodium, 732mg potassium, 54g total carbohydrate, 17g dietary fiber, 20g protein

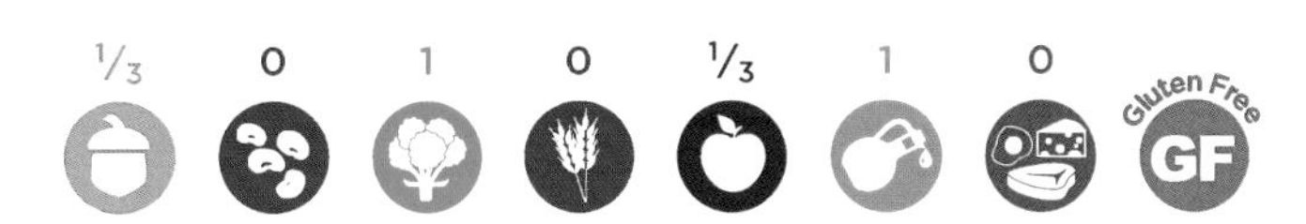

Serves 6

Tri-Colored Floret Salad

This delicious and colorful cruciferous-vegetable salad is loaded with sulfuraphanes, which are thought to have protective properties against cancer. Pair this salad with grilled chicken for a fresh, crunchy, nutritious supper.

4 cups broccoli florets, cooked and blanched
2 cups cauliflower florets, cooked and blanched
1 cup sunflower seeds
1/4 cup red or green onion, diced
1/4 cup Vegenaise mayonnaise substitute
2 tablespoons honey or agave nectar
2 tablespoons vinegar
1 cup dried cranberries

Preparation

1 In a large pot, cook broccoli and cauliflower in boiling water for 5 minutes. Drain and immediately cool under cold running water.

2 Mix sunflower seeds, onion, mayonnaise substitute, agave nectar, vinegar and cranberries in a large bowl. Fold in vegetables. Chill in refrigerator until ready to serve.

Per Serving: 225 calories, 10g total fat, 1g saturated fat, 0mg cholesterol, 37mg sodium, 154mg potassium, 31g total carbohydrate, 5g dietary fiber, 8g protein

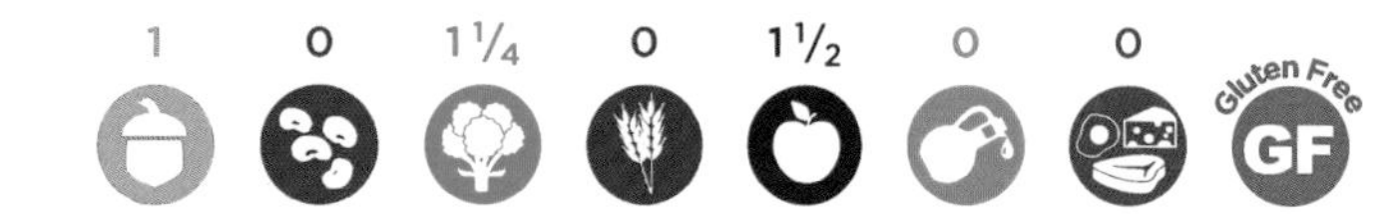

Serves 6

Triple Berry Salad with Strawberry Dressing

Did you know that a serving of eight strawberries contains more vitamin C than an orange? You can stock up on vitamin C as well as heart disease-fighting flavonoids with this sweet summer salad. Plus, it features romaine lettuce, which has more vitamins, protein and fiber than other varieties of lettuce.

6 cups romaine lettuce

2 Granny Smith apples, diced

4 celery ribs, diced

1 cup frozen peas, diced sugar peas, snap peas or green beans

1/4 cup dried blueberries or cherries

1/4 cup dried cranberries or 2 tablespoons currants or goji berries

1 8-ounce package blackberries or blueberries

1 8-ounce package raspberries, optional

1 tablespoon flaxseed meal

2 tablespoons sunflower seeds

1 cup walnuts, pecans or almonds

Dressing:

2 tablespoons raw cashews or blanched almonds

1/2 cup water

2 lemons juiced, 1 zested

1 shallot, optional

2 teaspoons honey or agave nectar

1/4 teaspoon ground pepper

1 teaspoon salt

1 16-ounce package of fresh strawberries, sliced, with 1 cup reserved on the side (substitute reserved strawberries with frozen strawberries or cherries)

Preparation

1. In a blender, purée the cashews, water, lemon juice, lemon zest, honey, salt and pepper, and reserved strawberries until smooth. Season to taste and set aside.

2. In a large bowl, toss lettuce, apples, celery, peas, dried blueberries, dried cranberries, and chill. Right before serving, toss with sliced strawberries, blackberries, raspberries, and dressing. Top with flaxseed meal, nuts and seeds.

Per Serving: 257 calories, 13g total fat, 1g saturated fat, 0mg cholesterol, 0mg sodium, 0mg potassium, 33g total carbohydrate, 11g dietary fiber, 0g protein

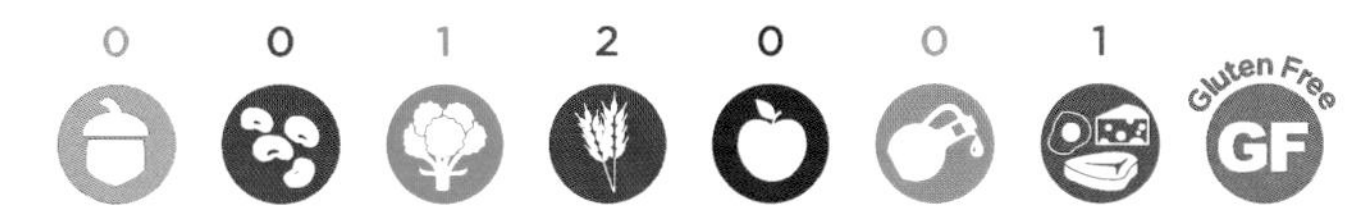

Serves 4

Tuna Pasta Salad

Consuming fish high in omega-3 fat such as tuna can increase levels of healthy HDL cholesterol and improve insulin sensitivity. Enjoy this scrumptious salad with sprouted grain toast.

Dressing:

1 tablespoon Dijon mustard

2 lemons, juiced and zested

1/4 teaspoon hot sauce or 1/8 teaspoon black pepper or crushed red pepper

1/4 cup chopped fresh parsley or basil

1/2 tablespoon tarragon

4 green or red onion, diced

2 tablespoons capers

1 tablespoon Vegenaise mayonnaise substitute

14-ounce canned tuna in water, or 1 pound ahi tuna, seared and sliced

4 cups cooked whole grain fusili, penne or bowtie pasta

1 diced bell pepper or 2 diced carrots

1 cup frozen green beans, thawed and diced

1/2 cup frozen peas, thawed

3 celery ribs, diced

1 cup cherry tomatoes, halved

Roasted pine nuts for garnish, optional

Preparation

1 In a large bowl, whisk together Dijon mustard, lemon juice, lemon zest, hot sauce, parsley, tarragon, onions, capers and mayonnaise substitute.

2 Add cooked pasta, tuna, bell pepper, green beans, peas, celery, and tomatoes, and toss. Top with pine nuts.

TIP

To make a Tuna Niçoise Sandwich, add 2 boiled eggs, diced, and olives instead of capers.

Per Serving: 273 calories, 2g total fat, 0g saturated fat, 13mg cholesterol, 335mg sodium, 145mg potassium, 55g total carbohydrate, 10g dietary fiber, 14g protein

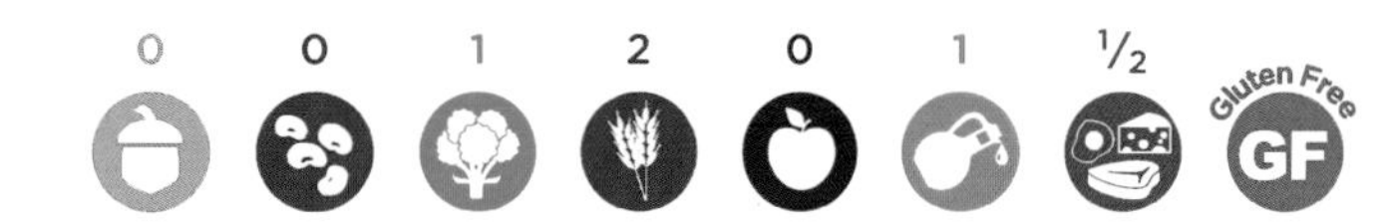

Serves 1

Tuna Salad and Egg Open-Faced Sandwich

Crunchy veggies in a creamy sauce mixed with hearty, protein-packed egg make the perfect lunch! Eggs are rich in vanadium, an essential nutrient that can help improve insulin sensitivity in people with prediabetes. Make this scrumptious tuna salad sandwich today!

1 hardboiled egg, sliced and set aside

1 celery rib, diced

1/2 tablespoon capers

1/2 green onion, sliced

2 tablespoons canned tuna in water, or diced smoked salmon

1/4 cup diced tomatoes

1 tablespoon Vegenaise mayonnaise substitute

1 tablespoon Tofutti sour cream substitute or plain nonfat Greek yogurt

1/2 teaspoon lemon juice or Dijon mustard

Hot sauce or sriracha to taste

1 slice toasted rye bread or sprouted grain toasts

Fresh parsley, dill or chives for garnish

Preparation

1 In a medium bowl, mix celery, capers, green onion, tuna, tomatoes, mayonnaise substitute, sour cream substitute, Greek yogurt, lemon juice and hot sauce.

2 Spread on bread and top with sliced egg and herbs.

TIP

If you prefer, mash the egg slices into the vegetable mixture.

Per Serving: 375 calories, 15g total fat, 3g saturated fat, 219mg cholesterol, 368mg sodium, 417mg potassium, 36g total carbohydrate, 7g dietary fiber, 21g protein

Serves 1

Veggie Melt Sandwich

This sandwich makes a great morning or midday meal! We've given you several options in the ingredient list; just choose your favorite option when building your Veggie Melt.

1 veggie chicken patty, veggie burger or egg white patty
2 slices sprouted grain bread, English muffin or flatbread
1 tablespoon Vegenaise mayonnaise substitute, Walnut Pesto, Garden Marinara Sauce, or hummus
1/2 cup baby greens, roasted bell peppers, portabellas, or summer squash
2 slices tomatoes
1 tablespoon shredded non-dairy rice cheese or 1/2 diced avocado
1/2 tablespoon pickled onions, jalapenos, or kosher pickles

Preparation

1. Make several for the week by laying out 12 slices of bread. Spread with mayonnaise substitute.
2. Pack on the greens and roasted vegetables.
3. Roll or top sandwiches and wrap individually for storage. Cook in the microwave or toast in oven for 7 minutes. Top with fresh tomatoes and avocado right before serving.

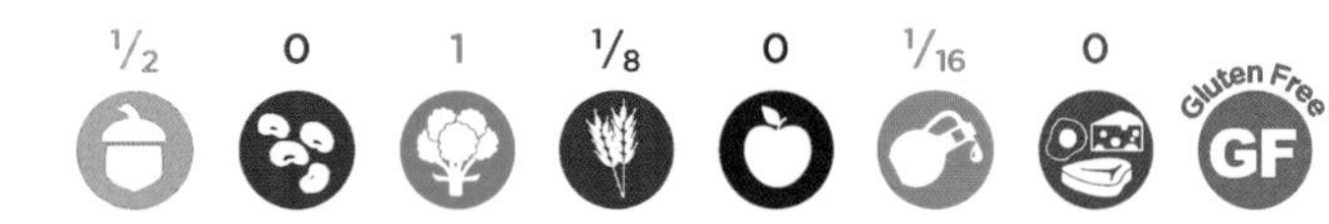

Serves 8

Wild Mushroom Soup

Rich, earthy and full of depth, this soup will satisfy the mushroom lover in any family. Wild mushrooms are an excellent way to add flavor to dishes without adding fat or calories. This soup combines several different mushrooms for extra texture and variety. Loaded with potassium, vitamin A, vitamin C and dietary fiber, this dish is a power-shot of nutrition.

1 pound fresh mushrooms, sliced

1 cup portabella mushrooms, diced

3 1/2 ounces fresh or dried shiitake mushrooms, de-stemmed and chopped

3 1/2 ounces fresh or dried oyster mushrooms, chopped

3 1/2 ounces of dried trumpet mushrooms

1 ounce dried porcini mushrooms

6 medium shallots, diced, or 1/2 small onion, diced, and 2 cloves minced garlic

4 celery ribs, diced

2 tablespoons Earth Balance or Benecol butter substitute, or olive oil

4 sprigs fresh thyme or 2 teaspoons dried thyme

1/8 teaspoon crushed red pepper

4 cups vegetable broth

1/2 cup uncooked quinoa

1 cup raw cashews puréed with 1 cup water

1 cup soy creamer

1 teaspoon salt and pepper to taste

1/2 cup chopped walnuts for garnish

4 cups chopped kale leaves, optional

Preparation

1. Cook dried mushrooms in vegetable broth in medium saucepan on medium-high heat until boiling. Reduce and cover with lid for 10 minutes. Remove mushrooms and drain broth through fine mesh screen or cheesecloth to remove sandy bits. Chop mushrooms by hand or in a food processor and set aside.

2. In a large pot over medium heat, melt butter substitute and sauté shallots until lightly golden. Add all the mushrooms and season with thyme, salt and pepper. Sauté for 5 minutes more. Add celery and sherry and allow to simmer for 5 minutes. Add vegetable and mushroom stock then uncooked quinoa and simmer for 20 minutes.

3. In blender, purée raw cashews, water and soy creamer until creamy and smooth. Whisk into soup. Fold in kale leaves and cook until tender, about 7 minutes. Ladle in bowls and serve with crushed walnuts.

Per Serving: 284 calories, 14g total fat, 2g saturated fat, 0mg cholesterol, 270mg sodium, 726mg potassium, 28g total carbohydrate, 5g dietary fiber, 10g protein

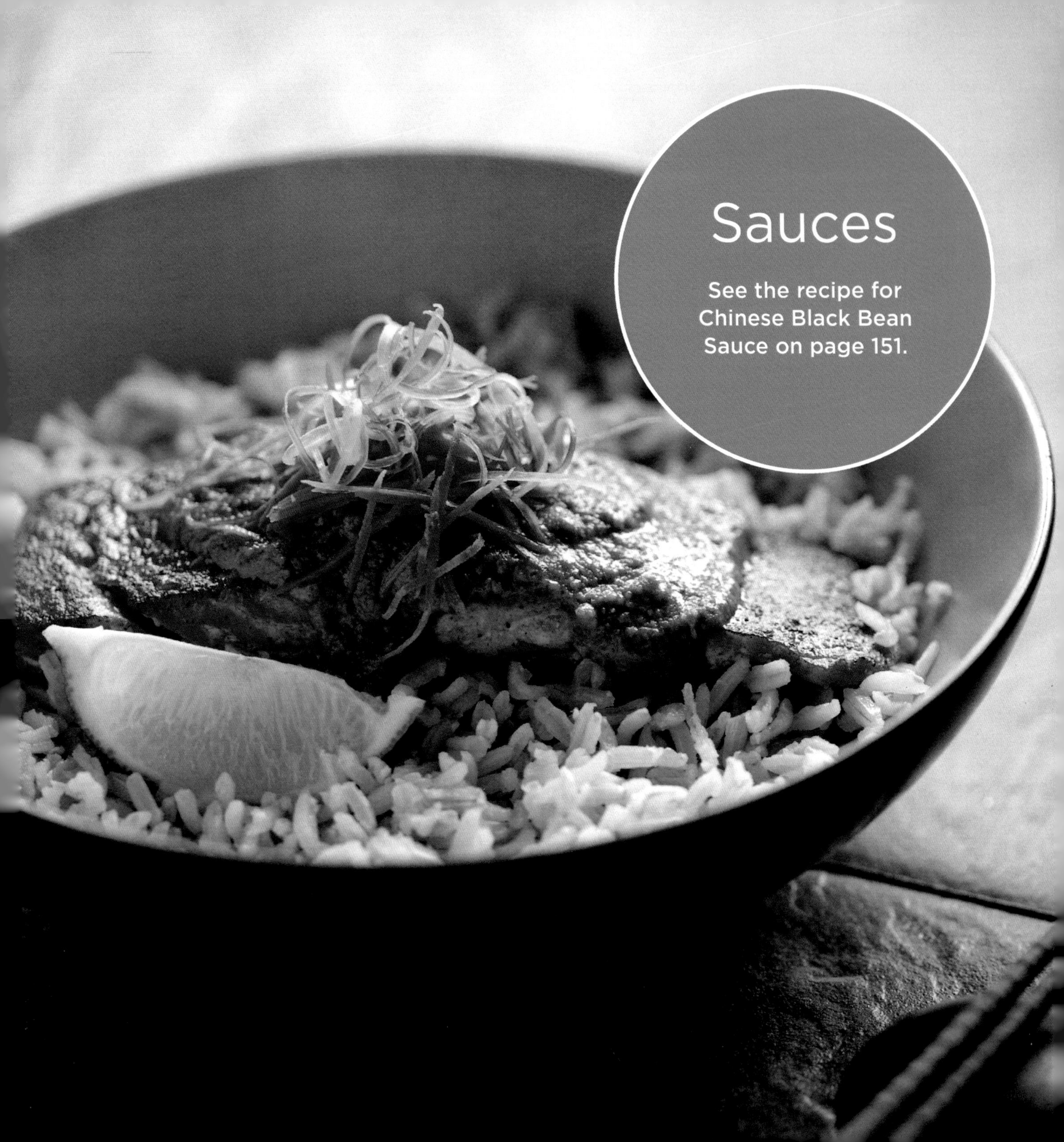

Sauces

See the recipe for Chinese Black Bean Sauce on page 151.

SAUCES

Recipe Index

Serves 6

Béchamel

This classic French sauce is made with cashews, which contain oleic acid, a heart-healthy monounsaturated fat that can help reduce high triglyceride levels, a condition associated with prediabetes. Béchamel sauce can be used as a base to make more interesting sauces. Simply prepare the Béchamel sauce and then add your desired ingredient at the end. Common ingredients include non-dairy cheese, herb blends, mustard, parsley, peppercorn or cooked mushrooms, onions and leeks.

$^{1}/_{2}$ container silken or soft tofu

1 container Tofutti cream cheese substitute

1 cup soy creamer or $^{1}/_{2}$ cup raw cashews puréed with $^{3}/_{4}$ cup water

1 tablespoon Dijon mustard

1 teaspoon garlic, chopped

1 tablespoon Earth Balance or Benecol butter substitute

$^{1}/_{4}$ teaspoon nutmeg

1 teaspoon salt

$^{1}/_{4}$ teaspoon white pepper or 1/8 teaspoon hot sauce

TIP

Warm this sauce gently on the stove with your favorite cheese or cheese substitute and mix with whole grain pasta for delicious macaroni and cheese. Or, layer with lasagna noodles, Swiss chard and mushrooms for a white lasagna. Another option: Spoon onto vegetable gratins and top with sprouted grain bread crumbs and a sprinkling of parmesan or rice cheese.

Preparation

1 Combine all ingredients in a blender and purée until smooth. Adjust salt for individual recipes and taste preference. Makes six $^{1}/_{2}$-cup servings.

Per Serving: 163 calories, 13g total fat, 4g saturated fat, 0mg cholesterol, 611mg sodium, 6g total carbohydrate, 0g dietary fiber, 5g protein

Serves 8

Chinese Black Bean Sauce

Steam-sauté your favorite vegetables and serve with this nutrient-rich sauce. The ginger in this recipe is packed with zinc, which can treat the symptoms of zinc deficiency, including skin lesions, hair loss and recurrent infections. Zinc may also improve sleep.

2 cloves garlic, chopped
1/2 teaspoon diced red chilies or 1/4 teaspoon crushed red pepper
1/2 cup diced onion or 1 small onion
1/2 cup cooked black beans
1 tablespoon sesame oil or olive oil
1 tablespoon rice wine vinegar
2 teaspoons Bragg Liquid Aminos or low-sodium soy sauce
2 tablespoons dates or raisins or 1/2 tablespoon sugar
3/4 cup water
1 tablespoon sesame seeds, optional
1/2 teaspoon dried ginger or 1 teaspoon fresh diced ginger, optional

Preparation

1. In small skillet, heat sesame oil and cook garlic, then add onion, red chilies and ginger, if using, and cook. Don't let vegetables brown. Add 1 teaspoon water to prevent browning.

2. Pour mixture from pan into a blender. Add water, vinegar, Bragg Liquid Aminos and dates, and purée all the ingredients until smooth and creamy.

3. Serve warm in 1/4-cup servings. Garnish with sesame seeds. Refrigerate in airtight container for up to two weeks.

Per Serving: 50 calories, 2g total fat, 0g saturated fat, 0mg cholesterol, 111mg sodium, 6g total carbohydrate, 1g dietary fiber, 1g protein

Serves 6

Chinese Stir-Fry Sauce

Ditch Chinese takeout and make your own stir-fry at home with this easy sauce! Ginger has been shown to effectively manage high levels of blood sugar by increasing the uptake of glucose in muscles. Fresh ginger root keeps for months, but dried ginger will do in a pinch.

½ cup low-sodium chicken broth or cold water
1 tablespoon cornstarch
4 tablespoons low-sodium soy sauce
½ teaspoon honey or agave nectar
2 tablespoons fresh ginger, minced, or 1 teaspoon ground ginger
1 tablespoon rice wine vinegar or lemon juice
1 teaspoon hot sauce or sriracha
1 tablespoon sesame or olive oil
2 cloves garlic, minced

Preparation

1 In a medium saucepan, warm sesame oil and lightly cook garlic for 1-2 minutes; do not let brown.

2 In a small bowl, combine chicken broth and cornstarch. Add soy sauce, honey, ginger, vinegar and hot sauce. Pour the contents of the bowl into the saucepan with garlic and cook for 2-3 minutes until slightly thickened. Remove from heat and toss with steam-sautéed vegetables, chicken or beef.

Per Serving: 37 calories, 2g total fat, 0g saturated fat, 0mg cholesterol, 209mg sodium, 3g total carbohydrate, 0g dietary fiber, 1g protein

Serves 6

Coconut Curry Sauce

This rich Asian curry is delectable! The coconut adds a punch of sweet flavor and a dose of calcium, potassium and magnesium. Plus, it's good for people with prediabetes, as a compound in curry called curcumin has been shown to improve blood glucose control.

1 tablespoon olive oil or coconut oil
1 cup onions or shallots, diced
2 garlic cloves, minced
2 teaspoons sriracha or 1/8 teaspoon crushed red pepper
4 teaspoons chopped fresh lemongrass
Juice of 1 lime
1 1/2 tablespoons mild curry powder blend
2 teaspoons low-sodium soy sauce or salt
2 tablespoons agave nectar or honey
1 can coconut milk

Preparation

1. Warm the oil in a medium saucepan and lightly cook minced garlic and onions for 1-2 minutes. Do not let it brown. Add curry powder and sauté with onions and garlic until fragrant, about 30 seconds. Add 2 tablespoons water, soy sauce, agave nectar, sriracha, lemongrass, and lime juice. Then simmer on medium-high for 2 minutes. Pour in coconut milk and simmer sauce on medium heat for 3-4 minutes until flavors have incorporated. Remove from heat and serve over chicken or seafood and steamed vegetables. Garnish with basil or cilantro.

Per Serving: 182 calories, 17g total fat, 13g saturated fat, 0mg cholesterol, 103mg sodium, 13g total carbohydrate, 1g dietary fiber, 13g protein

Serves 8

Creamy Garlic Alfredo with Cashews

Puréed cashews give this Alfredo sauce its creamy texture without the added cholesterol found in traditional Alfredo recipes. Cashews contain oleic acid, a healthy type of fat also found in olive oil that promotes cardiovascular health by reducing triglycerides. This sauce pairs well with shrimp, which is high in protein and low in fat.

2-3 cloves garlic or shallots, chopped
1 tablespoon Earth Balance butter substitute or olive oil
1/2 teaspoon lemon juice
1 cup raw cashews
1 cup water
1/4 teaspoon hot sauce or 1/8 teaspoon crushed red pepper
1 teaspoon salt
1/2 tablespoon brewer's yeast, optional

Preparation

1. In small skillet, melt butter substitute and cook garlic; don't let brown. Add 1 teaspoon of water if it begins to brown.

2. Pour contents from pan into a blender. Add raw cashews, water, lemon juice, hot sauce or crushed red pepper, salt, and brewer's yeast, if using, and purée all ingredients until smooth and creamy.

3. Season with salt. Serve warm. Keep refrigerated in airtight container for up to seven days.

Per Serving: 97 calories, 7g total fat, 1g saturated fat, 0mg cholesterol, 317mg sodium, 5g total carbohydrate, 1g dietary fiber, 3g protein

Serves 8

Creamy Garden Ranch Dip

Classic and healthy, this ranch dressing is perfect drizzled on salads or used as a dip for veggies. It has a hearty serving of lima beans–legumes packed with protein, magnesium and zinc. Replace your traditional ranch dressing with this healthy substitute!

1 clove garlic
1/4 teaspoon kosher salt
1/4 cup Vegenaise mayonnaise substitute
2 tablespoons Tofutti sour cream substitute or plain nonfat Greek yogurt
1/2 cup of lima beans or cannellini beans, drained and rinsed
1/4 cup fresh parsley, minced
2 tablespoons fresh dill, minced, or 1 tablespoon dry dill
1 tablespoon minced green onions
1/2 teaspoon ground pepper
1/2 teaspoon lemon juice or apple cider vinegar
1/4 teaspoon paprika
1/8 teaspoon cayenne pepper
1/4-1/2 cup water

Preparation

1 Put all the ingredients into blender and add 2 tablespoons water. Blend until beans are smooth and consistency is creamy.

2 Add more water and adjust seasoning if using for a dressing. Leave thick if using as a dip. Store in refrigerator for up to seven days. Can be used as a sandwich spread too!

Per Serving: 71 calories, 5g total fat, 1g saturated fat, 0mg cholesterol, 195mg sodium, 4g total carbohydrate, 1g dietary fiber, 1g protein

Serves 8

Creamy Herb Salad Dressing

This fresh take on dressing is loaded with bright flavors and has no added oil. Packed with fiber, this dressing incorporates healthful ingredients and shines with amazing, balanced flavors without the extra fat!

2 cloves garlic or shallots, chopped
1/8 teaspoon pepper, dried red chilies or hot sauce
1 tablespoon lemon juice and zest of half a lemon
1/4 cup fresh herbs (parsley, basil, oregano, mint, thyme) or 1 tablespoon dried herbs
3/4 cup water or more, depending on consistency
1/4 cup raw nuts (cashew, almond, or walnut)
1/2 teaspoon salt
1 teaspoon honey or 1 dried pitted date
1 tablespoon onion or green onion, diced, optional

Preparation

1. Pour all ingredients into a blender. Purée until smooth and creamy. Season with salt. Serve warm or cold. Store in a covered container in refrigerator for up to 10 days.

Per Serving: 45 calories, 4g total fat, 0g saturated fat, 0mg cholesterol, 151mg sodium, 3g total carbohydrate, 1g dietary fiber, 1g protein

Serves 4

Curry Dip

This spicy dip is a tasty addition to any party. Curry contains a compound called curcumin that fights inflammation and the development of diabetes. According to one study, curcumin improves the function of beta cells, which are the cells in the pancreas that release insulin. You'll love the warmth and creaminess of this delicious dip!

2 tablespoons plain nonfat Greek yogurt or soy yogurt

1 tablespoon Vegenaise mayonnaise substitute

1/4 teaspoon agave nectar or honey

1/2 tablespoon curry powder blend

Preparation

1 In a small bowl, mix the yogurt, Vegenaise, nectar and curry until blended well. Serve with a variety of raw, crunchy veggies.

Per Serving: 53 calories, 5g total fat, 1g saturated fat, 0mg cholesterol, 43mg sodium, 1g total carbohydrate, 0g dietary fiber, 1g protein

Serves 8

Fig-Balsamic Dressing

This savory dressing features Dijon mustard and figs and is delicious over roasted fall vegetables and salads. Figs have more fiber per serving than any other fresh or dried fruit, making this dressing both healthful and filling. With no added oil, this dressing is low in fat and high on flavor!

6 dried figs (1/2 cup)
1/4 cup balsamic vinegar
1 tablespoon Dijon mustard
1 shallot, quartered
1 teaspoon salt
1/2 teaspoon ground pepper
1/4 cup raw walnuts
1/2 cup water
1 tablespoon agave nectar or honey

TIP

To prepare roasted vegetables, wash and prepare vegetables and chop all to approximately the same size. Toss with olive oil and roast on a parchment- or foil-lined baking sheet in a preheated oven at 425 degrees for 20 minutes.

Preparation

1. Put all the ingredients in a blender and purée until smooth. Add water until dressing reaches desired consistency. Drizzle dressing over roasted winter vegetables such as sweet potatoes, acorn squash, butternut squash, cauliflower, fennel, carrots, and Brussels sprouts. Reserve some on the side for dipping.

Per Serving: 65 calories, 3g total fat, 0g saturated fat, 0mg cholesterol, 334mg sodium, 11g total carbohydrate, 1g dietary fiber, 1g protein

Serves 24

Garden Marinara Sauce

With low sodium and no sugar added, this is a marinara you can feel good about! Tomatoes are high in antioxidants, vitamins C and E, beta-carotene, and manganese, all of which support cardiovascular health, the immune system, bone development, and protein digestion. This scrumptious sauce is sure to become a family favorite!

1 teaspoon olive oil

2 15-ounce cans diced tomatoes

1 8-ounce can tomato sauce and 1 can water

1 tablespoon minced garlic

1 large onion, diced

2 tablespoons red wine vinegar

2 tablespoons Italian seasoning

4 finely diced carrots

1 32-ounce jar prepared low-sodium, no-sugar-added marinara

½ cup date pieces or finely diced dates

1 handful spinach, chopped

1 cup chopped fresh parsley, or ½ cup diced fresh parsley and ½ cup chopped fresh basil

Preparation

1. Heat 1 teaspoon olive oil in a large skillet. Add onions and carrots and cook until soft. Add garlic and spinach and cook until spinach is wilted, about 1-2 minutes.

2. Put mixture in a blender and add 1 can of tomato sauce. Blend and return mixture to the skillet. Add 2 cans of diced tomatoes. When it begins to boil, add vinegar and dried Italian seasoning. Turn down the temperature and simmer for 15 minutes.

3. Add whole jar of prepared marinara to the pot and stir in dates. Simmer on low heat for 15 minutes more.

4. Fold in diced spinach. Add fresh parsley and basil, if using, and allow to simmer for 10 minutes. Makes twenty-four ½-cup servings. Store in the freezer for up to three months.

Per Serving: 52 calories, 1.5g total fat, 0g saturated fat, 0mg cholesterol, 18mg sodium, 8.5g total carbohydrate, 1.5g dietary fiber, 1.5g protein

Serves 8

Green Poblano Sauce

This green chili enchilada sauce brightens any Mexican-style dish with fresh, vibrant flavor. Peppers are high in potassium, one of the most soluble minerals, meaning some of the potassium can be lost during cooking, particularly if the vegetable is boiled. Potassium-rich foods such as peppers are great for nerve and muscle health.

2 cloves garlic or shallots, chopped

½ cup diced onion or green onion

6 diced poblano peppers or 4 cans diced green chilies

½ teaspoon ground cumin

2 tablespoons lime plus zest from half a lime (peel with vegetable peeler), or sherry vinegar

½ cup spinach

½ cup diced cilantro or mint or both

¾ cup water or more

2 tablespoons olive oil

1 teaspoon salt

1 teaspoon honey or 1 dried pitted date

Preparation

1. In a small skillet, heat 1 tablespoon olive oil and sauté garlic and onions. Add diced poblano peppers and cumin and cook down with 2 tablespoons of water. Continue adding a little water to steam-sauté until peppers are cooked through, about 7 minutes.

2. Pour all the ingredients into the blender. Purée until smooth and creamy while adding the last tablespoon of olive oil.

3. Season with salt. Serve warm or cold. Keep refrigerated and tightly covered for seven to 10 days.

Per Serving: 50 calories, 4g total fat, 1g saturated fat, 0mg cholesterol, 300mg sodium, 5g total carbohydrate, 1g dietary fiber, 1g protein

Serves 6

Lemongrass Sauce

Try this full-flavored Vietnamese sauce on a bed of steam-sautéed vegetables with lean meat. Lemongrass has anti-inflammatory properties that are important for cardiovascular health.

2 stalks fresh lemongrass or zest of 3 limes
6 cloves garlic, minced
2 tablespoons Asian fish sauce (substitute with low-sodium soy sauce or 3 anchovies)
1 tablespoon low-sodium soy sauce
4 teaspoons honey or agave nectar
1 teaspoon sriracha or 1/2 teaspoon crushed red pepper
1 tablespoon sesame oil or olive oil

Preparation

1. In a medium saucepan, warm sesame oil and lightly cook minced garlic for 1-2 minutes; do not let brown. Add 2 tablespoons water, minced lemongrass, fish sauce, honey and crushed red pepper. Simmer on medium-high for 2 minutes.

2. Remove from heat and serve over grilled meat and steamed vegetables or as a dipping sauce. Serve the sauce with lime wedges for extra flavor!

Per Serving: 42 calories, 2g total fat, 0g saturated fat, 0mg cholesterol, 538mg sodium, 5g total carbohydrate, 0g dietary fiber, 1g protein

Serves 8

Mushroom Sauce

Our version of this classic mushroom sauce doesn't have loads of sodium and fat typically found in canned-mushroom-soup recipes. The fresh mushrooms used in this recipe are nutritious, containing protein, fiber and vitamins C, D, B6 and B12. This delicious sauce makes a great topping for vegetables and meat dishes.

1 cup raw cashews
1/2 cup water
1 tablespoon Dijon mustard
1/2 cup soy creamer
1 teaspoon minced shallots
2 tablespoons Earth Balance butter substitute
1 pound diced mushrooms
2 pinches nutmeg
1 teaspoon salt and pepper to taste
1/4 cup water

Preparation

1 Sauté mushrooms with water for 3 minutes. Add butter substitute and shallots and cook for 3 minutes. Set aside. Purée cashews, Dijon mustard and soy creamer in a blender. Add mushroom mixture and purée.

Per Serving: 210 calories, 16g total fat, 3g saturated fat, 0mg cholesterol, 73mg sodium, 11g total carbohydrate, 2g dietary fiber, 7g protein

Serves 8

Romesco Sauce

Romesco is a classic Spanish roasted red pepper sauce that is full of flavor and easy to make. Almonds are a great source of potassium, which aids in glucose metabolism. A deficiency can result in changes in the central nervous system, muscle weakness and bone fragility. Serve with roasted vegetables, red potatoes or asparagus spears, or as a sandwich spread.

1 slice whole grain bread

2 cloves garlic, peeled and chopped

1 teaspoon paprika

1/2 cup raw almonds or hazelnuts or cashews

1 tablespoon tomato paste

2 roasted red peppers, or 1 8-ounce jar roasted red peppers

1/4 cup sherry or red wine vinegar

1/2 teaspoon salt and pepper to taste

1/8 teaspoon crushed red pepper

2 tablespoons extra-virgin olive oil

3/4 cup water, plus more to taste

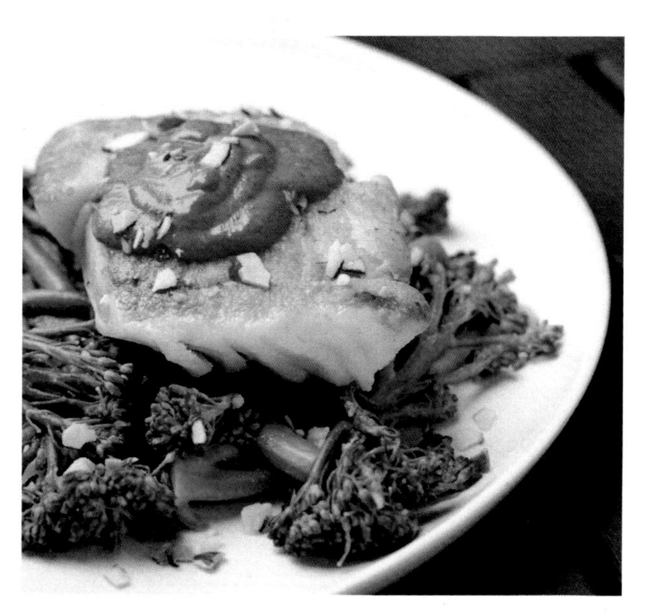

Preparation

1 Tear bread in pieces and place all ingredients into blender with water. Purée until smooth. Add more water if it's too thick and pasty; thicken with more nuts or bread if too thin.

2 Season with salt. Serve warm. Keep refrigerated in airtight container for up to seven days.

Per Serving: 88 calories, 7g total fat, 1g saturated fat, 0mg cholesterol, 100mg sodium, 85mg potassium, 5g total carbohydrate, 1g dietary fiber, 2g protein

Serves 8

Salsa Caliente

This cooked salsa is made with diced tomatoes sautéed in olive oil. Tomatoes contain lycopene, and cooking them actually increases the amount of lycopene available to the body. Olive oil helps the absorption of lycopene. Serve with baked corn tortillas and guacamole over rice and beans for a nutritious meal high in fiber and protein. It's so good you will never want to eat store-bought salsa again!

2 tablespoons olive oil
1 diced onion
2 pounds tomatoes, roughly diced with skin
2 diced poblano peppers or 1 diced jalapeno (adjust to your heat preference)
1 diced yellow or green bell pepper
1 tablespoon vinegar (apple cider, red wine or white vinegar)
1/2 tablespoon salt

Preparation

1 In a small skillet, heat 1 tablespoon of olive oil and sauté the onions. Add diced peppers, tomatoes, vinegar and salt and cook down for 10-15 minutes.

2 Pour all the ingredients into the slow cooker and cook on high for 4-6 hours or overnight.

3 Mash all the ingredients with a potato masher, fork or with an immersion blender, keeping it slightly chunky. Serve warm or cold. Store in a covered container in the refrigerator for 10-12 days, or you can freeze for up to a year.

Per Serving: 80 calories, 4g total fat, 1g saturated fat, 0mg cholesterol, 444mg sodium, 407mg potassium, 9g total carbohydrate, 3g dietary fiber, 2g protein

Serves 6

Sesame-Ginger Sauce

A savory sauce for stir-fry and other Asian dishes, this Sesame-Ginger Sauce is both healthy and delicious. It contains tahini, a butter made from sesame seeds that can be found in the ethnic foods aisle-or near peanut butter-in a grocery store. Use fresh ginger instead of dried ginger–it has a stronger aroma and delivers a more intense, zesty flavor.

½ cup tahini

2 tablespoons water

3 tablespoons Bragg Liquid Aminos or low-sodium soy sauce

½ tablespoon sesame oil

1-2-inch piece of fresh ginger, peeled and diced

⅛ teaspoon cayenne pepper or red chili flakes

2 lemons, zested and juiced

Preparation

1. Combine lemon zest, tahini, water, soy sauce, sesame oil, ginger, pepper, and lemon juice in a blender and mix until smooth. Transfer to a jar until ready to serve. Garnish with scallions.

Per Serving: 137 calories, 12g total fat, 2g saturated fat, 0mg cholesterol, 136mg sodium, 7g total carbohydrate, 1g dietary fiber, 4g protein

Serves 6

Sesame-Lime Sauce

This flavorful and healthy sauce balances traditional Asian flavors and makes a light dressing for a salad or rice bowl. Limes are considered to be a diabetes superfood: their peels contain high levels of soluble fiber that can help stabilize blood glucose levels by slowing down your body's absorption of sugar. Using both the juice and the zest of the lime, as this recipe does, brings the most benefits.

1 tablespoon sesame oil

2 tablespoons Bragg Liquid Aminos or low-sodium soy sauce

2 limes juiced, 1 zested

1 teaspoon honey or agave nectar

1 teaspoon sriracha hot sauce or 1/4 teaspoon crushed red pepper

1 tablespoon toasted sesame seeds

2 tablespoons water

Preparation

1 In a blender, combine all ingredients except water. Add 2 tablespoons water and season to taste. Toss with salad or top over an entrée.

Per Serving: 39 calories, 3g total fat, 0g saturated fat, 0mg cholesterol, 118mg sodium, 3g total carbohydrate, 0g dietary fiber, 1g protein

Serves 6

Sesame-Shallot Sauce

Shallots, a relative of the onion, are an excellent source of vitamin C, folic acid, potassium, iron and protein. Use this recipe as a salad dressing or in your favorite stir-fry.

3 tablespoons rice vinegar

3 teaspoons agave nectar

6 tablespoons water

6 teaspoons sesame oil

6 teaspoons low-sodium soy sauce or Bragg Liquid Aminos

6 teaspoons raw sesame seeds

3/4 teaspoon crushed red pepper or 1 1/2 teaspoon sriracha hot sauce

6 tablespoons shallots

Preparation

1. In a blender, purée all ingredients. Pour over a salad.

Per Serving: 77 calories, 6g total fat, 1g saturated fat, 0mg cholesterol, 134mg sodium, 6g total carbohydrate, 0g dietary fiber, 1g protein

Serves 8

Sherry-Dijon Vegetable Dressing

With zero added oil, this sherry-Dijon dressing is low in "bad" fat. Cashews offer a dose of healthy fat that promote cardiovascular health and add creamy texture and nutty flavor! This delicious dressing also features walnuts, which are high in antioxidants and can help prevent certain types of cancer.

1/2 tablespoon Italian seasoning
2 tablespoons Dijon mustard
1/4 cup lemon juice and 1 lemon peel
1/2 cup sherry vinegar
1 date or 1/2 tablespoon honey or agave nectar
1 shallot, quartered
1 teaspoon salt
1 teaspoon ground pepper
1/2 cup walnuts or raw cashews
1 cup water

TIP

Substitute Italian seasoning with herbs de Provence or fresh herbs like basil, parsley, cilantro or chives for a different flavor.

Preparation

1 Put all the ingredients in a blender and purée until smooth. Add more water if it's too thick. Makes eight 1/4-cup servings. Drizzle over grilled vegetables. Store in airtight container in refrigerator for seven to 10 days.

Per Serving: 67 calories, 5g total fat, 0g saturated fat, 0mg cholesterol, 355mg sodium, 69mg potassium, 5g total carbohydrate, 1g dietary fiber, 1g protein

Serves 8

Walnut Pesto

Try this divine, nutrient-rich, high-protein version of the classic pesto. Walnuts contain a powerful antioxidant called melatonin, which promotes restful sleep. The nut is also rich in gamma-tocopherol, a form of vitamin E that helps fight breast, prostate and lung cancers. Freeze in ice cube trays or store in a jar so it's ready to use. It tastes great on fresh bread or pasta.

1 1/4 cups spinach leaves, packed and stemmed
1/4 cup extra-virgin olive oil
1 cup non-dairy rice mozzarella
1/2 cup canned cannellini beans
1 cup walnut pieces
2 medium garlic cloves
2 tablespoons lemon juice
3/4 teaspoon salt
1/4-1/2 cup water, reserved
2 tablespoons brewer's yeast, optional

Preparation

1 Place all the ingredients except water in a food processor or blender and pulse a few times. Scrape the sides of the container and slowly add water until the mix reaches a slightly loose consistency. Add water until desired consistency is reached. Store in refrigerator for up to seven days.

Per Serving: 221 calories, 19g total fat, 2g saturated fat, 0mg cholesterol, 378mg sodium, 209mg potassium, 7g total carbohydrate, 3g dietary fiber, 8g protein

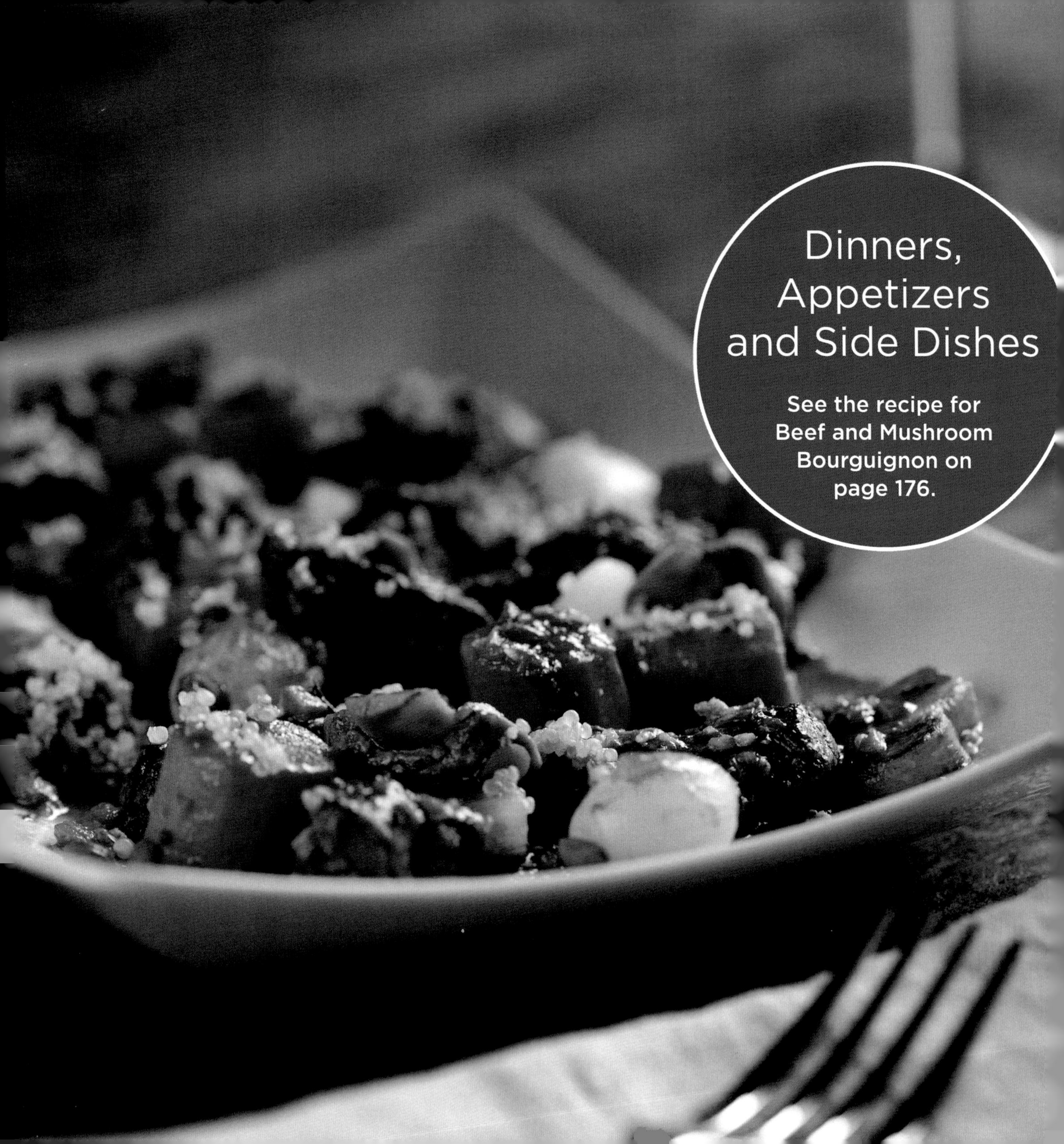

Dinners, Appetizers and Side Dishes

See the recipe for Beef and Mushroom Bourguignon on page 176.

Recipe Index

Appetizers

Many of the recipes in this book can be used as delicious, show-stopping appetizers to serve at celebrations and gatherings. Once you find recipes you like, think of other ways you can use them: topped on salad or served with rice and pasta–the possibilities are endless!

Here are a few appetizers you can make using our recipes...

Hot Artichoke-Spinach Strudel

1. Prepare our Hot Artichoke-Spinach Dip.

2. Place three sheets of frozen phyllo dough on top of each other. Cut the layered sheets into 3 long strips.

3. Place a rounded 1/2 tablespoon of Hot Artichoke-Spinach Dip on one end of the dough and fold over into a triangle. Spray or brush the dough lightly with olive oil and fold the triangle over until the end of the dough strip.

4. Repeat until all the phyllo pastry is used up. Brush the triangles with olive oil. Bake at 425 degrees for 12-15 minutes until lightly golden.

Mediterranean Pinwheels

1. Prepare our Garlic Lemon Hummus.

2. Spread 1 tablespoon of Garlic Lemon Hummus on 1/2 of a whole grain tortilla.

3. Add julienned carrots, sprouts, cucumber (seeded and thinly sliced lengthwise) and sliced sundried tomatoes. Roll tightly and set into a parchment-lined baking sheet. Continue rolling these until vegetables and tortillas are used up.

4. Tightly wrap in plastic wrap and refrigerate for up to 4 hours before serving. To serve, slice both ends off and slice 2-inch pinwheels down the length of the tortilla.

5. Stick a toothpick through each pinwheel and lay on a large tray on flat side. Serve with more Garlic Lemon Hummus garnished with cilantro and pine nuts.

Mini Meatballs

1. Prepare our Garlicky Meatloaf, adding 1 more egg to the recipe. Instead of building a loaf, you'll make balls instead.

2. Scoop out 1 tablespoon and roll into a ball and place onto an ungreased parchment-lined baking sheet with a lip. Continue with the rest of the meat.

3. Bake at 375 degrees for 15-20 minutes. Serve with the Easy Marinara Sauce as a dip. Garnish with diced parsley or chives.

Skewered Winter Fruit Kabobs with Creamy Coconut-Pineapple Sauce

1. Prepare our Gingered Fruit Salad, cutting fruit (except oranges) into 1-inch chunks. Peel and section oranges. Substitute red grapes or strawberries for the cranberries.

2. Prepare Coconut-Pineapple Sauce. Set aside to chill in the refrigerator.

3. Skewer strawberry or red grape first, then pineapple, Asian pear, orange wedge and apple. Set skewered fruit onto a lined baking sheet. Cover

tightly with plastic wrap and refrigerate until ready to serve.

4. Place Coconut-Pineapple Sauce in a bowl and transfer skewers onto a platter. Garnish sauce with orange zest and mint leaf. Can be made up to six hours ahead.

Stuffed Tomatoes and Cucumber

1. Prepare our Lemony Chicken Salad.

2. Cut the tops off cherry or Roma tomatoes and scoop put seeds. Cut English cucumber in 1-inch rounds and hollow out the center.

3. Put Lemony Chicken Salad into the hollowed-out tomatoes and cucumbers. Garnish with lemon zest and parsley.

You can also use Lemony Chicken Salad to make Stuffed Puff Pastry:

1. Roll out pastry until it's about 1/4-inch thick. Wrap Lemony Chicken Salad in the puff pastry and baked at 425 degrees for 12 minutes.

Sweet Potato Bites

1, Prepare our Curry Dip.

2. Cut 2 pounds sweet potatoes into 1/2 inch discs, brush both sides with olive oil and roast in the oven at 425 degrees for 20 minutes until roasted lightly browned. Cool and remove from pan.

3. Dollop curry yogurt on top and garnish with diced chives, or dollop Romesco Sauce on top and garnish with diced chives and capers.

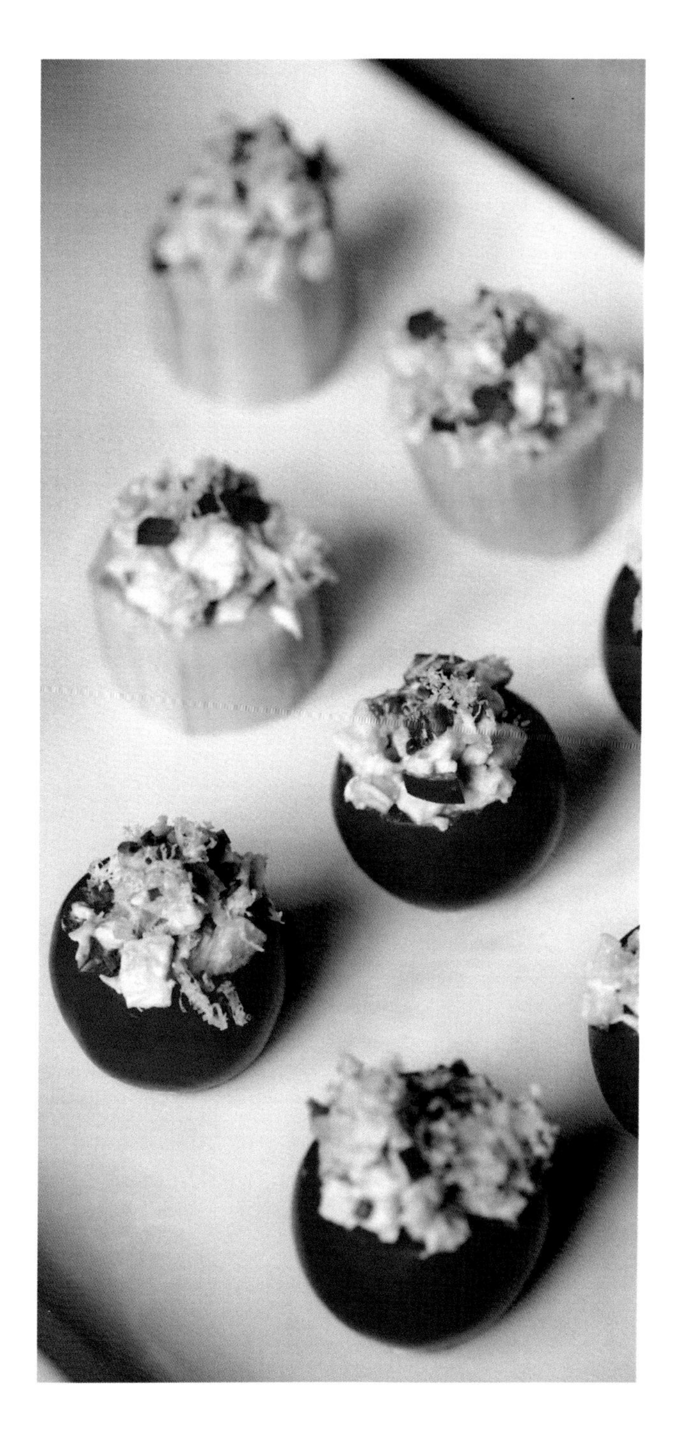

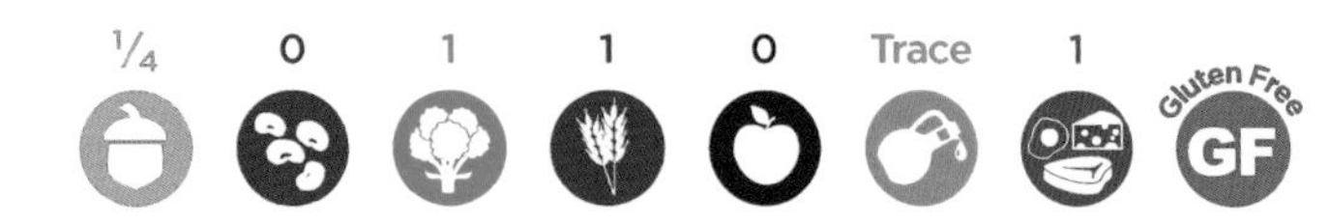

Serves 4

Baked Red Snapper with Béchamel

Red snapper is high in omega-3 fatty acids that help boost good cholesterol and reduce inflammation. It's also an excellent source of vitamin B12, selenium, phosphorus and protein. Make this delicious dish today!

1 pound red snapper fillet, divided into 4 servings
1 teaspoon olive oil
1 pinch salt and ground pepper
1/4 cup white wine
2 tablespoons almond slivers
1 cup Béchamel Sauce (recipe in Sauces section)
PAM cooking spray
2 tablespoons parsley, chopped
1 lemon, sliced
2 cup brown rice, cooked
4 cups baby greens, such as arugula, chard or spinach

Preparation

1. Preheat oven to 400 degrees and grease baking pan with PAM. Brush both sides of fish filets with olive oil and season with salt and pepper.

2. Place red snapper in baking pan and pour white wine into pan. Bake in oven for 7 minutes and remove from oven.

3. Pour Béchamel Sauce over red snapper and sprinkle with almond slices. Return to oven and bake for an additional 15 minutes until sauce is bubbly. Remove from oven and garnish with parsley and lemon slices.

4. To serve, lay 1 cup baby greens on each plate, then spoon on hot rice and gently lay a serving of fish on top. Spoon remaining sauce onto fish or serve on the side.

Per Serving: 282 calories, 6g total fat, 2g saturated fat, 46mg cholesterol, 137mg sodium, 13mg potassium, 27g total carbohydrate, 3g dietary fiber, 27g protein

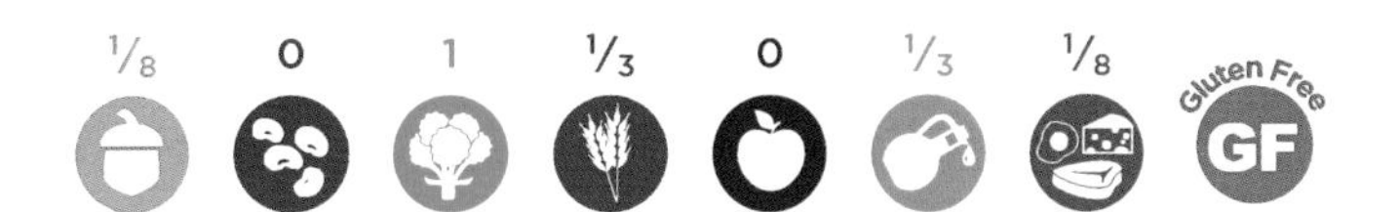

Serves 6

Baked Vegetable Risotto

This quick risotto recipe is a snap to make, since it doesn't require 40 minutes of constant stirring over the stove like the traditional risotto recipes. Our oven-baked version uses brown rice instead of starchy white short-grain rice. Brown, red and black rice (sometimes called "forbidden rice") are nutrient dense whole grains that can help prevent blood sugar spikes.

2 1/2 cups cooked brown rice, whole grain quinoa or faro

2 tablespoons Earth Balance butter substitute

1/4 cup chopped onions

1/2 cup chopped colored bell peppers (red, yellow and green)

1/4 cup chopped mushrooms

1/2 cup diced zucchini

1/2 cup frozen green beans or peas

1 cup soy creamer

3 tablespoons heavy cream

2 tablespoons white wine or cooking sherry

1/2 cup shredded non-dairy rice mozzarella

Salt and ground pepper to taste

Preparation

1. Heat the butter substitute in a pan. Add the onions and sauté until they turn translucent. Add the bell peppers and sauté until they become soft. Add mushrooms and cook for 5 minutes.

2. Add diced zucchini. Add the rice and wine and then simmer for a few minutes. Add soy creamer and 1/4 cup cheese and mix well.

3. Put the mixture in a greased baking dish and sprinkle remaining cheese on top. Bake in oven at 400 degrees for 15 minutes. Remove from oven and fold in the heavy cream. Season with salt and pepper, and serve hot.

Per Serving: 225 calories, 6g total fat, 1g saturated fat, 0mg cholesterol, 99mg sodium, 118mg potassium, 27g total carbohydrate, 3g dietary fiber, 4g protein

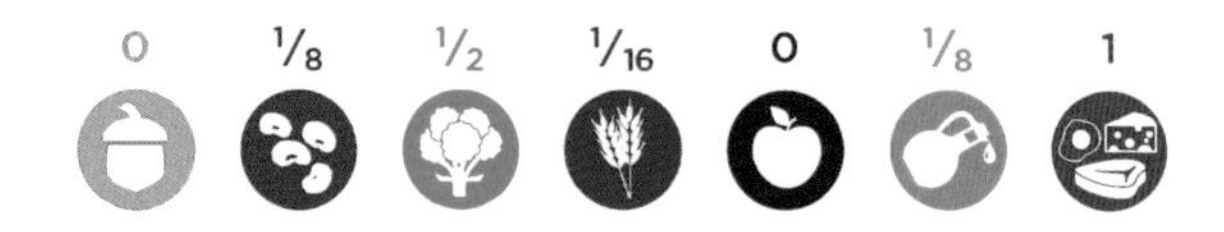

Serves 8

Beef and Mushroom Bourguignon

This rich, luxurious dish is a healthier take on the iconic French classic. Lean beef is a good source of linoleic omega-6 fats, which can't be made by the body and need to be supplemented in a healthy, balanced diet.

1 tablespoon olive oil or grapeseed oil
2 pounds beef round steak, cubed, or cubed stew meat
1 package veggie beef tips
1 large onion, diced
4 carrots, diced
3 celery ribs, diced
½ cup uncooked quinoa or brown rice
½ cup uncooked lentils
2 10-ounce cans low-sodium vegetable broth or water
1 tablespoon tomato paste
2 garlic cloves, minced
4 teaspoon dried thyme
2 teaspoon dried rosemary
1 teaspoon salt
½ teaspoon ground pepper
2 whole bay leaves
1 ½ pounds white pearl onion, frozen
1 pound fresh mushrooms, sliced
½ cup Burgundy wine or red wine

Preparation

1. Brown beef cubes in medium saucepan with olive oil. Place browned beef cubes in crockpot.
2. Add diced onion, garlic, mushrooms, carrot, celery, and 2 tablespoons water to saucepan and cook for 7 minutes.
3. Add tomato paste, thyme and rosemary. Season vegetables and meat with salt and pepper. Add uncooked lentils and quinoa to crockpot. Pour vegetables on top.
4. Add vegetable broth and wine, and mix well. Add bay leaf and pearl onions. Cover and cook on low for 8-10 hours.
5. Before serving, add veggie beef tips and warm through. Serve with mashed potatoes and vegetables.

Per Serving: 372 calories, 9g total fat, 1g saturated fat, 40mg cholesterol, 170mg sodium, 321mg potassium, 21g total carbohydrate, 8g dietary fiber, 39g protein

0 ½ ½ 0 0 0 1

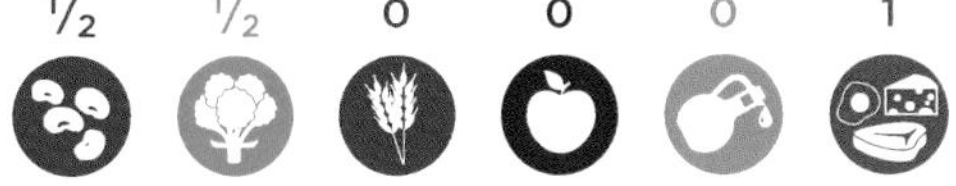
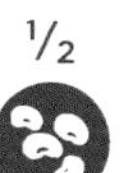
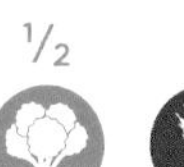
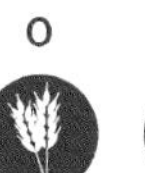
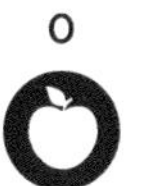
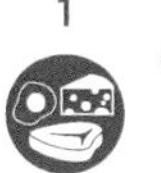
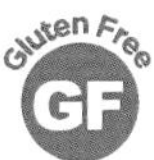

Gluten Free GF

Serves 8

Beef Enchiladas with Hatch Rojo Sauce

Canned enchilada sauce makes a nice shortcut when preparing this dish. We enrich the recipe with puréed tomatoes and carrots, which fortifies the meal with vitamins C and A. Our enchiladas contain 40% less fat than a traditional enchilada recipe, but remains full-flavored, delicious and satisfying.

1 pound lean ground beef
1 large onion, chopped
2 cloves garlic, minced
2 tablespoons chili powder blend
1 can diced artichokes
1 cup julienned carrots
1 cup frozen chopped spinach
1 package veggie beef crumbles
1 15-ounce can veggie chili or black beans
1 can fire-roasted red enchilada sauce
1 14.5-ounce can crushed low-sodium tomatoes
12-16 corn tortillas
16 ounces cottage cheese
1 cup shredded non-dairy rice cheese
1 green onion, diced
1 tablespoon sliced olives

Preparation

1 Preheat oven to 375 degrees. Brown beef in large skillet with 1 tablespoon water until evaporated. Crumble meat with potato masher and add onion, garlic and chili powder. Sauté until onion is cooked through, about 7 minutes.

2 Add diced artichokes, carrots and spinach, and cook for another 7 minutes. Remove from heat and fold in chili and veggie beef crumbles and set aside.

3 In a pitcher or bowl, mix enchilada sauce and crushed tomatoes. Pour 1 cup of the sauce into the meat mixture. Stir to combine. Set the rest of the sauce aside. Warm tortillas in the microwave with damp towel until pliable.

TIP

For traditional rolled enchiladas, fill each tortilla with 1 teaspoon cottage cheese and 1 tablespoon of meat filling and roll, then set with seam down into lightly sprayed dish. Continue rolling enchiladas to fill bottom of the pan. Pour 1 cup sauce over rolled enchiladas and spread to cover. Repeat with another layer of rolled enchiladas. Press down and pour remaining sauce all over to cover the enchiladas. Top with veggie cheese. Place casserole on foil-lined baking sheet and bake for 30 minutes. Top with diced scallions and sliced olives and serve.

4 Lightly spray cooking oil onto two 9x9-inch baking dishes or a large 9x13-inch baking dish. Pour 2 cups of sauce or more to cover the bottom of the dish.

5 Add the following layers: tortillas, sauce, meat, tortillas, sauce, cottage cheese, tortillas, sauce, meat, tortillas, sauce and, lastly, rice cheese. Bake in oven for 25-30 minutes. Top with diced scallions and sliced olives and serve.

Per Serving: 353 calories, 10g total fat, 3g saturated fat, 40mg cholesterol, 374mg sodium, 484mg potassium, 40g total carbohydrate, 9g dietary fiber, 28g protein

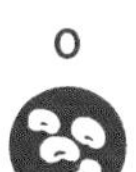 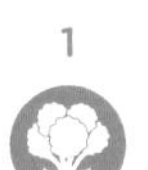 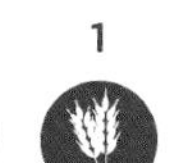 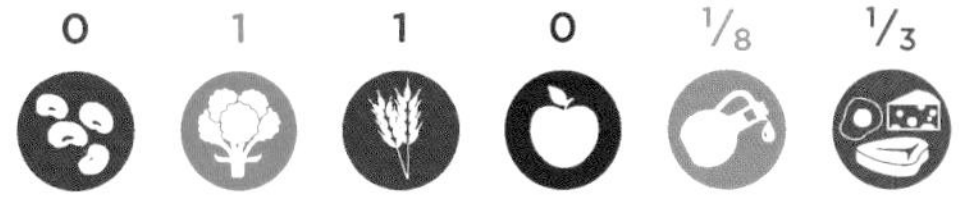  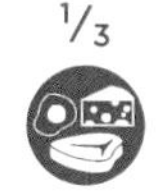 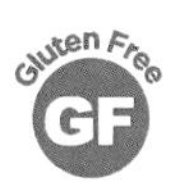 

1/2 0 1 1 0 1/8 1/3 Gluten Free GF

Serves 6

Chinese Cashew Chicken

There's no reason to order Chinese takeout once you get familiar with this easy, healthy recipe! Cashews contain less fat than most other popular nuts, including peanuts, pecans, almonds and walnuts. They are high in dietary fiber, making them a nutritious addition to this stir-fry recipe. Serve with brown rice and wilted spinach for a nutrient-rich, delicious meal.

1/2 cup low-sodium chicken broth or water

1 tablespoon cornstarch

4 tablespoons low-sodium soy sauce

1/2 teaspoon honey

1 teaspoon ground ginger or 2 tablespoons fresh ginger, minced

1 teaspoon red pepper sauce or hot sauce

1 tablespoon vegetable oil

1/2 pound boneless skinless chicken breast, cut into 1-inch pieces, or beef eye round, sliced

1 package veggie chicken strips, diced, or veggie beef tips

2 cloves garlic, minced

1 cup raw cashews

1 large red or green bell pepper, cut into 1-inch pieces

1 medium onion, diced

2 cups sliced mushrooms

2 carrots, sliced

1 pound green beans or snow peas

1 8-ounce can sliced water chestnuts, drained

2 green onions, sliced for garnish

3 tablespoons dry roasted cashews for garnish, optional

3 cups cooked short-grain brown rice

TIP

Steam vegetables ahead of time or buy frozen vegetables and thaw for a quick shortcut.

Preparation

1. In a small saucepan, mix cornstarch, chicken broth, soy sauce, honey, ginger, and hot sauce. Cook on medium heat until thickened, about 4 minutes. Remove from heat.

2. In a large wok, heat vegetable oil and add garlic, then raw cashews, stirring constantly until lightly golden. Add onions, bell peppers, chicken, mushrooms and 2 tablespoons water and cook until water is evaporated.

3. Add carrots, green beans and water chestnuts to the wok. Add 2 tablespoons water and steam-sauté until carrots and green beans are tender, about 7-8 minutes.

4. Add diced veggie chicken and pour reserved sauce over the mixture. Warm through. Serve over a bed of cooked brown rice. (Each serving of rice is ½ cup.) Garnish with sliced green onions and more cashews if desired.

Per Serving: 425 calories, 15g total fat, 3g saturated fat, 23mg cholesterol, 512mg sodium, 314mg potassium, 45g total carbohydrate, 6g dietary fiber, 28g protein

0  0 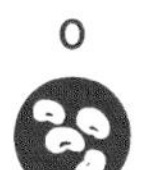 ½ 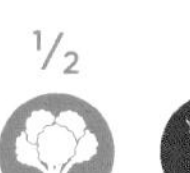 0 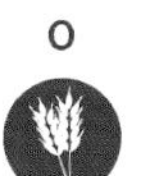 0  ½  0 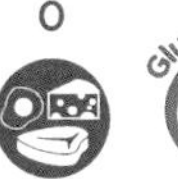 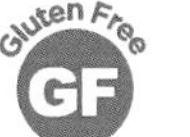

Serves 4

Crispy Kale Chips

Craving something salty and crunchy? These chips make a perfect snack! Kale is chock-full of vitamins and minerals and is very low in calories. This quick and easy recipe is tasty enough for kids and is an excellent substitution for potato chips.

1 large bunch kale
½ tablespoon olive oil spray
¼ teaspoon sea salt

Preparation

1 Preheat oven to 350 degrees. Line baking sheet with foil and spray lightly with olive oil.

2 Wash kale leaves and press to dry or spin in a salad spinner. Tear leaves off the hardy stems into roughly 2-inch pieces. Spread onto baking sheet, making sure they do not touch.

3 Spray kale leaves with olive oil and sprinkle with salt. Then massage the leaves a bit with your hands. Set pan in oven and roast about 10-12 minutes. As it bakes, the kale will shrink and get crispy. Do not let the leaves brown-it will make them bitter. Take out of the oven and serve immediately.

TIP

For other flavor versions, sprinkle with chili powder, garlic powder or your favorite seasoning.

Per Serving: 22 calories, 1g total fat, 0g saturated fat, 0mg cholesterol, 135mg sodium, 152mg potassium, 4g total carbohydrate, 1g dietary fiber, 1g protein

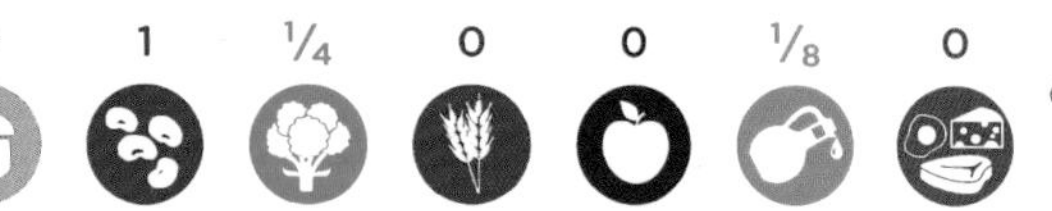

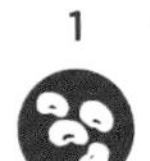
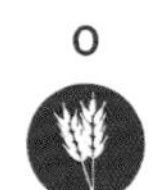
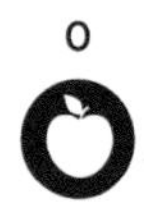

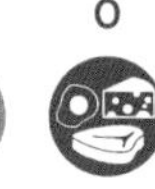
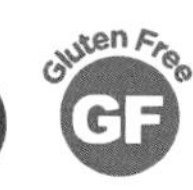

Serves 8

Edamame Pea Dip

Our Edamame Pea Dip is high in fiber, has bright flavor and is easy to prepare. Edamame contains folic acid, an important vitamin found in high amounts in beans and also green leafy vegetables. This recipe uses edamame that are blanched-a cooking method that helps retain nutrients in vegetables. Try this fresh take on dip-you'll love it!

1 cup frozen edamame

1 1/2 cups frozen peas

1 large diced shallot or 1/4 red onion, diced

1 garlic clove

2 tablespoons water

2 tablespoons olive oil

1 lemon or lime, juiced and zested (peel zest with vegetable peeler)

1 teaspoon salt

1/4 teaspoon pepper

2 tablespoons fresh parsley or mint for garnish

Preparation

1 Cook edamame in boiling water until bright and firm, about 3 minutes. Remove with a slotted spoon. Add frozen peas to water and cook for 1 minute. Put edamame and peas into colander and run under cold water until they are cool.

2 Place in a blender or food processor and add remaining ingredients. Pulse and blend until roughly combined but not puréed.

3 Season and garnish with parsley or mint. Serve with sprouted grain toast, crackers or vegetables.

Per Serving: 84 calories, 5g total fat, 1g saturated fat, 0mg cholesterol, 328mg sodium, 23mg potassium, 7g total carbohydrate, 3g dietary fiber, 4g protein

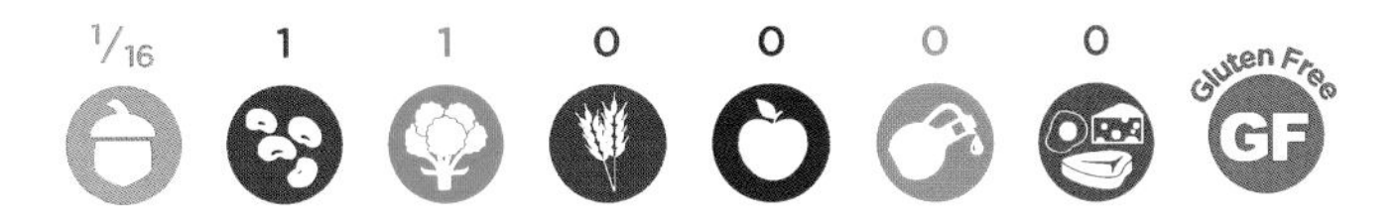

Serves 16

Fresh Garlic-Lemon Hummus

Eating just one-third cup of beans per day can boost your health, studies say. Beans may improve blood sugar levels and insulin secretion, and lower levels of LDL ("bad") cholesterol, total cholesterol and triglycerides. This delicious hummus is more affordable than store-bought hummus, plus it's a snap to make!

2 cans chickpeas, 1 can drained, liquid reserved from the other

2 cloves garlic

1 lemon, juiced and zested (peel zest with vegetable peeler and drop in blender)

1 jalapeno, seeded and sliced

1/4 cup tahini paste 1/4 bunch cilantro, washed and roughly chopped

1 handful baby spinach

Preparation

1. Purée all ingredients in blender. Add water to thin the mixture if it's too thick. Serve with whole grain crackers, fresh or steamed vegetables or as a sandwich spread.

TIP

To change things up, add 2 sun-dried tomatoes and half a jar of roasted red bell peppers in place of spinach and cilantro.

Per Serving: 77 calories, 3g total fat, 1g saturated fat, 0mg cholesterol, 49mg sodium, 36mg potassium, 10g total carbohydrate, 3g dietary fiber, 3g protein

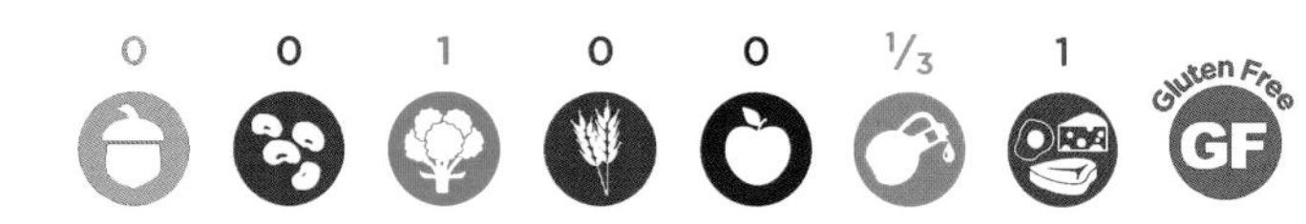

Serves 6

Green Chile Chicken Enchiladas

The dark green poblanos used in this recipe are mild to medium in spice compared to the hotter varieties of peppers. This sauce is made healthier by using non-fat Greek yogurt, a sour cream substitute, that's high in calcium and protein and contains healthy probiotics for improved digestive health.

1 pound poblano chile peppers or green chile peppers

1 tablespoon Earth Balance or Benecol butter substitute

1 tablespoon olive oil

1 onion, diced

5 tomatillos, diced, or can of tomatillo salsa

5 cloves garlic, finely chopped

1/2 teaspoon salt

1/2 cup Tofutti sour cream substitute or plain nonfat Greek yogurt

3 cups low-sodium chicken broth, divided

12 corn tortillas

2 1/2 cups chicken breasts cooked, shredded and diced (season with a little chile powder and cumin and roast in oven)

2 cups non-dairy rice cheddar or mozzarella

1/2 bag frozen chopped spinach (about 1 1/2 cup) or 3 cups fresh spinach

1 can artichoke hearts, diced

1/2 cup chopped cilantro for garnish

1 sliced avocado for garnish

Preparation

1 Preheat oven to 400 degrees. Stem, seed and chop chiles. Heat olive oil and butter substitute in a large frying pan over medium heat. Add garlic and cook until fragrant, about 30 seconds.

2 Add onions, chiles, salt, and pepper. Cook, stirring occasionally, for about 3 minutes. Add tomatillos and 1 cup chicken broth and simmer until reduced by one-third, about 10 minutes. Whisk in sour cream substitute.

3 Meanwhile, prepare tortillas: In a small frying pan, bring remaining 2 cups chicken broth to a gentle simmer. Working one at a time, quickly dip tortillas into broth to barely soften. Transfer each tortilla to a large baking sheet (you may need 2 or 3 sheets). Do not overlap or tortillas will stick.

4. Divide 1 1/4 cups cheese equally among tortillas and top each with shredded chicken, artichokes and spinach, dividing evenly. Wrap tortilla around filling and transfer, seam-side down, to a 9x13-inch baking dish.

5. Pour chile sauce over enchiladas and top with remaining 3/4 cup rice cheese. Bake until rice cheese is bubbling and browned, 15 to 20 minutes. Serve with sliced avocados and cilantro.

Per Serving: 330 calories, 11g total fat, 2g saturated fat, 50mg cholesterol, 400mg sodium, 765mg potassium, 32g total carbohydrate, 8g dietary fiber, 28g protein

Grilled Summer Vegetables

Basic grilled vegetables are a nutritious, tasty addition to any meal. Eating a variety of vegetables will nourish your body with protein, fiber, and vitamins-nutrients that are essential for good health. Not sure how to grill veggies? It's easier than you think!

Use any combination of seasonal vegetables such as asparagus, red bell peppers, poblano peppers, zucchini, yellow squash, red onion, mushrooms, tomatoes, corn, and red potatoes. About 1 1/2 cups of vegetables makes one serving, but eat as many vegetables-and as many different types-as you want!

Preparation

1. Clean and chop asparagus, red bell peppers, poblano peppers, zucchini, yellow squash, red onion, mushrooms, tomatoes, or corn. Lightly spray or brush vegetables with olive oil. Grill the vegetables in a grilling basket on high heat for 7 minutes, stirring occasionally. Remove from grill.

2. Slice or cube potatoes and grill on high heat for 15-20 minutes until fork tender. Toss vegetables with dressing and reserve some on the side for dipping.

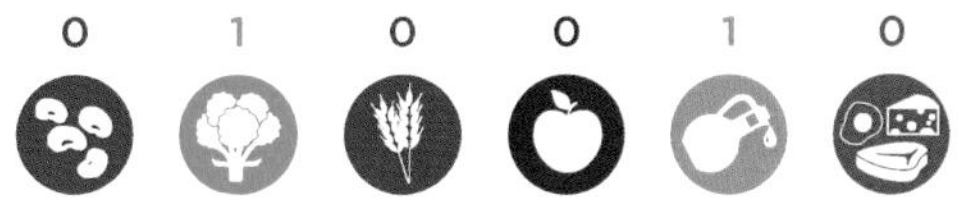

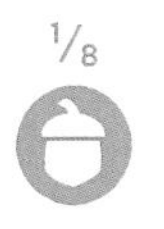
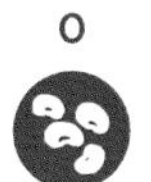

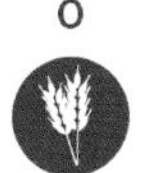

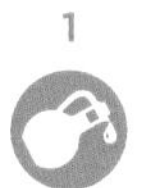
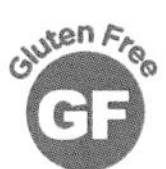

Serves 8

Haricot Vert with Mushroom Sauce and Crispy Shallot Topping

A holiday staple at any buffet table, this version is healthier since it's without the loads of sodium and fat found in canned mushroom soup. Don't just save this dish for the holidays-make it as frequently as you can!

1 pound diced mushrooms

1 teaspoon minced shallots, plus 2 minced shallots, plus 6 shallots, sliced into rings

1/4 cup water

2 tablespoons Earth Balance butter substitute

1 cup raw cashews

1 tablespoon Dijon mustard

1/2 cup soy creamer

2 pinches nutmeg

2 pounds haricot verts or green beans, trimmed

1 red bell pepper, diced

2 teaspoons salt

1/8 teaspoon pepper, plus more to taste

2 tablespoons water

4 tablespoons cornstarch with 3 tablespoons water

1/2 cup cornmeal

Preparation

1 Sauté mushrooms with 1/4 cup of water for 3 minutes. Add 2 tablespoons butter substitute and 1 teaspoon minced shallots and cook for 3 minutes. Set aside. Purée cashews, Dijon, soy creamer and nutmeg in a blender. Add mushroom mixture and purée.

2 Steam-sauté the green beans, red bell pepper and 2 minced shallots. Season with 1 teaspoon salt and pepper to taste. Fold in the mushroom sauce and pour into a baking dish. Set aside.

3 To make shallot topping, mix cornstarch, 2 tablespoons water, 1 teaspoon salt and pepper. Dip 6 sliced shallots in the cornstarch mixture. Dredge shallots in seasoned mixture. Fry shallots in 1/2 cup coconut or grape seed oil. Drain on paper towels.

4 Top green beans with shallot topping and bake at 375 degrees for 25-30 minutes.

Per Serving: 225 calories, 13g total fat, 3g saturated fat, 0mg cholesterol, 482mg sodium, 117mg potassium, 22g total carbohydrate, 3g dietary fiber, 5g protein

0 0 1/4 0 0 1/2 1/4

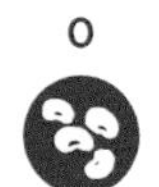
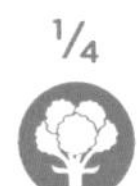
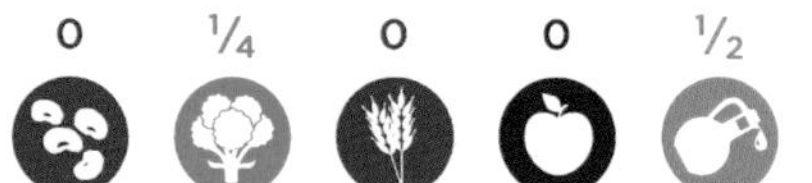

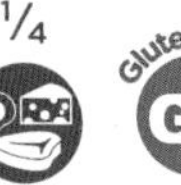

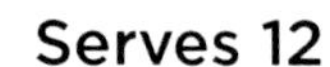

Serves 12

Hot Artichoke-Spinach Dip

This recipe is a healthy alternative to a classic favorite. Artichokes contain a high amount of antioxidants and are rich in the phytochemical cynarin, which aids in digestion by stimulating bile production. Omit the parmesan cheese for a non-dairy dip that's low in fat and cholesterol.

1/4 cup grated parmesan cheese

2 cups shredded non-dairy rice mozzarella

1/2 cup Tofutti sour cream substitute

1/4 teaspoon ground pepper

1 tablespoon Earth Balance butter substitute

4 shallots, diced, or 1 medium onion and 3 cloves garlic, crushed

1 teaspoon hot sauce

1 14-ounce can artichoke hearts, drained and chopped

1 tub Tofutti cream cheese substitute

10 ounces frozen chopped spinach, thawed, drained and squeezed dry

1 tablespoon parsley for garnish

Preparation

1 Preheat oven to 350 degrees. Combine 2 tablespoons parmesan cheese, 1 1/2 cups rice cheese, sour cream substitute, and ground pepper in a large bowl, and stir until well blended.

2 In a small skillet, melt butter substitute and sauté shallots or onions and garlic, about 3 minutes. Add hot sauce, artichoke hearts, spinach and cream cheese until incorporated. Remove from heat and pour into bowl with cheeses.

3 Stir to combine ingredients and spoon mixture into a 1 1/2-quart baking dish. Sprinkle with remaining rice cheese and parmesan cheese and bake at 350 degrees for 30 minutes or until bubbly and golden brown.

4 Garnish with parsley and serve with baked tortilla chips, toasted wheat baguette or whole wheat pita crisps.

Per Serving: 144 calories, 9g total fat, 3g saturated fat, 2mg cholesterol, 492mg sodium, 108mg potassium, 10g total carbohydrate, 2g dietary fiber, 7g protein

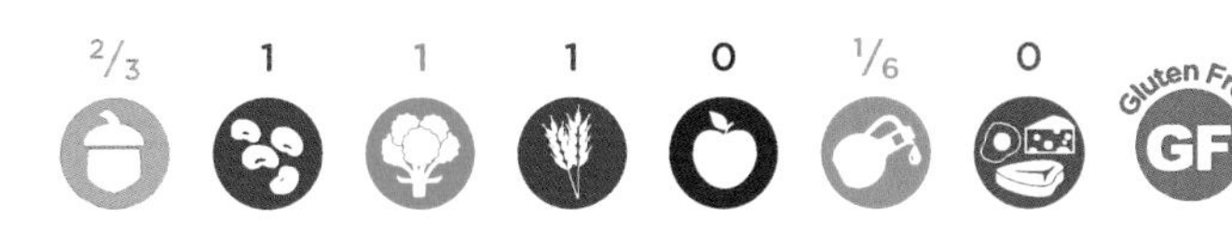

Serves 6

Indian Chana Masala

This delicious, classic Indian recipe uses canned garbanzo beans, also called chickpeas. Research shows there's little difference in the nutritional value between canned garbanzo beans and home-cooked ones. Stock your pantry with these healthy beans so that you have several delicious meal options always available. Enjoy this savory dish served over steaming hot brown rice.

1 tablespoon olive oil
1 onion, diced
1/4 teaspoon crushed red pepper
2 tablespoons fresh ginger, minced
4 cloves garlic, minced
1 tablespoon curry powder blend or garam masala
1/4 diced jalapeno, add more for greater spice
2 15-ounce cans garbanzo beans
2 15-ounce cans crushed tomatoes or 2 1/2 cups diced fresh tomatoes
1/2 cup water
4 cups chopped baby spinach or kale
1/4 cup raw cashews puréed with 1/4 cup water
1 bunch cilantro, chopped
5 cups cooked brown rice (add cinnamon stick while steaming for more flavor)

Preparation

1. In a large wok or pot, heat oil until lightly smoking. Add onion, crushed red pepper, ginger, garlic and jalapenos. Cook for 30 seconds.

2. Add garbanzo beans and curry powder. Cook for 2 minutes, stirring constantly.

3. Add tomatoes, water, spinach and cashew purée. Cook 4 minutes. Remove from heat. Finish with cilantro and serve with rice.

Per Serving: 254 calories, 5g total fat, 1g saturated fat, 0mg cholesterol, 126mg sodium, 286mg potassium, 49g total carbohydrate, 10g dietary fiber, 9g protein

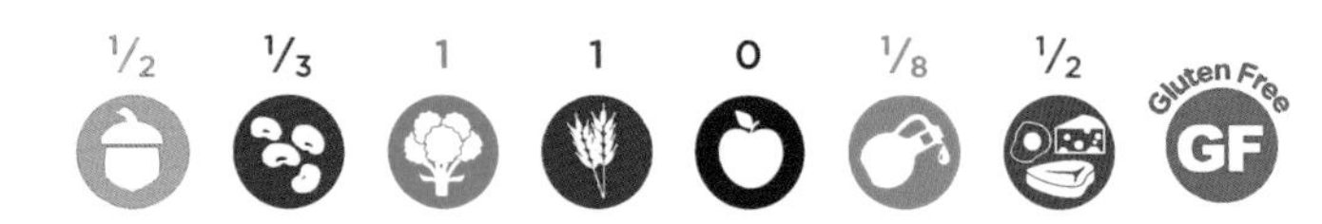

Serves 8

Indian Rogan Josh with Cinnamon Basmati Rice

"Rogan josh" is an exotic dish that originates from the state of Kashmir, bordering India and Pakistan. This rich and delicious dish is made with roasted spices, tomato and puréed almonds. Nuts impart a delicious, creamy flavor as well as a healthy dose of fiber and nutrients. Quick tip: If you have a pressure cooker, this meal can be prepared in just 35 minutes.

1 pound lean eye round beef, trimmed and cut into chunks 1 package veggie beef tips

1 tablespoon vegetable oil

2 teaspoons paprika 1 teaspoon turmeric 1 teaspoon ground coriander 1 teaspoon cumin 1/8 teaspoon cayenne pepper

4 green cardamom pods, crushed, or 1/2 teaspoon ground cardamom 2 cans garbanzo beans, drained

4 peeled carrots, diced

3 celery ribs, diced

1 red or green bell pepper, diced

1 cup chopped kale or spinach 3 tablespoons uncooked quinoa (use rice or bread crumbs in a pinch)

1 cup water

2 teaspoons garam masala or curry powder blend 1 12-ounce can petite diced or crushed tomatoes (use spaghetti sauce in a pinch)

2 cloves garlic, peeled

1 large onion, chopped

1 2-inch piece ginger root

1/2 cup almonds or cashews puréed with 3/4 cup water, or 1 cup soy creamer

2 cups brown basmati rice

1 small cinnamon stick or 1/2 teaspoon ground cinnamon

2 tablespoons chopped cilantro

Cilantro sprigs for garnish

Preparation

1 In a bowl, toss beef and veggie beef with vegetable oil. Add spices (paprika, turmeric, coriander, cumin, cayenne, and cardamom) to meat mixture. Place in crockpot. Pour in garbanzo beans and mix. Toss vegetables in and combine, and then pour in 1 cup water.

2 In a blender, combine garam masala, tomatoes, garlic, onions, ginger and soy creamer, and purée until smooth. Pour over meat and vegetable mixture in crockpot. Add quinoa. Cook on low for 8 hours or overnight.

3 Cook basmati rice according to package instructions. Place a cinnamon stick in the pot with the rice to infuse while cooking.

4 Remove lid of crockpot and check for stew consistency. Cook over stove on simmer until curry is nicely thickened. Stir in chopped cilantro just before serving. Spoon curry over cinnamon basmati rice and garnish with cilantro sprigs.

Alternative cooking method:

1 In a pressure cooker, heat oil over medium heat. Add tomato mixture and cook for 5 minutes. Stir in meat and marinade. Stir in water and vegetables.

2 Lock the lid in place and bring cooker up to full pressure over medium-high heat. Reduce heat to medium-low, just to maintain even pressure, and cook for 20 minutes. Remove from heat and release pressure quickly. The beef should be fork tender. If not tender, return to full pressure and cook for another 5 minutes. Release pressure quickly.

3 Remove lid and bring to boil. Reduce heat and simmer curry until nicely thickened. Stir in cilantro just before serving. Garnish with cilantro sprigs.

Per Serving: 445 calories, 9g total fat, 1g saturated fat, 30mg cholesterol, 325mg sodium, 413mg potassium, 59g total carbohydrate, 12g dietary fiber, 32g protein

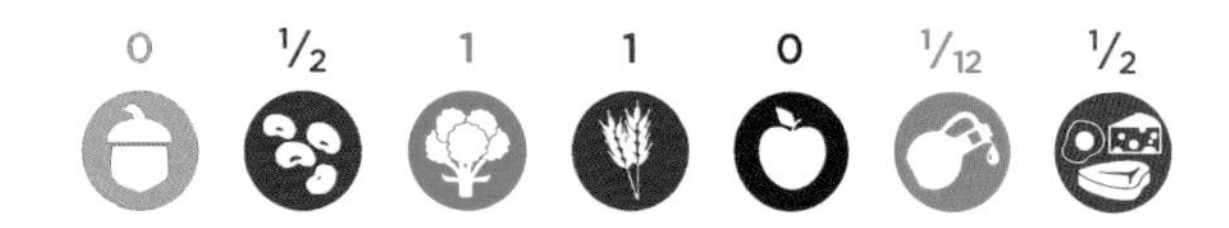

Serves 6

Italian Chicken Cacciatore

This classic Italian family favorite loses none of its depth and flavor in this healthy rendition. Our chicken cacciatore uses navy beans, but other types of white beans such as cannellini or Great Northern beans can be substituted in a pinch. Serve with spinach greens for a complete protein-rich meal!

1 large onion, thinly sliced

1 red or green bell pepper, finely chopped

3 peeled carrots, diced small

3 celery stalks, diced

6 ounces sliced mushrooms

1 pound chicken breasts

1 bag veggie chicken strips

3 garlic cloves, minced

2 teaspoons dried oregano or 1 tablespoon fresh oregano

1 teaspoon dried basil or 1/2 tablespoon fresh basil

2 tablespoons fresh parsley, optional

1/2 teaspoon ground celery seed, optional

1 teaspoon salt

1/2 cup dry white or red wine or balsamic vinegar

1 can petite diced low-sodium tomatoes

1/2 6-ounce can low-sodium tomato paste

1 can low-sodium navy or butter beans

1 tablespoon olive oil

1/4 teaspoon crushed red pepper, optional

3 cups cooked brown rice pasta, cooked brown rice or millet polenta

Preparation

1 Place onions, bell peppers, carrots, celery and mushrooms in the bottom of the crockpot. Add the chicken pieces.

2 In a mixing bowl, combine garlic, oregano, basil, parsley, celery seed, salt, wine, tomatoes, tomato paste, beans, olive oil and crushed red pepper. Pour that mixture over the chicken. Cook on low heat for 7-9 hours or high heat for 4 hours.

3 Serve over pasta, rice or millet polenta with spinach greens.

Per Serving: 296 calories, 4g total fat, 0g saturated fat, 43mg cholesterol, 528mg sodium, 782mg potassium, 28g total carbohydrate, 9g dietary fiber, 33g protein

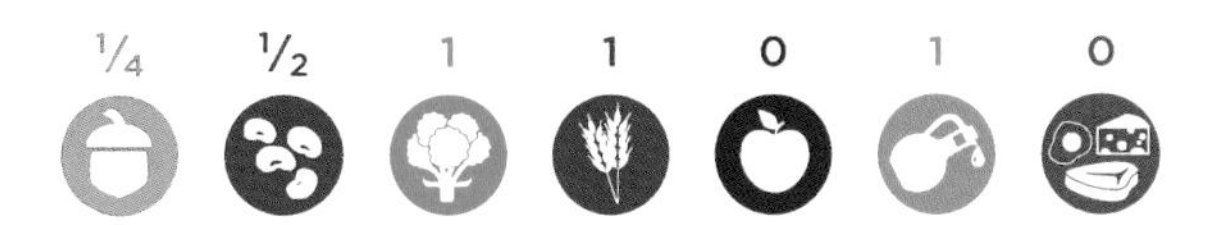

Serves 6

Italian Whole Grain Pasta Bowl

Hearty and full of different flavors and textures, you'll never tire of this delicious pasta! To maximize health benefits, eat a combination of raw and cooked vegetables every day. This guilt-free pasta also is high in fiber and protein. Serve it warm or cold.

Dressing:

1/2 cup Walnut Pesto (recipe in the Sauces section)

2 tablespoons water

1 lemon, juiced

1/4 cup chopped parsley

1/8 teaspoon crushed red pepper, optional

6 cups cooked whole grain pasta (fusili, bowtie or penne)

2 cups diced fresh green beans or haricot verts

1 cup frozen peas or edamame

1 can cannellini beans or navy beans

1 cup diced tomatoes or halved cherry tomatoes

1/4 cup toasted pine nuts or crushed walnuts for garnish

1/2 cup shredded non-dairy rice mozzarella for garnish

Preparation

1. In a large pot, cook pasta according to package instructions.

2. In a medium-sized pot, bring 1 cup water to boil, add green beans and steam for 3 minutes. Add frozen peas and continue to steam additional 4 minutes. Drain vegetables and pasta.

3. In a large bowl, combine Walnut Pesto, water, lemon juice, parsley, and crushed red pepper. Then pour in pasta, cooked vegetables, tomatoes, and cannellini beans, and stir to coat with dressing. Season with salt and garnish with pine nuts and mozzarella.

Per Serving: 315 calories, 8g total fat, 1g saturated fat, 0mg cholesterol, 223mg sodium, 299mg potassium, 51g total carbohydrate, 10g dietary fiber, 17g protein

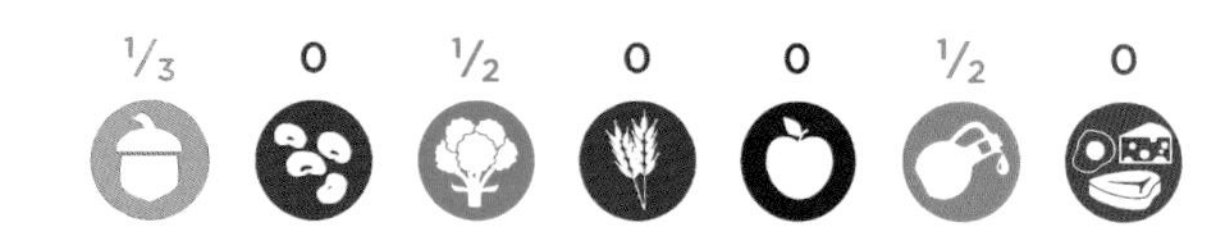

Serves 12

Kale, Carrot and Herb Strudel

Kale is a superfood that's rich in nutrients and low in calories. Boiling kale causes it to lose most of its nutrients; opt to stream, roast, microwave or sauté to retain the health benefits. This festive puff pastry is a simple, quick appetizer that'll steal the show at your next party! Can be served warm or cold.

2 sheets of frozen puff pastry, thawed for 30-45 minutes

1 1/2 tablespoons Earth Balance butter substitute

1 large onion, minced, or 4 minced shallots

4 cloves garlic, minced

1/4 cup pine nuts

1 large bunch kale, torn from stems, or Swiss chard

1 cup julienned or shredded carrot

2 tablespoons fresh dill

1 lemon, zested and juiced

1/2 teaspoon salt

1/8 teaspoon ground pepper or crushed red pepper

1/2 cup grated non-dairy rice mozzarella

1/4 cup minced fresh parsley

Preparation

1. Preheat oven to 375 degrees. Turn thawed pastry onto parchment-lined baking sheet and roll out with a rolling pin until the pastry is 1/4-inch thick or less. You will need two sheets.

2. Heat butter substitute in a medium skillet and add onion and garlic and sauté until golden. Add pine nuts until fragrant. Roll kale leaves, slice into strips and sauté. Add carrots and 2 tablespoons water and steam-sauté for 5 minutes. Stir in parsley, dill, lemon juice, lemon zest, salt and pepper. Remove from heat.

3. Sprinkle mozzarella down the middle of the puff pastry. Then spread kale and carrots on top of cheese. Fold one side of pastry over the veggies and fold the other side on top and pinch the corners. Cut pastry into 12 slices with a sharp knife.

4. Repeat process on the other puff pastry sheet. Bake for 20-25 minutes until golden. Serve warm or at room temperature on a platter and garnish with parsley and pine nuts.

Per Serving: 206 calories, 13g total fat, 6g saturated fat, 0mg cholesterol, 298mg sodium, 49mg potassium, 20g total carbohydrate, 2g dietary fiber, 5g protein

0 0 1/2 0 0 1/4 0

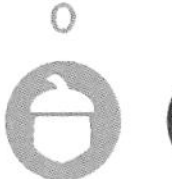 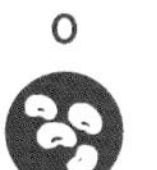 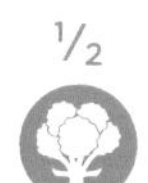 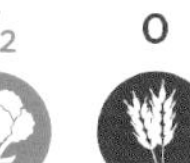 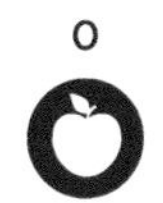  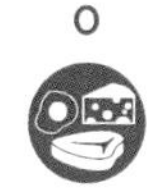 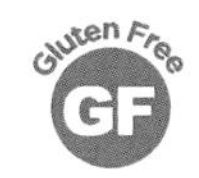

Serves 8

Lemon-Glazed Sweet Potatoes

Forget the traditional holiday sweet potatoes and try this full-flavored recipe instead. Sweet potatoes contain natural sugars that are slowly released into the bloodstream, helping to ensure a balanced and regular source of energy. We omit the brown sugar and marshmallows and use agave nectar, which can help prevent the blood sugar spikes that cause fatigue and weight gain.

2 pounds sweet potatoes, peeled and cut into 1-inch discs
2 tablespoons Earth Balance butter substitute
2 tablespoons of agave nectar or honey
1/2 cup fresh lemon juice
1/8 teaspoon ground cinnamon
1/2 teaspoon kosher salt

Preparation

1. Preheat oven to 325 degrees. Grease 9x13-inch pan with butter substitute. Arrange sweet potato discs in a single layer.

2. Whisk agave nectar, lemon juice, cinnamon and salt in a bowl and pour over the potatoes. Cover and bake in the oven for 30-45 minutes until tender.

3. Remove foil and cook for another 20-30 minutes until glaze thickens and is syrupy.

Per Serving: 146 calories, 3g total fat, 1g saturated fat, 0mg cholesterol, 126mg sodium, 558mg potassium, 29g total carbohydrate, 4g dietary fiber, 2g protein

0 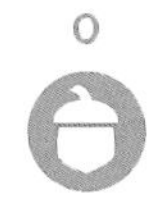 0 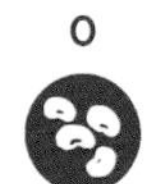 1  0 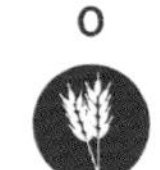 0  1/4  0 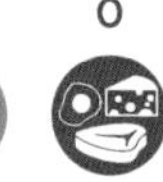 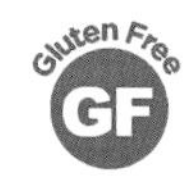

Serves 8

Mashed Red Potatoes with Herbs

Replace your regular mashed potato recipe with this healthy substitute. Red potatoes contain five times as much of the antioxidant anthocyanins compared to Russet potatoes. This recipe is cholesterol-free, low fat, high fiber and, most of all, delicious!

8 -10 medium red potatoes

1/2 cup soy creamer

2 tablespoons plain nonfat Greek yogurt, Tofutti sour cream substitute or 2 tablespoons puréed raw cashews

2 tablespoons Earth Balance or Benecol butter substitute

1 1/2 teaspoon salt to taste

Ground pepper to taste

1/4 cup herbs (dill, basil, oregano, thyme, chives, mint, parsley, or garlic)

Preparation

1 Quarter and boil potatoes in salted water until tender, about 30 minutes. Drain water from pot and add butter substitute, Greek yogurt and soy creamer.

2 Mash with potato masher for desired consistency. Add herbs, salt and pepper.

Per Serving: 150 calories, 4g total fat, 1g saturated fat, 0mg cholesterol, 471mg sodium, 721mg potassium, 27g total carbohydrate, 3g dietary fiber, 4g protein

¼ ¼ ⅙ 0 0 0 ¼

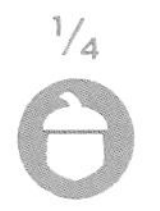
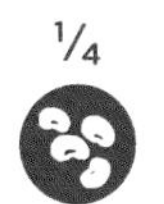

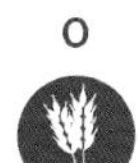
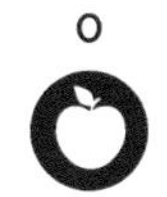
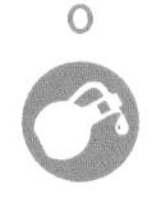
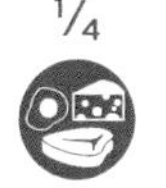
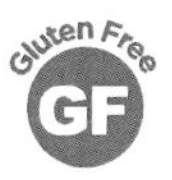

Serves 16

Mediterranean Tri-Color Paté

This paté is a party show-stopper! It's extra delicious when served with a fresh whole grain baguette or sprouted grain crackers. Beans add protein and fiber while walnuts offer a dose of melatonin, a powerful antioxidant that promotes sleep.

2 garlic cloves

1 cup fresh basil leaves

1 cup baby spinach

¼ cup pine nuts

¼ cup walnuts

¼ cup parmesan

7 ounces roasted fresh red bell pepper or 1 7-ounce jar roasted red bell peppers, drained

1 cup crumbled feta cheese

¼ cup blanched almonds or pine nuts

2 15-ounce cans butter beans or cannellini beans, drained and rinsed thoroughly

1 lemon, juiced and zested

2 cloves garlic

1 tablespoon fresh oregano or 1 teaspoon dried oregano

Preparation

1. Line loaf pan with plastic wrap, leaving 4 inches hanging over the sides.
2. Blend or process garlic, basil, spinach, pine nuts, walnuts and parmesan until smooth. Gently spoon pesto layer into lined loaf pan.
3. Rinse blender or processor and purée bell pepper, feta cheese and almonds. Spoon contents over the pesto layer, gently spreading to the edges.
4. Rinse blender or processor and purée butter beans, lemon juice, lemon zest, garlic, and oregano. Spoon contents over the pepper layer. Fold plastic wrap over the paté and refrigerate until ready to serve.
5. To serve, gently unwrap the plastic wrap and allow it to hang off the sides. Invert rectangular platter on top of loaf pan and flip over. Tap the top of the loaf pan all around to loosen the paté. Remove loaf pan and peel off plastic wrap.

Per Serving: 109 calories, 6g total fat, 2g saturated fat, 9mg cholesterol, 247mg sodium, 37mg potassium, 9g total carbohydrate, 3g dietary fiber, 6g protein

0 ½ ½ ¼ 0 ¼ ¼

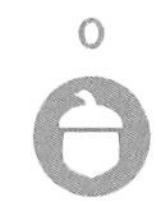  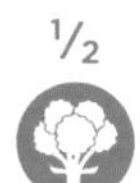 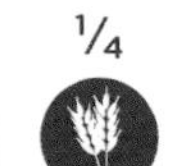 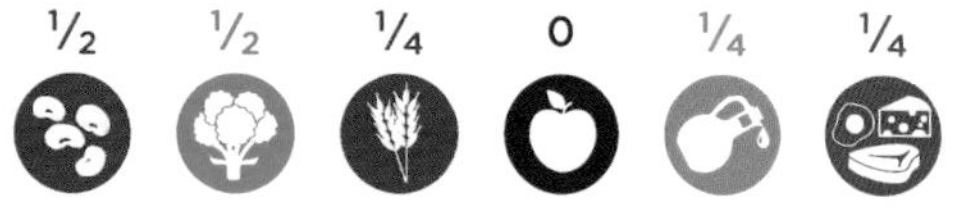   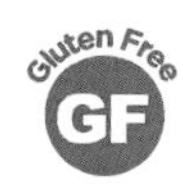

Serves 8

Mexican Tamale Pie

This fun dish features tamale ingredients rearranged in casserole form. Made with beef, millet and other iron-rich ingredients, our Mexican Tamale Pie can help prevent iron-deficient symptoms, such as fatigue. Serve it over a bed of spinach with Greek yogurt and avocado slices.

⅓ pound lean ground beef (90% lean)
1 package veggie meat crumbles
2 carrots, diced
1 bell pepper, diced
2 celery ribs, diced
1 chopped onion
2 cups finely diced kale or spinach
1 15-ounce can crushed tomatoes (use tomato sauce in a pinch)
1 teaspoon garlic powder or 1 clove garlic, minced
½ teaspoon chili powder
2 teaspoon oregano
1 teaspoon ground cumin
1 can black beans, drained
½ cup water
1 dash salt and pepper
1 cup dried polenta
½ cup millet
2 tablespoons Earth Balance or Benecol butter substitute
Ground pepper to taste
1 cup shredded non-dairy rice cheddar or mozzarella
1 tablespoon green onions
Sliced black olives for garnish, optional
Spinach greens
Avocado slices
Fresh cilantro sprigs

TIP

Make the sauce in the crockpot with an additional cup of water overnight or while at work. Prepare the millet polenta mixture and assemble to bake.

Preparation

1. In a small skillet, cook beef and onion over medium heat until meat is no longer pink; drain. Stir in the garlic, cumin, oregano, chili powder, pepper until fragrant, about 2 minutes. (Or, substitute 1 tablespoon taco seasoning in place of spices.)

2. Add vegetables and sauté for 5 minutes. Stir in tomatoes and black beans with 1/2 cup water and simmer for 30 minutes to incorporate the flavors. Remove from heat.

3. In a small saucepan, boil millet covered for 20 minutes. In medium saucepan, boil 3 cups water and whisk in dried polenta until incorporated. Turn heat to medium and fold in butter substitute and cooked millet.

4. Preheat oven to 375 degrees. In a 9x13-inch casserole dish, lightly spray or brush with olive oil and place thin layer of millet polenta mixture on the bottom.

5. Layer meat and vegetable filling on the millet polenta, then top with the rest of the millet polenta. Garnish with rice cheese and green onions.

6. Bake tamale pie for 20-25 minutes. Serve on top of spinach greens with sliced avocados and cilantro.

Per Serving: 339 calories, 8g total fat, 2g saturated fat, 12mg cholesterol, 441mg sodium, 910mg potassium, 46g total carbohydrate, 9g dietary fiber, 23g protein

0	0	0	1/2	0	1/4	0	
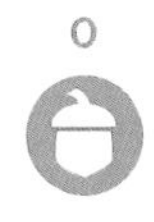	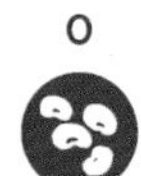	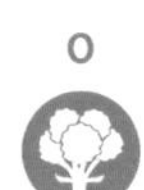	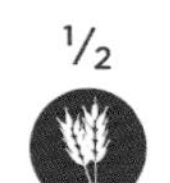	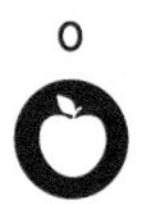		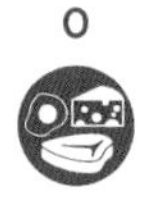	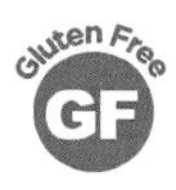

Serves 8

Millet Polenta

This dish is a perfect accompaniment to our Italian Chicken Cacciatore. Millet is one of the highest sources of iron, containing higher levels than kale and spinach. Iron deficiency can result in anemia, so be sure to get your daily recommended amount of the mineral.

1 cup dried bulk polenta
1/2 cup millet
2 tablespoons Earth Balance or Benecol butter substitute
1 1/2 teaspoons salt to taste
Ground pepper to taste

Preparation

1 In a small saucepan, boil millet with 1 1/2 cup lightly salted water, covered for 20 minutes.

2 In medium saucepan, boil 3 cups water and whisk in polenta until incorporated. Turn heat to medium and fold in butter substitute. Fold in cooked millet. Add salt and pepper.

Per Serving: 137 calories, 3g total fat, 1g saturated fat, 0mg cholesterol, 183mg sodium, 0mg potassium, 23g total carbohydrate, 2g dietary fiber, 3g protein

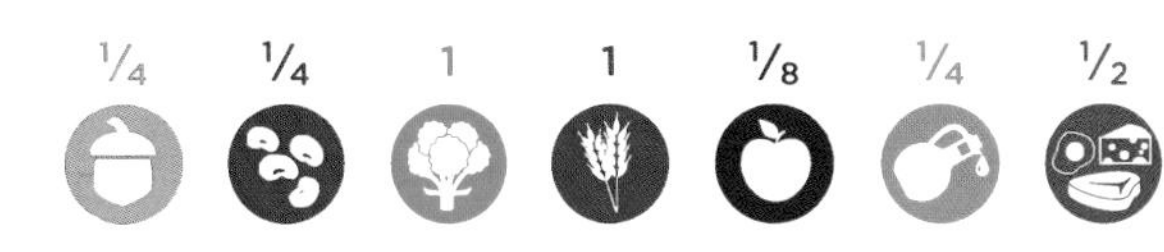

Serves 8

Moroccan Beef Stew with Apricots

This rich savory and Moroccan stew is balanced with braised sweet apricots. Substitute the lemon peel for the traditional preserved lemons if you can find them. If the classic Moroccan spice ras el hanout is not available, use the spice blend included in this recipe. Kale is high in vitamin C, an antioxidant essential to good health. Great served over brown rice pasta for a gluten-free dinner, or with crusty flatbread and whole wheat couscous.

2 tablespoons olive oil, divided

3/4-1 pound beef chuck, trimmed and cut into 3/4-inch cubes

1 package of veggie beef tips

1/2 teaspoon ground pepper, divided, plus more to taste

3 cloves garlic, finely chopped

3 large carrot, chopped

3 celery ribs, chopped

1 large yellow onion, chopped

4 tablespoons ras el hanout or Moroccan Spice Blend (see recipe to the right)

3 cups beef stock

3 cups water

2 15-ounce cans chickpeas, rinsed and drained

6 cups kale leaves, chopped

1/2 cup uncooked quinoa

1 cup diced apricots

6 tablespoon chopped cilantro, for garnish, optional

1 large lemon, cut into 6 wedges

1/2 cup sliced almonds, roasted

Moroccan Spice Blend:

4 teaspoons ground cumin

4 teaspoons sweet paprika

2 teaspoons ground cinnamon

2 teaspoons ground ginger

Preparation

1 Heat 1 tablespoon oil in a large Dutch oven or heavy pot over medium-high heat. Add beef and 1/4 teaspoon pepper and cook, stirring occasionally, until no juices remain and meat is browned, about 10 minutes.

2 Add remaining 1 tablespoon oil, garlic, carrot, celery, and onion, and cook until vegetables are softened, about 6-8 minutes. Stir in ras el hanout or Moroccan Spice Blend and cook, stirring constantly, for 1 minute.

3 Add beef stock, water and chickpeas; bring to a boil, scraping up any browned bits. Reduce heat to medium-low, cover, and simmer until beef is just tender, about 45 minutes; skim off and discard any foam on surface while cooking.

4 Add quinoa, kale, veggie meat, 1/2 teaspoon pepper and continue to cook, covered, until quinoa is al dente, 10 to 20 minutes more.

5 Season to taste with salt and pepper, then ladle stew into bowls over brown rice pasta or couscous and garnish with cilantro, almonds and lemon wedges.

Alternative Cooking Method:

1 After Step 2, pour contents into slow cooker and cook on low for 6-8 hours, then add beef stock, water and chickpeas, bring to a boil, scraping up any browned bits. Add quinoa, kale, veggie beef, 1/4 teaspoon pepper and diced apricots, and continue to cook. Keep covered.

Per Serving: 431 calories, 24g total fat, 5g saturated fat, 41mg cholesterol, 267mg sodium, 643mg potassium, 36g total carbohydrate, 9g dietary fiber, 25g protein

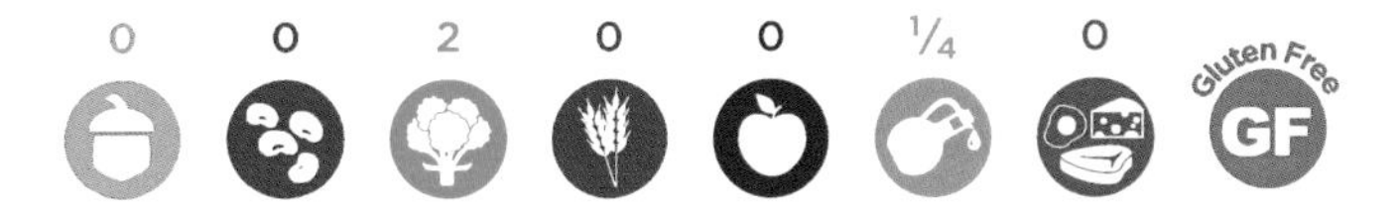

Serves 4

Moroccan Roasted Carrots

Pair this vegetable dish with any dinner. The Moroccan spice ras el hanout or a curry blend can be substituted in place of the spices listed below in these delicious and flavorful roasted carrots. Vitamin A, found in carrots, and cumin help reduce inflammation.

8 carrots, sliced into 1/4-inch rounds
1 tablespoon olive oil
2 cloves garlic, minced
1/2 teaspoon cumin
1/2 teaspoon paprika
1/4 teaspoon allspice or cinnamon
1 teaspoon salt
1 lemon, halved and juiced

Preparation

1 Preheat oven to 425 degrees. Toss carrots with olive oil, garlic, cumin, paprika, allspice, and salt.

2 Roast on foil-lined pan for 20 minutes. Sprinkle with lemon juice before serving.

Per Serving: 107 calories, 4g total fat, 1g saturated fat, 0mg cholesterol, 591mg sodium, 27mg potassium, 18g total carbohydrate, 0g dietary fiber, 2g protein

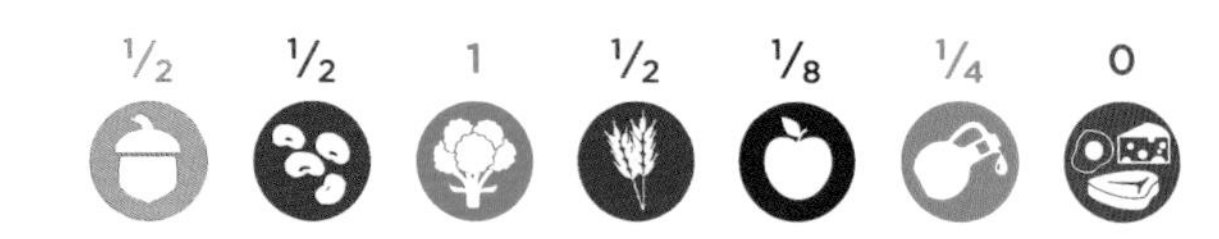

Serves 8

Moroccan Roasted Vegetable Tagine

Brightly colored and slowly cooked, this succulent vegetable dish from North Africa will tantalize your tastebuds. Our tagine serves up loads of protein with the inclusion of sweet potato, chickpeas, quinoa, and couscous. Sweet potatoes are also high in vitamin A, which can boost vision health.

2 tablespoons olive oil

1 medium yellow onion, diced

1/2 teaspoon ground pepper

2 teaspoons ras el hanout or curry powder blend (use garam masala in a pinch)

1 cinnamon stick

2 teaspoon fresh ginger, grated

3 medium cloves garlic, thinly sliced

4 peeled carrots, diced

2 peeled sweet potatoes, diced

1 cup canned diced tomatoes in juice

1 can chickpeas, drained

4 cups vegetable broth, plus 3 cups for couscous

1 pinch saffron threads, optional

1 medium head cauliflower, diced large

1 1/4 cup green olives, such as picholine, pitted and halved

1 preserved lemon, seeded and finely chopped, or 1 lemon, zested and juiced

1/2 cup dried currants, chopped apricots or dried goji berries

2 cups dry quinoa cooked with 2 cups water

3 cups dry couscous

2 tablespoons olive oil

1 cup slivered almonds or roasted pine nuts for garnish

1/2 cup sliced scallions for garnish

Preparation

1 Heat olive oil in a large Dutch oven or heavy-bottomed pot with a tight-fitting lid over medium heat. When oil shimmers, add onion and season with pepper. Stir occasionally until soft and translucent, about 5 minutes.

2 Stir in ras el hanout and cinnamon stick, and toast until aromatic, about 1 minute. Add ginger and garlic, and cook until just softened, about 1 minute more.

3 Add carrots, sweet potatoes, tomatoes and chickpeas. Season with pepper and cook until slightly tender, about 5 minutes.

4. Add 4 cups vegetable broth and saffron and stir to combine. Bring mixture to a simmer and cook, covered, until vegetables are almost cooked but still raw in the center, about 7 minutes.

5. Add cauliflower, olives, preserved lemon, and currants, and simmer, stirring occasionally, until cauliflower is just tender, about 10 minutes more. Taste tagine and adjust seasoning if necessary.

6. Cook quinoa in medium saucepan for 20 minutes. Set aside.

7. Place couscous in a large bowl or baking dish. Bring 3 cups vegetable broth to a boil. Pour broth over couscous and let stand until water is absorbed, about 5 minutes.

8. Add olive oil to couscous, season to taste with salt and pepper, and stir briefly to combine. Combine the cooked quinoa and couscous and top with tagine, almonds and scallions. Serve with Greek yogurt or whole milk yogurt on the side.

Per Serving: 201 calories, 5g total fat, 1g saturated fat, 0mg cholesterol, 151mg sodium, 607mg potassium, 36g total carbohydrate, 8g dietary fiber, 6g protein

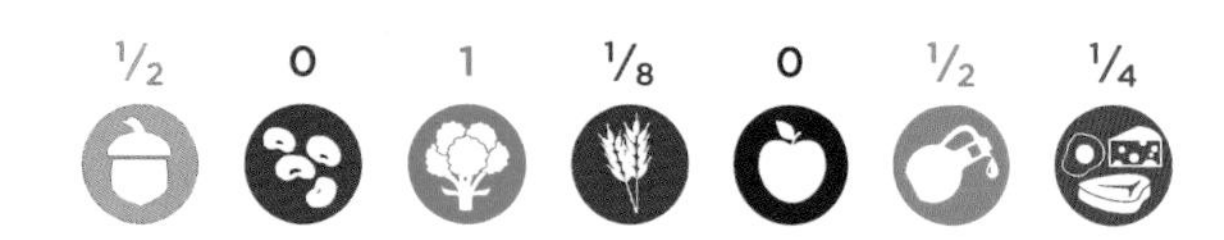

Serves 8

Moussaka

Moussaka is the Greek version of lasagna featuring the amazing eggplant. High in potassium, copper, folate, magnesium and fiber, eggplant also contains flavonoids and phenols that fight cancer and protect against various diseases. This dish tastes great served over steaming hot brown rice pasta.

1/2 cup sprouted grain bread crumbs, optional

3 tablespoons shredded non-dairy rice mozzarella

1 tablespoon chopped parsley for garnish

1 package brown rice pasta (elbow or fusili)

Eggplant:

2 large eggplants (about 2 3/4 pounds), unpeeled and cut lengthwise into 1/2-inch slices

2 tablespoons extra-virgin olive oil, sprayed or brushed on eggplant

1 pinch salt and freshly ground pepper

Meat sauce:

1/2 tablespoon extra-virgin olive oil

3 cloves garlic, minced

1 medium yellow onion, chopped

1 tablespoon water

1/2 pound ground beef

1 teaspoon dried oregano

1/2 teaspoon ground allspice

2 pinches ground cloves

2 cinnamon stick, broken in half

1 pinch ground pepper

2 carrots, diced

2 celery ribs, diced

1 cup finely chopped kale or spinach

1 package veggie beef crumbles

1 24-ounce can crushed tomatoes

2 bay leaves

Custard sauce:

1 tablespoon Earth Balance or Benecol butter substitute

1 tablespoon cornstarch

1 1/2 cups soy creamer

1 cup raw cashews puréed with 1 cup water

1 pinch salt

1 pinch ground nutmeg

Preparation

For the eggplant:

1 Preheat the oven to 425 degrees. Brush the eggplant slices on both sides with the oil and lay on a large (or two small) foil-lined baking sheet. Season with salt and pepper. Bake until the eggplant is soft, about 15-20 minutes. Set aside and cover.

For the meat sauce:

1. Heat the oil in a large pot over medium-high heat. Add garlic and cook, stirring frequently, until fragrant, about 1 minute. Add onion and cook, until lightly browned, about 4 minutes.

2. Add the beef, oregano, allspice, cloves, and cinnamon. Break the meat up into small pieces and season with pepper to taste. Cook, stirring occasionally, for about 2 minutes. Lower the heat to medium and cook, stirring, until just cooked but still slightly pink inside, about 1 minute more.

3. Add carrots, celery and kale until kale is wilted. Add the veggie beef, tomatoes and bay leaves and bring to a simmer. Cover and cook until the sauce is thickened and fragrant, about 30 minutes.

Alternative Cooking Method:

1. Place all the ingredients in crockpot and cook on low for 6-8 hours or overnight and continue with recipe below.

For the custard sauce (Béchamel):

1. Melt the butter substitute in a medium saucepan over medium heat. Whisk in the cornstarch until smooth. Stir while cooking for 1 minute. Remove pan from heat and add the soy creamer, salt, and nutmeg. Return to the heat and while whisking constantly, bring to a boil. Reduce heat and simmer for 2 minutes. Whisk in puréed raw cashews and warm on low until sauce is thick and creamy.

To assemble Moussaka:

1. Lower the oven to 350 degrees. Brush a 9x13-inch casserole dish with oil. Scatter the breadcrumbs over the bottom of the pan. Lay half of the eggplant in the pan, overlapping the slices if needed. Cover with half of the meat sauce and smooth with a rubber spatula. Repeat with the remaining eggplant and meat sauce. Pour the custard sauce over the layered mixture and smooth with a rubber spatula. Top with the rice mozzarella and bake, uncovered, until lightly browned and the custard sets, about 1 hour. Cook pasta according to package directions 15 minutes before serving. Remove the Moussaka from the oven and let rest for 10 minutes. Use a slotted spoon or spatula to serve. Serve on top of cooked pasta. Garnish with fresh parsley.

Per Serving: 362 calories, 15g total fat, 3g saturated fat, 18mg cholesterol, 322mg sodium, 1075mg potassium, 31g total carbohydrate, 11g dietary fiber, 22g protein

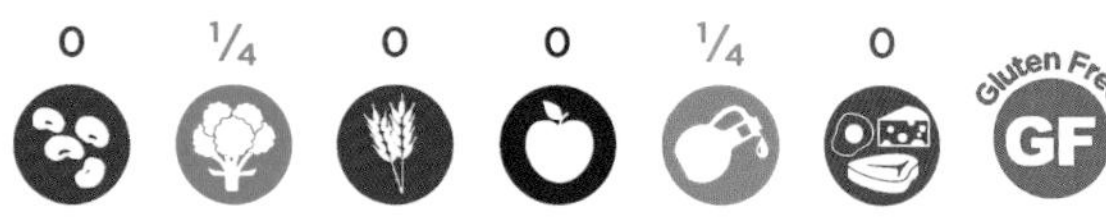

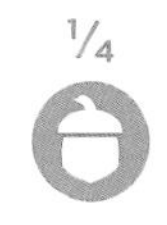
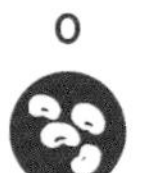
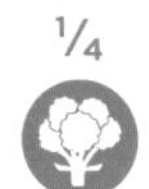
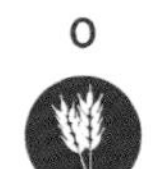

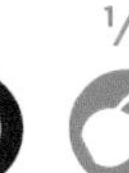
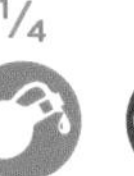
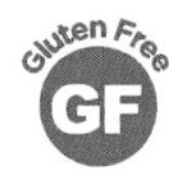

Serves 8

Mushroom Paté with Sherry and Thyme

Mushrooms can nourish your body with a punch of nutrition: They're packed with selenium, riboflavin, vitamin B, potassium, and vitamin D. Plus, the beta-glucans in mushrooms may help enhance your immune system! Make this sophisticated appetizer for special occasions, or use it as a sandwich spread throughout the week.

2 tablespoons Earth Balance or Benecol butter substitute

4 shallots, diced

16 ounces fresh mushrooms

1/8 teaspoon hot sauce

1 tablespoon sherry

1/2 teaspoon thyme

1 cup raw cashews

1/3 cup water

1/4 cup parsley for garnish

Preparation

1. In a medium skillet, melt butter substitute and sauté shallots for 2 minutes.
2. Add mushrooms, hot sauce, sherry, thyme and cashews and sauté until mushrooms are cooked, about 4-5 minutes.
3. Pour mushroom mixture into a blender and add water. Purée until smooth. Season to taste and pour into eight individual ramekins to serve. Garnish with parsley. Serve with pumpernickel bread toasts, sliced wheat baguette or whole wheat pita crisps, or gluten-free bread or crackers.

Per Serving: 111 calories, 8g total fat, 1g saturated fat, 0mg cholesterol, 46mg sodium, 89mg potassium, 7g total carbohydrate, 1g dietary fiber, 3g protein

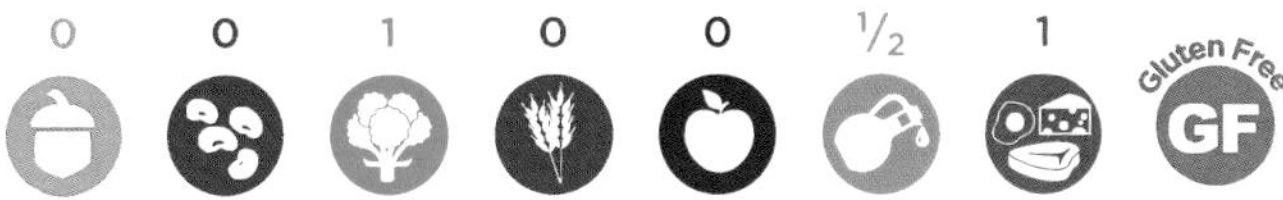

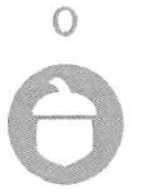
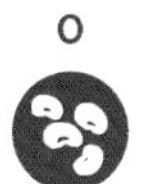

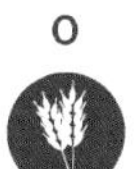
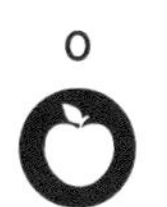

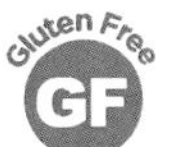

Serves 8

Oven-Roasted Halibut with Romesco Sauce

Halibut contains selenium, an essential mineral found in seafood that plays an important role in protecting your cells against the effects of free radicals. The antioxidant action of selenium can even help prevent heart disease, an associated condition of prediabetes and diabetes. Serve this beautiful dish with roasted red potatoes or quinoa. If you're a salmon lover, feel free to swap out the halibut with salmon.

8 halibut fillets, 3- to 4-ounces each, with skin
1 pinch salt and ground pepper
2 tablespoons canola oil
8 cups spinach
2 garlic cloves, minced
1 lemon, juiced
1 tablespoon olive oil
1 cup Romesco Sauce (recipe in Sauces section)

Preparation

1. Pat the halibut fillets dry with paper towel. Season the halibut with salt and pepper. Heat the canola oil over medium-high heat in a large oven-proof frying pan until lightly smoking.
2. Add fish skin side down, and shake pan so that fish are moving and not sticking to the surface. Reduce heat to med-low and cook for 3 minutes, or until fish is slightly raw on top. Turn fish over and cook for 30 seconds. Remove from pan and let it rest.
3. In hot sauté pan, add olive oil, and garlic. Cook for a few seconds. Add spinach and toss until just wilting. Add lemon juice and a pinch of salt. Toss.
4. Serve halibut on bed of spinach and top with warm Romesco Sauce.

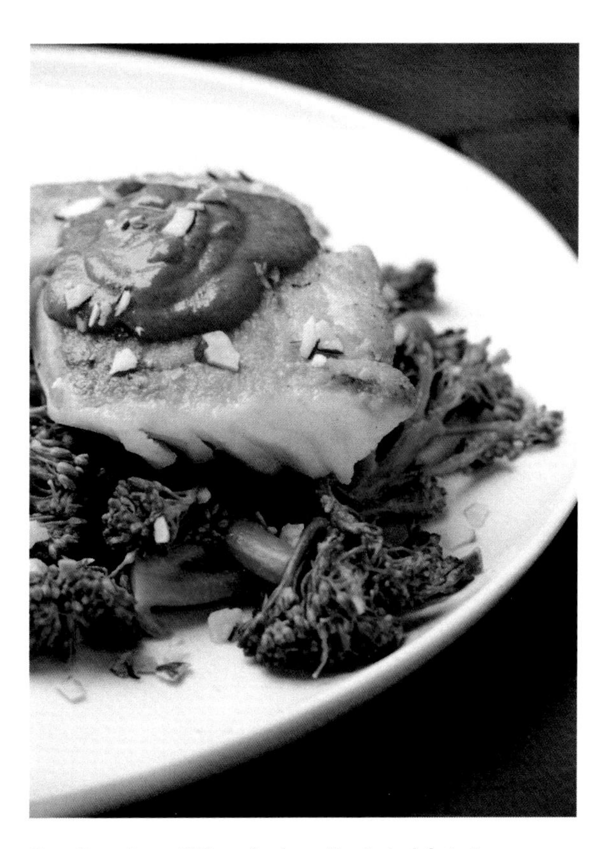

Per Serving: 156 calories, 7g total fat, 1g saturated fat, 36mg cholesterol, 121mg sodium, 679mg potassium, 2g total carbohydrate, 1g dietary fiber, 24g protein

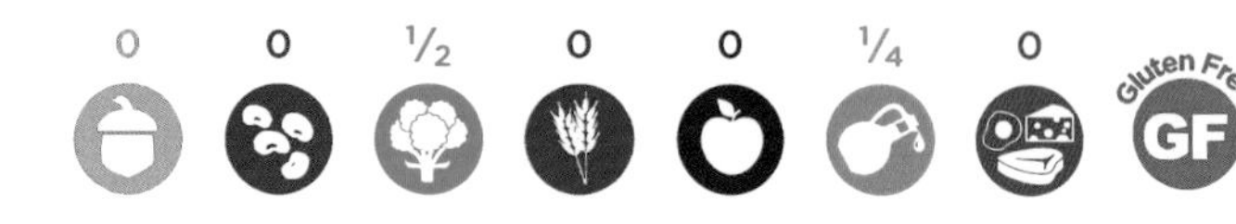

Serves 4

Oven-Roasted Sweet Potatoes with Curry Dip

Crunchy sweet potato "fries" get an instant and tasty kick with this creamy curry dip. Sweet potatoes make a great high-fiber and nutrient-rich snack or side dish. Loaded with flavor and vitamins, this starchy vegetable is high in fiber and vitamin A, which is important for vision health. Cauliflower–low in fat and carbohydrates and high in fiber, folate and vitamin C–can be substituted for sweet potatoes and roasted the same way. Double the recipe and enjoy the dish again later in the week.

2 medium sweet potatoes, peeled and sliced thin

1 tablespoon olive oil

1 pinch salt

1/8 teaspoon cayenne pepper

1/2 tablespoon curry powder blend

Fresh lime juice, optional

See Curry Dip recipe in Sauces section

Preparation

1 Preheat oven to 425 degrees. Mix sweet potatoes with the olive oil, then add the salt, cayenne pepper, curry powder and lime juice, and mix so that the spices coat each potato.

2 Roast sweet potatoes on foil-lined baking sheet for 25 minutes until they reach the desired crispy texture. Serve with Curry Dip.

Per Serving: 107 calories, 6g total fat, 3g saturated fat, 0mg cholesterol, 125mg sodium, 25mg potassium, 12g total carbohydrate, 2g dietary fiber, 1g protein

$^1/_4$ 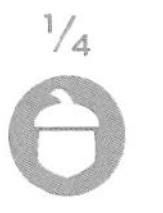 0 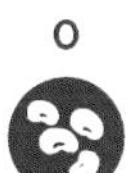 $^1/_2$  $^1/_2$ 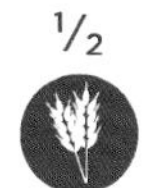 0 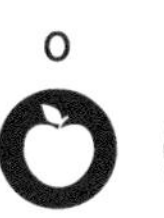 $^2/_3$ 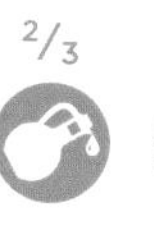 $^1/_2$ 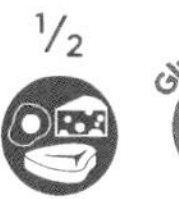 Gluten Free GF

Serves 6

Pad Thai

Fresh and exciting, this dish is exactly how you would find it in Bangkok, except with more vegetables. The peanut flavor allows the Pad Thai to sing, and makes it nutritious too: Peanut butter contains vitamin E, which is also found in green leafy vegetables and other seeds and nuts. To give the meal an extra nutrition boost, serve over wilted spinach. Your family is sure to want seconds of this savory, famous noodle dish!

12 ounces brown rice fettuccine or linguine

4 tablespoons olive oil

4 garlic cloves, finely chopped

2 tablespoons tamarind powder

2 tablespoons light soy sauce

2 tablespoons packed light brown sugar or honey

1 tablespoon tomato paste

1 tablespoon ketchup

3 anchovies or 2 tablespoons veggie or regular fish sauce

2 tablespoons peanut butter

$^1/_2$ tablespoon paprika

1 tablespoons sriracha, hot sauce or ground chile pepper

$^1/_2$ pound diced chicken breasts

1 package veggie chicken strips

4 large shallots, diced

4 large eggs, optional

1 bunch scallions, sliced into 1-inch pieces

2 cups finely sliced cabbage

1 cup julienned carrots

2 cups frozen or fresh green beans, blanched and diced

$^1/_2$ cup roasted peanuts or cashews, coarsely chopped, for garnish

$^1/_2$ cup cilantro leaves for garnish

Preparation

1 In a large pot, bring water to a boil, add fettuccine and cook for 10 minutes. Drain noodles and rinse with cold water.

2 In a small pan, heat $^1/_2$ tablespoon oil and brown the garlic. Add 1 tablespoon water and stir in tamarind powder until dissolved.

3 Stir in soy sauce, brown sugar, tomato paste, ketchup, anchovies, peanut butter, sriracha, and paprika, stirring until sugar has dissolved.

4 Cut the chicken into 1-inch cubes and pat very dry. Heat 2 tablespoons of oil in wok over high heat and fry chicken until edges are browned. Then add shallots over medium-low heat, stirring frequently, until lightly browned.

5 Crack eggs, if using, into mixture and scramble with 1 teaspoon salt. Keep mixture moving. Break into chunks with spatula.

6 Stir fry scallions, and remaining shallots until softened, about 1 minute. Add cooked noodles and sauce, and stir fry over medium heat (use 2 spatulas if necessary) 3-5 minutes. Add sauce and simmer, turning noodles over to absorb sauce evenly, until noodles are tender, about 4-6 minutes.

7 Fold in vegetables and continue to stir fry in a little water until cabbage is wilted and noodles are tender, about 6 minutes, and transfer to a large shallow serving dish.

8 Sprinkle Pad Thai with peanuts and cilantro leaves and serve with lime wedges and extra sriracha or chile paste if desired.

TIP

The trickiest part is soaking the noodles, which should be somewhat flexible and solid, not completely expanded and soft. When in doubt, under-soak. You can always add more water to the pan, but you can't take it out. Shrimp can be substituted. For kids, omit the ground chile pepper.

Per Serving: 547 calories, 23g total fat, 3g saturated fat, 157mg cholesterol, 411mg sodium, 421mg potassium, 49g total carbohydrate,5 dietary fiber, 18g protein

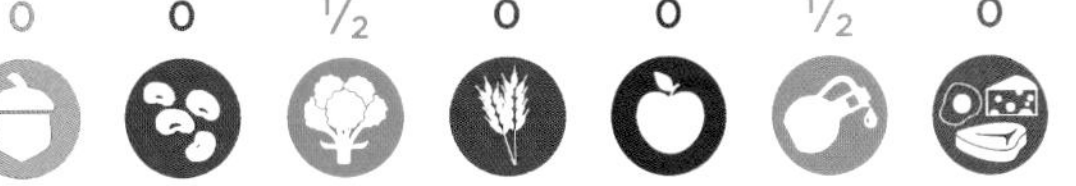
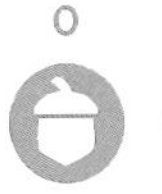
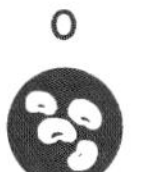

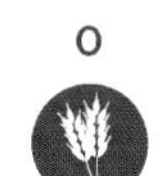
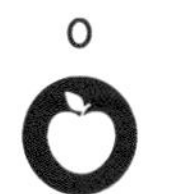

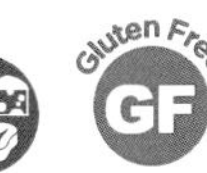

Serves 6

Roasted Brussels Sprouts with Pickled Radishes

If Brussels sprouts haven't been on your menu in a while, this dish may change that! Brussels sprouts are a cruciferous vegetable known for their high fiber and heart-healthy benefits. This recipe is prepared with garlic, which also has cardio-protective benefits and may help regulate blood sugar. Crunchy and flavorful, this side dish goes great with meatloaf, chicken potpie and just about any fish dish.

1 pound Brussels sprouts, halved or quartered
2 tablespoons olive oil
1 pinch salt and pepper
1/8 teaspoon crushed red pepper
1 minced garlic clove
1/2 teaspoon nutmeg
6-8 fresh radishes, halved
1 tablespoon Earth Balance butter substitute
1 tablespoon vinegar or champagne vinegar
1 teaspoon sugar
1 pinch salt
1 pinch ground pepper
2 tablespoon fresh parsley, chopped

Preparation

1 Preheat oven to 425 degrees. Toss Brussels sprouts with olive oil, salt, pepper, red pepper, garlic and nutmeg. Pour Brussels sprouts onto greased baking sheet and roast for 20 minutes.

2 In a medium saucepan, melt butter substitute and add radishes, sugar, vinegar, salt and pepper, and braise for 5-7 minutes until radishes are pink. Toss radishes with Brussels sprouts, and sprinkle with parsley to serve.

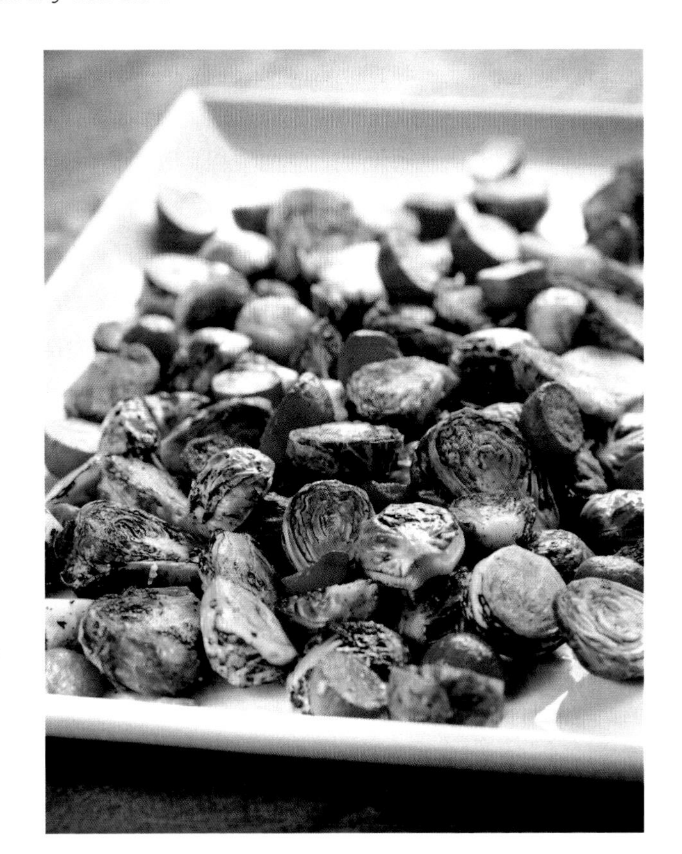

Per Serving: 84 calories, 7g total fat, 1g saturated fat, 0mg cholesterol, 134mg sodium, 185mg potassium, 5g total carbohydrate, 2g dietary fiber, 2g protein

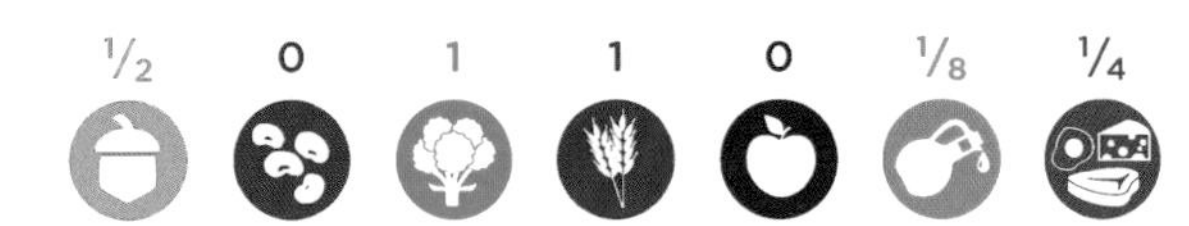

Serves 8

Roasted Stuffed Pumpkin with Gruyère

Give your holiday a nutritious boost and serve this roasted stuffed pumpkin. The traditional Turkey Day stuffing gets a healthy makeover with sprouted grain bread free of fat-loaded butter and turkey stock. Here's the best part: Our Roasted Stuffed Pumpkin with Gruyère is just as mouthwatering as the unhealthy stuffing you know and love. Delicious and healthy, this dish is sure to steal the show at any holiday table!

1 pumpkin, about 2 ½ or 3 pounds

Salt and freshly ground pepper

6 slices sprouted grain bread, diced into small chunks

1 tablespoon olive oil or Earth Balance butter substitute

2-4 garlic cloves, coarsely chopped

2 tablespoons diced shallots or onions

1 pound sliced mushrooms

4 celery stalks, diced

¼ cup fresh chives or sliced scallions

1 tablespoon minced fresh thyme or 1 teaspoon dried thyme

1 tablespoon cooking sherry or white wine

1 teaspoon salt

1 cup raw cashews puréed with 1 cup water, or 1 ½ cup soy creamer

1 pinch freshly grated nutmeg

¼ pound Gruyère, Emmenthal or cheddar cheese, diced into ½-inch chunks

¼ cup water

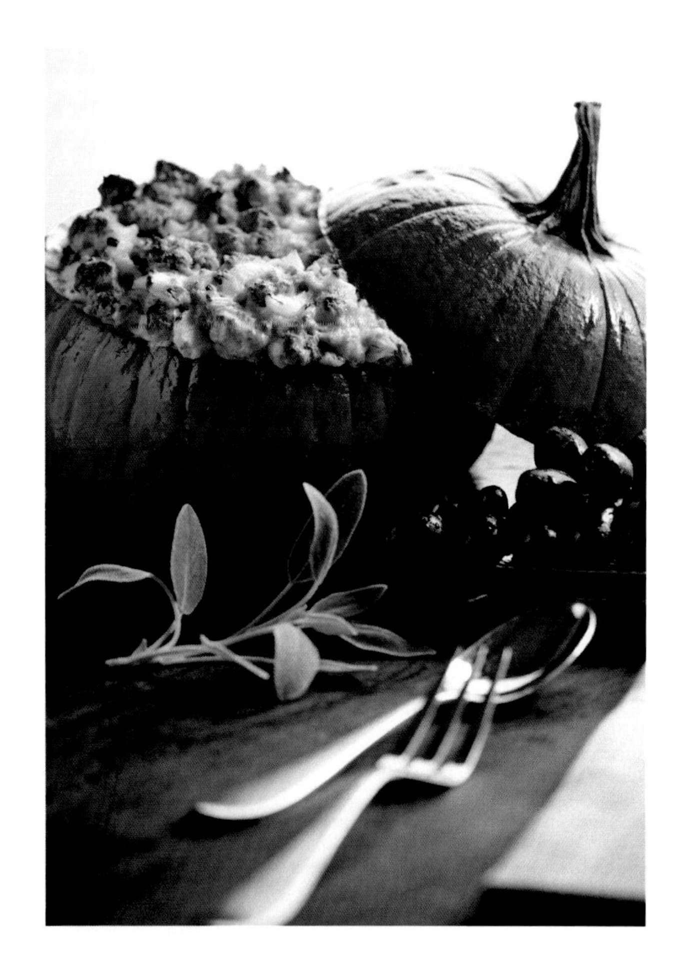

Preparation

For the pumpkin:

1. Cut a cap out of the top of the pumpkin (think Halloween Jack-o'-lantern). It's easiest to work your knife around the top of the pumpkin at a 45-degree angle. You want to cut off enough of the top to make it easy for you to work inside the pumpkin. Clear away the seeds and strings from the cap and from inside the pumpkin. Season the inside of the pumpkin generously with salt and pepper and place pumpkin on baking sheet or in a large round pie plate.

For the stuffing:

1. Preheat oven to 350 degrees. In a large skillet, heat oil and sauté garlic and shallot for 1 minute. Add mushrooms and 2 tablespoons water, and sauté until mushrooms are slightly cooked. Add celery, thyme, chives and sherry. Sprinkle with salt and sauté until celery is tender, about 7 minutes. Do not let brown. Add another 2 tablespoons of water to keep the vegetables moist and prevent them from browning.

2. Add mixture to bread crumbs in a large bowl and season with pepper. Fold in cheese, nutmeg and puréed raw cashews or soy creamer.

3. Fill pumpkin with stuffing, cover the top of the pumpkin with foil and bake for 2 hours. After 1 hour, remove foil and place pumpkin cap on baking sheet next to pumpkin and bake for the remaining hour. Allow pumpkin to cool for 10 minutes before serving. Garnish with more diced chives and serve, either by spooning out contents or slicing whole pumpkin into 8 pieces.

Per Serving: 200 calories, 12g total fat, 3g saturated fat, 10mg cholesterol, 337mg sodium, 120mg potassium, 17g total carbohydrate, 3g dietary fiber, 10g protein

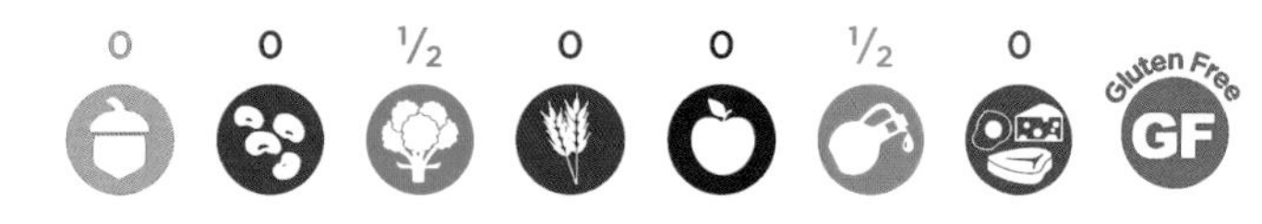

Serves 8

Roasted Vegetable Lasagna with Italian Turkey Sausage

This Italian favorite is made more nutrient-rich by substituting one layer of noodles with roasted eggplant. Eggplant is high in potassium, copper, folate, magnesium, and fiber, and contains flavonoids and phenols that fight viruses and harmful bacteria. Your family will love this healthier version of the saucy, layered classic dish!

1 package whole grain or gluten-free brown rice lasagna noodles

2 medium eggplant, sliced

2 large red bell peppers, diced

1 peeled sweet potato, diced

2 cups diced carrots

1 package or 8 ounces sliced mushrooms

½ pound asparagus, cut, or ½ cup frozen green beans

2 cups baby spinach greens

1 tablespoon olive oil, plus olive oil spray

1 quart marinara (homemade or store-bought)

1 can fire-roasted diced tomatoes

2 tablespoons balsamic vinegar

1 tablespoon agave nectar or honey

2 tablespoons fresh parsley, chopped, or 1 tablespoon dried parsley

2 tablespoons fresh basil, sliced, or 1 tablespoon dried basil

1 teaspoon hot sauce or ¼ teaspoon crushed red pepper

1 package shredded non-dairy rice mozzarella

8 ounces cottage cheese

1 pound Italian turkey sausage

2 cloves minced garlic or 1 tablespoon prepared garlic

½ package veggie crumbles

Preparation

1. Preheat oven to 425 degrees. Soak four lasagna noodle sheets in warm water and set aside.

2. Prepare vegetables to roast. Toss carrots, mushrooms, sweet potatoes, asparagus (but not green beans) and red bell peppers with 1 tablespoon olive oil and place on foil-lined baking sheet. Lightly salt.

3. Ribbon-peel eggplant and slice in ¼-inch slices. Lightly spray foil-lined baking sheet with olive oil and lay slices on pan. Lightly spray olive oil on top of eggplant and sprinkle with ¼ teaspoon salt.

4 Place both baking sheets of vegetables in oven to roast for 20 minutes. Remove from heat and put the diced vegetables into a large bowl. Toss in green beans. Reserve eggplant and spinach for later.

5 Reduce oven temperature to 350 degrees. Meanwhile, warm marinara in medium saucepan and add diced tomatoes, vinegar, agave, parsley, basil, and hot sauce. Stir in 2 tablespoons to ½ cup water to thin the sauce (since noodles aren't boiled first, the sauce has to be a little thinner than usual).

6 In a small bowl, mix half a package of mozzarella with cottage cheese and set aside.

7 Remove turkey sausage from casing and cook in a dry medium skillet with ½ tablespoon water. Cook until water is evaporated and meat begins to brown.

8 Add garlic and cook for 1 minute. Remove from heat and combine with roasted vegetables. Pour this into the sauce and combine.

9 Lightly spray two 9x9-inch baking dishes or a large 9x13-inch baking dish. Pour 2 cups marinara sauce or more to cover the bottoms of the lasagna pans. Line with one layer of noodles. If noodles are firm, cut or break to fit in pan. Pour 1-2 cups marinara sauce over noodles to cover.

10 Add roasted diced vegetables and cover with marinara sauce. Then add one thick layer of spinach greens. Top with cottage cheese mixture.

11 Add roasted eggplant in a single layer over the cottage cheese. Pour remaining sauce generously over eggplant and top with remaining mozzarella. Place lasagna on foil-lined baking sheet.

12 The lasagna is best made one day in advance–it enhances the flavor! After the lasagna is prepped, bake in 350-degree oven for 50 minutes. Cover and store in the fridge. The next day, warm leftovers in 325-degree oven for 15 minutes. Let cool for 10 minutes before serving.

Per Serving: 200 calories, 12g total fat, 3g saturated fat, 10mg cholesterol, 337mg sodium, 120mg potassium, 17g total carbohydrate, 3g dietary fiber, 10g protein

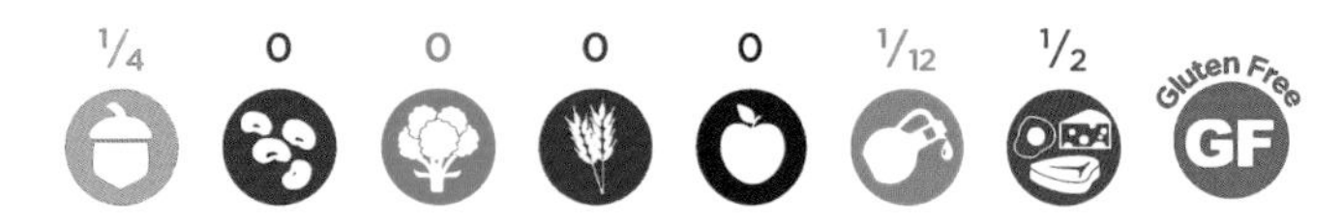

Serves 6

Sake-Poached Salmon with Sesame-Ginger Sauce

This simple and delicious dish is loaded with flavor and protein-rich sesame seeds. Salmon contains niacin, an important vitamin that helps repair DNA and has a special role in insulin response. Serve chilled.

3 cups sake

1 cup plus 2 tablespoons water

1 2-inch piece fresh ginger, peeled and diced

1/4 teaspoon ground pepper or 1/8 teaspoon crushed red pepper

1/2 tablespoon sesame oil

1/2 lemon, juiced, plus 2 lemons, juiced and zested (use vegetable peeler to zest)

1 1/2 pounds boneless, skinless salmon fillet, cut into six 2-ounce servings

1/2 cup tahini

3 tablespoons Bragg Liquid Aminos or low-sodium soy sauce

1/2 tablespoon sesame oil

1/2 inch diced ginger

1/8 teaspoon cayenne pepper or crushed red pepper

1 pinch salt

4 scallions sliced for garnish

1/2 cup diced cilantro for garnish

1/2 tablespoon sesame seeds for garnish

Preparation

1 Combine sake, water, ginger and pepper in a covered pan and cook for 10 minutes to infuse the water with flavor; reduce heat to lowest setting, carefully slide salmon into the water. Cover and poach until fish is just cooked through, about 5 to 7 minutes. Remove the fish with a slotted spoon and cool completely before transferring to an airtight container. Sprinkle with lemon juice and add about 1/2 cup of the poaching liquid to the container to keep the fish moist. Chill in the refrigerator until ready to serve.

2 To make Sesame Ginger Sauce, combine lemon juice and zest, tahini, 2 tablespoons water, Bragg Liquid Aminos, sesame oil, ginger, cayenne pepper, and salt in a blender and blend until smooth. Transfer to a jar until ready to serve.

3 To serve, place the cold salmon on a bed of baby spinach or steamed bok choy and then drizzle the Sesame-Ginger Sauce over the top and serve brown rice on the side. Garnish with scallions, cilantro and sesame seeds.

Per Serving: 403 calories, 18g total fat, 3g saturated fat, 31mg cholesterol, 368mg sodium, 366mg potassium, 14g total carbohydrate, 1g dietary fiber, 16g protein

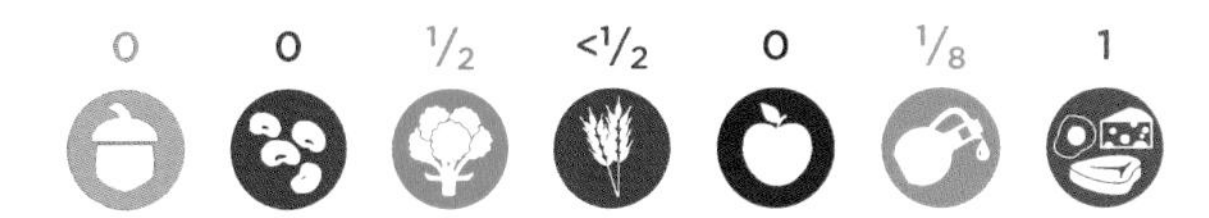

Serves 8

Savory Italian Meatloaf

This healthy rendition gives you all the comfort of the classic dish with less fat and fewer calories. Easy to make, our meatloaf is perfect for any day of the week and features a tasty Easy Marinara Sauce. Vitamin B5 is commonly found in whole grain products, mushrooms and kale, which is used in this recipe.

1 1/2 slices sprouted grain bread, diced

1/2 cup onion, diced small

1 tablespoon olive oil

2 celery ribs, diced small

1/2 cup carrots, diced small

2 garlic cloves, minced

24 ounces ground turkey

2 egg whites

2 teaspoons mustard

1 1/2 teaspoons salt

1 teaspoon ground pepper

1/2 teaspoon hot sauce or 1/8 teaspoon crushed red pepper

2 teaspoons thyme, chopped

Easy Marinara Sauce:

1 small onion, diced small

1 tablespoon olive oil

3 garlic cloves, minced

1 15-ounce can chopped tomato

3 sprigs fresh thyme or 1 tablespoon dried thyme

1 tablespoon oregano

1 tablespoon basil, lightly chopped

Preparation

1. Preheat oven to 375 degrees. In saucepan, sauté onions with olive oil until soft. Add celery and carrots. Cook until soft, about 9 minutes. Add garlic and cook until fragrant. Remove from heat and cool.

2. Once chilled, add vegetables to the turkey along with eggs, bread, mustard, salt, pepper, hot sauce and thyme. Mix together and shape into two large loaves or 4-6 individual loaves. Bake in oven for 30-40 minutes. Serve with Easy Marinara Sauce.

For Easy Marinara Sauce:

1. Sauté onion in olive oil until soft and translucent. Add garlic and cook until fragrant. Add remaining ingredients except basil. Cook on low heat for 30 minutes. Remove from heat and stir in basil and salt and pepper to taste.

Per Serving: 188 calories, 8g total fat, 2g saturated fat, 60mg cholesterol, 547mg sodium, 199mg potassium, 9g total carbohydrate, 2g dietary fiber, 18g protein

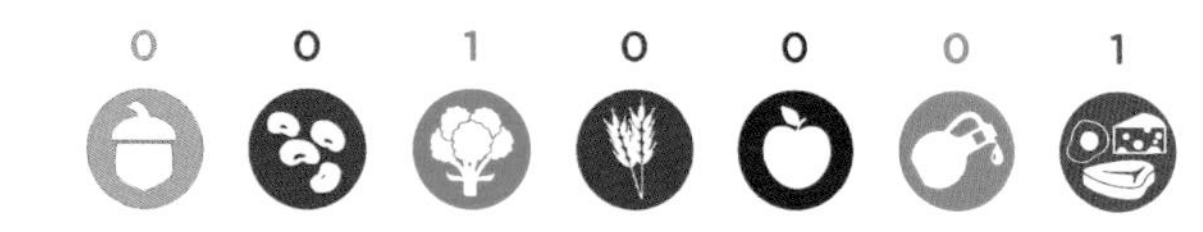

Serves 4

Spring Vegetable Tart

Beautiful and delicious, this spring tart is made with asparagus, which is high in insoluble fiber, slowing the uptake of sugar into the bloodstream. Eat this gorgeous, tasty tart cold or warm and serve with a salad or as an appetizer.

1 sheet frozen puff pastry, thawed

1 cup shredded non-dairy rice mozzarella

20 thin asparagus spears, trimmed, or 1/8-inch sliced yellow squash and tomatoes

1 large shallot, finely diced

1/2 cup Egg Beaters or egg whites

2 tablespoons soy milk or soy creamer

1/2 teaspoon plus 1/8 teaspoon salt

1/4 cup grated parmesan, manchego or fontina cheese

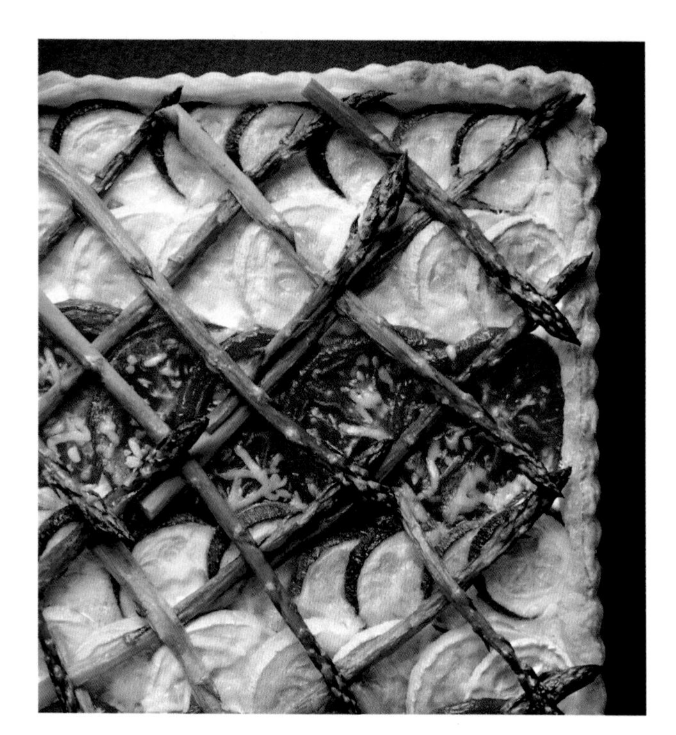

Preparation

1 Preheat oven to 400 degrees. Line rimmed baking sheet with parchment paper and lay puff pastry on top. Fold over sides to make a 1-inch rim and pierce pastry with a fork.

2 Sprinkle with mozzarella and layer vegetables on top in a pretty design. Sprinkle diced shallots on top. Bake for 15 minutes.

3 While baking, mix Egg Beaters with soy milk or soy creamer, and salt. Pour mixture over tart and sprinkle with parmesan. Bake until pastry is puffed and golden, about 10-12 minutes. Let tart stand for 10 minutes before serving.

Per Serving: 355 calories, 20g total fat, 10g saturated fat, 5mg cholesterol, 629mg sodium, 66mg potassium, 31g total carbohydrate, 3g dietary fiber, 16g protein

0 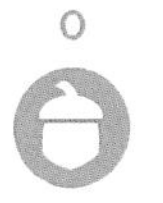 0 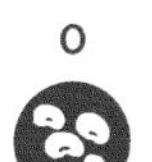 1 1/3 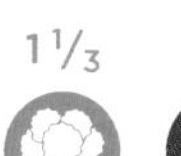 0 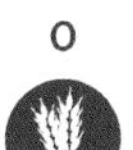 0 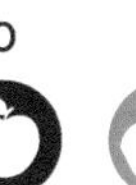 1/8  0 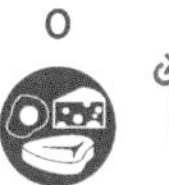 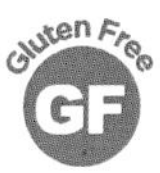

Serves 8

Summer Corn Succotash

Succotash highlights the best of summer's garden bounties. Corn is a major source of the essential B vitamins responsible for maintaining nerve health and cognitive function. It's also rich in thiamin and niacin... and delicious to boot! Bring this succotash to a potluck and be prepared to share the recipe.

6 ears fresh corn with husks
1 tablespoon olive oil
2 tablespoons diced shallots or onion
1 cup diced cherry tomatoes
1 diced green, red or poblano pepper, optional
4 tablespoons white or apple cider vinegar
1/2 tablespoon honey or agave nectar
1 teaspoon salt
1/2 teaspoon pepper
1/2 cup fresh basil, sliced
1 cup shelled edamame, optional

Preparation

1 Microwave or boil corn in hot water for 5-7 minutes until fragrant. Allow corn to cool down, then cut corn off the cob.

2 Warm skillet with olive oil and sauté shallots for 3 minutes, adding a tablespoon of water at a time to prevent browning. Add tomatoes and fresh peppers, and cook for another 3 minutes with vinegar, honey, salt and pepper.

3 Fold corn and edamame into the skillet. Remove from heat and fold in fresh basil. Serve immediately before basil begins to brown.

Per Serving: 118 calories, 4g total fat, 1g saturated fat, 0mg cholesterol, 307mg sodium, 236mg potassium, 19g total carbohydrate, 3g dietary fiber, 5g protein

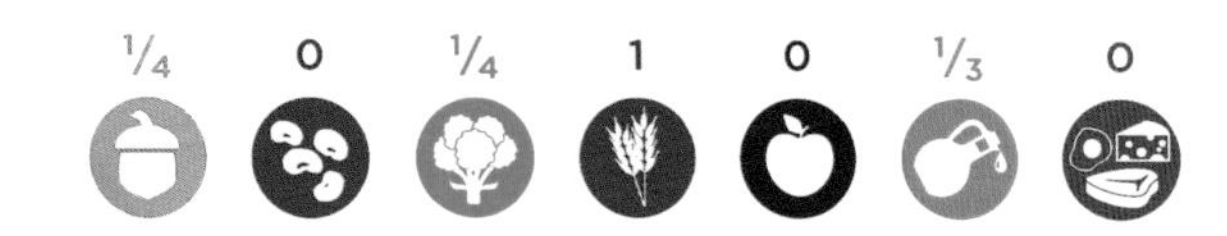

Makes 6

Sweet Potato Biscuits

Sweet potatoes are the oldest vegetable known to man and rich in vitamin A and beta carotene. The vegetable can also improve insulin resistance. Using quinoa flour makes for a whole grain and nutrient-rich biscuit that tastes delicious. To make a healthy version of the classic biscuits and gravy, top these biscuits with Béchamel sauce. Try this simple, tasty biscuit today!

- 1 medium baked sweet potato puréed or 1 cup canned sweet potato or pumpkin
- 2 cups quinoa flour, or half unbleached flour and half spelt flour
- 1 tablespoon baking powder
- 1/4 teaspoon baking soda
- 1 teaspoon salt
- 1/2 teaspoon nutmeg
- 1/4 cup plus 1 teaspoon Earth Balance butter substitute or olive oil
- 2 tablespoons maple syrup or agave nectar
- 1/4 cup chopped walnuts or pecans, optional

Preparation

1. Preheat oven to 375 degrees. Pulse ingredients together in a food processor until crumbly. Pour mixture in bowl and fold in nuts.

2. Turn the dough onto a floured board. Sprinkle a little flour on top and pat dough into a rectangle about 3/4-inch thick. Cut into 6 squares or use biscuit cutters. Place biscuits on a lightly greased baking sheet and bake for 12-15 minutes.

3. To dress these biscuits, press a piece of fresh sage or thyme onto the top of each biscuit right before baking.

1/4 0 1/2 1/8 0 1 1/3

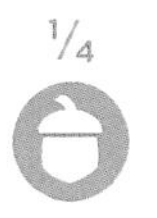 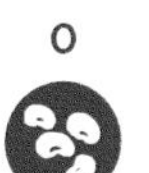  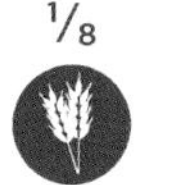 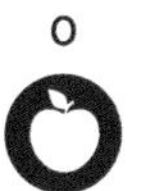 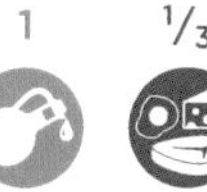 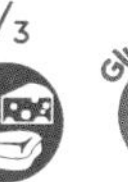 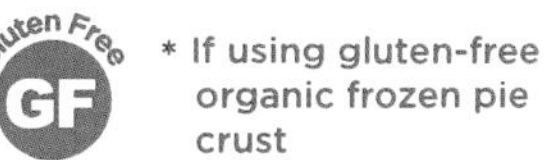

Serves 6

Tarragon Chicken Potpie

Our heart-healthy recipe uses low-cholesterol chicken breasts that pair marvelously with tarragon, a pungent herb that contains compounds known to help lower blood glucose levels. This warm comfort dish is filling and scrumptious!

- 1 medium onion, diced, or 1 leek, sliced (white part only)
- 1 shallot, diced, or 1/2 teaspoon garlic
- 4 large carrots, cut into 1/2-inch pieces, or 2 cups julienned carrots
- 3 celery ribs, diced
- 4 teaspoons dried tarragon, optional
- 3 tablespoons Earth Balance or Benecol butter substitute
- 1 cup chopped steamed kale or 1/2 cup chopped frozen spinach
- 1/4 cup cooked quinoa
- 1 1/2 cup frozen petite peas
- 1/2 pound boiled chicken breast, shredded and chopped
- 1/2 package of veggie chicken strips, diced
- 1 rounded tablespoon cornstarch
- 1 cup soy creamer or 1/2 cup puréed raw cashews
- 1 teaspoon salt
- 1/2 teaspoon hot sauce or 1/8 teaspoon ground pepper
- 4 sheets phyllo dough or 1 gluten-free pie crust

Preparation

1 Preheat oven to 425 degrees. In a medium saucepan, boil 4 cups of water, add chicken breast and boil until it floats, 12-15 minutes. Remove immediately to cool and set aside chicken broth.

2 Sauté onions in a large wok or Dutch oven with 1 tablespoon butter substitute. Add shallot, carrot, celery and dried tarragon to pan to combine flavors. Cook with 2 tablespoons water for 12 minutes until vegetables are slightly tender.

3 In a skillet, steam-sauté kale in 1/2 tablespoon of water until wilted, about 1 minute or less, then add to pot of vegetables. Stir in cooked quinoa and frozen peas. Remove from heat and set aside.

4 In small saucepan, melt 2 remaining tablespoons of butter substitute and whisk in cornstarch. Slowly add 1 cup chicken broth and cook until thickened.

5. Whisk in soy creamer and cook until thickened. Depending on consistency, add more chicken broth if too thick. Pour sauce over vegetables and fold in diced chicken and diced veggie chicken strips.

6. Pour into square 9x13-inch pan and cover with sheets of phyllo dough. Fold and push dough to fit pan; no need to trim. Fold and wrinkle on top for a fancy look.

7. Bake for 20 minutes until phyllo is golden. Serve warm over wilted spinach and brown rice.

Per Serving: 247 calories, 12g total fat, 2g saturated fat, 15mg cholesterol, 662mg sodium, 210mg potassium, 23g total carbohydrate, 4g dietary fiber, 11g protein

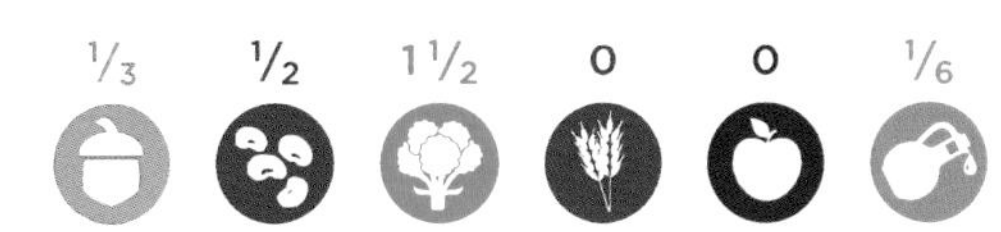

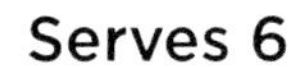

Serves 6

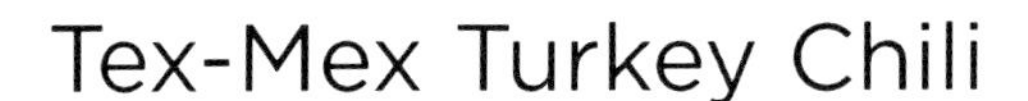

Tex-Mex Turkey Chili

Get your veggies and plenty of flavor too! Tomatoes are full of vitamin C, iron and vitamin E, and the beans make this dish a source of magnesium and potassium, important nutrients for people with prediabetes.

- 1 tablespoon olive oil
- 16 ounces ground turkey breast or frozen veggie beef crumbles
- 1 tablespoon minced garlic
- 1 medium onion, diced
- 2 teaspoons chili powder or chili blend
- 2 teaspoons ground cumin
- 1 15-ounce can diced tomatoes, plus 1 can water
- 2 tablespoons tomato paste or ½ cup (8 ounces) tomato sauce
- 4 finely diced carrots
- 1 15-ounce can black or navy beans
- 1 cup chopped kale or baby spinach
- 2 tablespoons chia seeds
- 1 teaspoon salt
- 2 tablespoons diced scallions or chives for garnish

Preparation

1. In a large saucepan or pot, add olive oil and when oil shimmers, crumble up ground turkey and brown lightly.

2. Add onions and garlic with 2 tablespoons of water and steam-sauté for 3 minutes. Add chili powder, cumin and a pinch of salt and sauté until fragrant. Do not let brown.

3. Add more water a tablespoon at a time. Add diced tomatoes with water, tomato paste, carrots and beans, and simmer on medium-high for 15 minutes until carrots are tender.

4. Fold in kale and chia seeds. Season lightly with salt and simmer for another 10 minutes. Serve hot with scallions on top.

Per Serving: 239 calories, 5g total fat, 1g saturated fat, 37mg cholesterol, 482mg sodium, 543mg potassium, 24g total carbohydrate, 9g dietary fiber, 24g protein

1/2 0 1/2 0 0 1/2 0

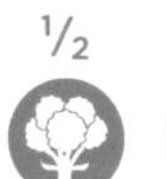
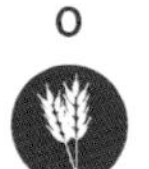
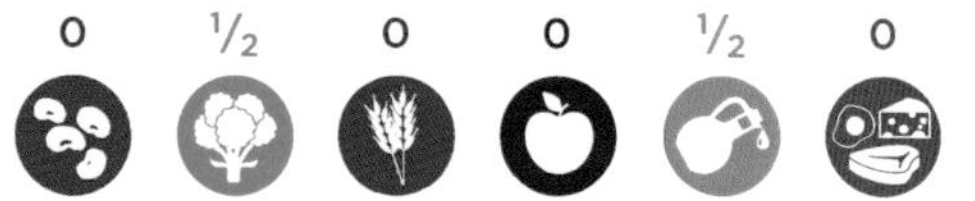

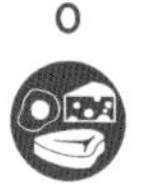
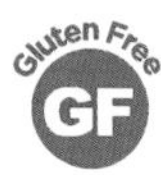

Serves 12

Thyme Potato Gratin

This delicious side dish is always a favorite for any occasion, but especially the holiday season! Potassium-rich potatoes and magnesium-packed cashews make this dish super nutritious and delicious.

4 pounds of red potatoes, washed and cut into 1/4 inch discs
3 cups water
1 cup soy milk
1 tablespoon Earth Balance or Benecol butter substitute
4 sprigs of fresh thyme or 1/2 teaspoon dried thyme
1 teaspoon plus 1/4 teaspoon salt
1/2 cup grated parmesan or Jarlsberg cheese
See Béchamel Sauce recipe in Sauces section

Preparation

1 Preheat oven to 375 degrees. In a large Dutch oven or pot, boil water and add potatoes. Stir in soy milk, butter substitute, thyme and 1 teaspoon salt. Cook for 15-20 minutes until potatoes are tender.

2 Grease large casserole dish with olive oil and pour 1 cup Béchamel Sauce on the bottom. Using a slotted spoon, layer potatoes on top of sauce.

3 Sprinkle 1/4 teaspoon salt and 1/8 teaspoon pepper over potatoes and drizzle 1 cup Béchamel Sauce. Layer with potatoes and sauce, then sprinkle with parmesan. Repeat and top with cheese. Bake uncovered for 40 minutes. Broil to brown cheese on top.

Per Serving: 183 calories, 9g total fat, 3g saturated fat, 2mg cholesterol, 387mg sodium, 516mg potassium, 20g total carbohydrate, 2g dietary fiber, 6g protein

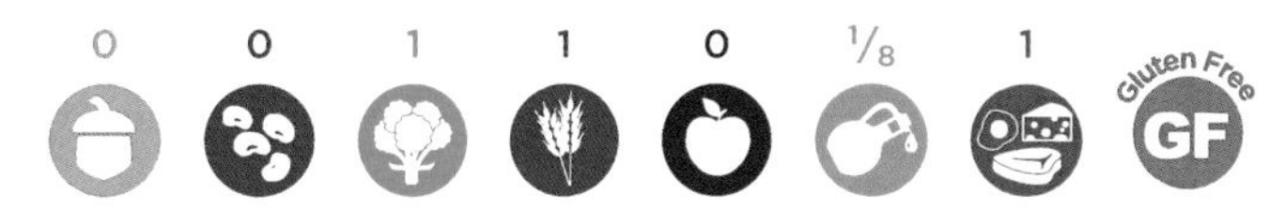

Serves 6

Vietnamese Coconut Curry Chicken

Fresh Southeast Asian ingredients like lemongrass, basil and coconut milk set this golden coconut curry apart from Indian curry. This recipe uses both chicken breasts and vegetarian chicken pieces so that you get delicious flavors with 30% less cholesterol. Serve it with brown rice for a rich, delicious supper.

1 tablespoon olive oil

2 medium onions, diced

2 garlic cloves, crushed

1/8 teaspoon crushed red pepper

4 teaspoons chopped fresh lemon grass or zest of 1 lime

2 tablespoons mild curry powder blend

2 pounds chicken breasts, chopped

1 bag veggie chicken pieces

1 red or green bell pepper, diced

2 sliced carrots

4 red potatoes, diced

2 tablespoons agave nectar or honey

1 can coconut milk

1/2 cup chicken stock or water

2 cups green beans

1 cup frozen peas

1/2 cup fresh basil leaves for garnish

3 cups cooked brown rice

Preparation

1. Heat the oil in a pan and fry the onion for about 5 minutes or until soft. Add garlic, crushed red pepper, ginger lemongrass and curry powder. Add chicken and braise on all sides, coating well with curry mixture. Cover and cook for 5 minutes over low heat.

2. Remove lid, add carrots, bell peppers and potatoes and honey or agave and stir well. Pour in coconut milk and stock and bring to a boil. Reduce heat and simmer uncovered for another 20 minutes then add green beans and peas.

3. Cook another 10 minutes or until potatoes are tender. Serve over brown rice and top with basil.

Per Serving: 513 calories, 13g total fat, 4g saturated fat, 87mg cholesterol, 168mg sodium, 608mg potassium, 54g total carbohydrate, 7g dietary fiber, 46g protein

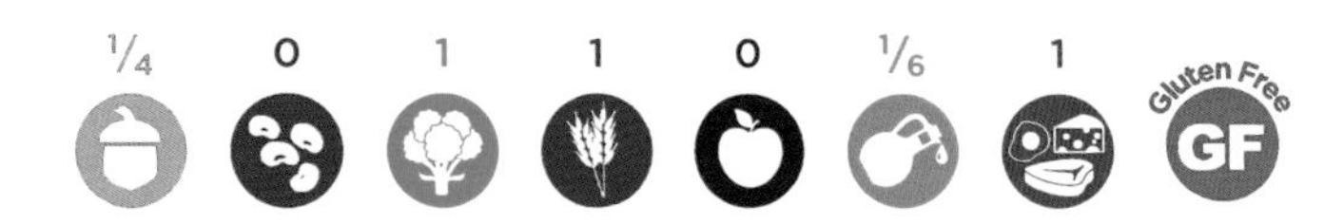

Serves 6

Vietnamese Lemongrass Beef

Lemongrass is an amazing super-herb that has been used for hundreds of years for both culinary and medicinal purposes. In this classic Vietnamese recipe, minced lemongrass is used to marinate and flavor beef. It has a distinct flavor that when crushed or cut releases the essential oil citral, which has antioxidant and disease-preventing properties. Serve over steaming hot short-grain brown rice.

2 stalks fresh lemongrass or zest of 3 limes
6 garlic cloves, minced

2 tablespoons Asian fish sauce, low-sodium soy sauce or 3 anchovies

1 tablespoon low-sodium soy sauce

4 teaspoons honey or agave nectar

1 tablespoon sesame oil

1 pound eye round steak, sliced

1 package veggie beef tips, halved or sliced

1 cup sliced or julienned carrots

1 pound chopped bok choy, blanched broccoli florets or green beans

1 pound seedless European cucumber, halved and cut into 1/4-inch pieces, optional

1/2 cup fresh basil leaves (preferably Thai basil), washed well and dried

1/2 cup fresh mint leaves, optional

1/2 cup fresh cilantro leaves, optional

Preparation

1 Thinly slice lower 6 inches of lemongrass stalks, discarding remainder of stalks. In a food processor or blender, finely grind together sliced lemongrass and garlic. Add fish sauce, soy sauce, honey and sesame oil and blend well. In a large resealable plastic bag, combine marinade and steak and seal bag, pressing out excess air. Marinate steak, turning bag once or twice, and store in fridge for at least 4 hours or overnight.

2 In a large wok or skillet, add beef and stir fry until slightly cooked. Remove and set aside.

3 Add carrots and bok choy in the wok with 2-3 tablespoons water and simmer until cooked through, approximately 7-10 minutes. Add veggie beef with vegetables until warmed through, about 3 minutes.

4 Pour in reserved beef until combined and remove from heat. Serve on top of cooked brown rice and place sliced cucumbers next to the rice. Top beef and vegetable mixture with basil and other herbs or lime wedge.

Per Serving: 258 calories, 8g total fat, 1g saturated fat, 20mg cholesterol, 404mg sodium, 337mg potassium, 29g total carbohydrate, 5g dietary fiber, 19g protein

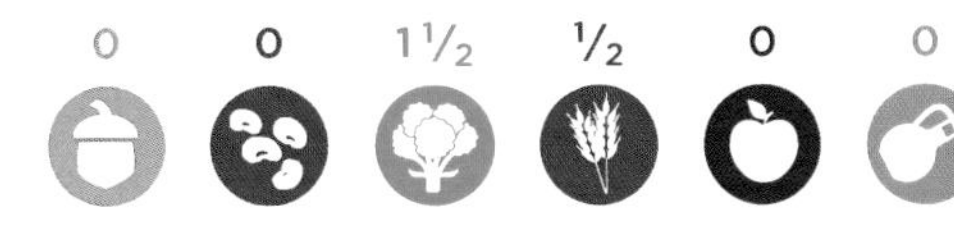

Serves 4

Vietnamese Pho

The national dish of Vietnam, pho is a complex, lip-smacking soup that will fill your stomach and win your taste buds! Our low-fat version is all about the rich beef broth, which is infused with delicious spices. Vegetables and tofu swim in the silky broth, resulting in a nutritious soup that's low in cholesterol and high in flavor.

1 pound dried shiitake mushrooms

1 pound beef long bones or neck bones rinsed with water

2 medium onions, 1 roasted

1 1-inch piece ginger, peeled and roasted

4 star anise

5 cloves

1 stick cinnamon

1 tablespoon sugar

2-4 tablespoons regular or veggie fish sauce, or 4 mashed anchovies

1 teaspoon salt

2 cups blanched vegetables (julienned carrots, kale, and broccoli)

1 16-ounce package brown rice or whole grain noodles (fettuccine, linguine or pho)

1/2 pound thinly sliced eye round beef and sliced tofu (firm, fried or seasoned)

1 yellow onion, thinly sliced

1 scallion, sliced

1/2 cup fresh cilantro

1/2 cup fresh Thai basil, optional

Sliced jalapenos, optional

Lime wedges, optional

1 cup mung bean sprouts, optional

Sriracha and hoisin sauce, optional

Preparation

1 In a large stockpot, bring 6 quarts water to a boil. Add mushrooms. Bring to a boil for 5 minutes. Add beef bones. Skim foam as it cooks.

2 To roast ginger, hold the piece with tongs directly over an open flame or place it directly on a medium-hot electric burner. While turning, char until the edges are slightly blackened and ginger is fragrant, about 7 minutes each side. Roast the onion in the same way. Add ginger and onions to the soup.

3 Add fish sauce and sugar. Wrap the star anise, cloves and cinnamon in a spice bag (or piece of cheesecloth) and add to the broth.

4. Remove the mushrooms, cool and slice. The broth needs to cook for 2-4 hours total (remove spice bag after 2 hours). Before serving, remove and discard both the spice bag and onions.

5. Add the salt and continue to simmer, skimming as necessary, until you're ready to assemble the dish. The broth will taste a little salty but will be balanced once the noodles and accompaniments are added.

6. Boil 2 liters of water in a large pot. Add noodles and cook for 5-7 minutes until tender. Pour noodles into a colander and rinse with cold water to blanch. Place the cooked noodles in large individual bowls.

7. Blanch raw vegetables 7 minutes before serving. Bring the broth to a rolling boil; ladle about 2-3 cups into each bowl. Drop beef and sliced tofu into hot soup. Garnish with yellow onions, scallions and cilantro.

8. Serve immediately, inviting guests to garnish the bowls with bean sprouts, basil, jalapenos, lime and sriracha.

Per Serving: 482 calories, 9g total fat, 3g saturated fat, 35mg cholesterol, 819mg sodium, 243mg potassium, 75g total carbohydrate, 8g dietary fiber, 23g protein

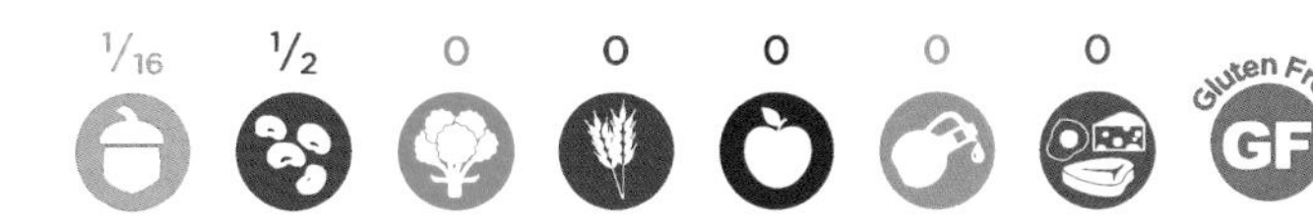

Serves 8

White Bean Paté

This divine mixture is a perfect spread for toast and works as a filling snack. Butter beans, also known as lima beans, contain molybdenum, which breaks down sulfites in the body. Foods containing sulfites–such as vinegar, wine, eggs, pickles and dried fruits–need this essential mineral to be metabolized properly. Protein-rich legumes also help lower cholesterol and regulate blood glucose levels, so stock up on canned beans today!

1 can butter beans

2 tablespoons tahini

1/2 tablespoon fresh lemon juice

1 pinch salt

Preparation

1. Drain butter beans in a small bowl. Add tahini and mash with a fork. Sprinkle with fresh lemon juice and salt to taste.

2. Spread paté on toast and top with sliced tomatoes, avocado, sprouts or baby spinach. If you have fresh basil or cilantro, feel free to add some for extra flavor!

Per Serving: 55 calories, 2g total fat, 0g saturated fat, 0mg cholesterol, 69mg sodium, 128mg potassium, 8g total carbohydrate, 2g dietary fiber, 3g protein

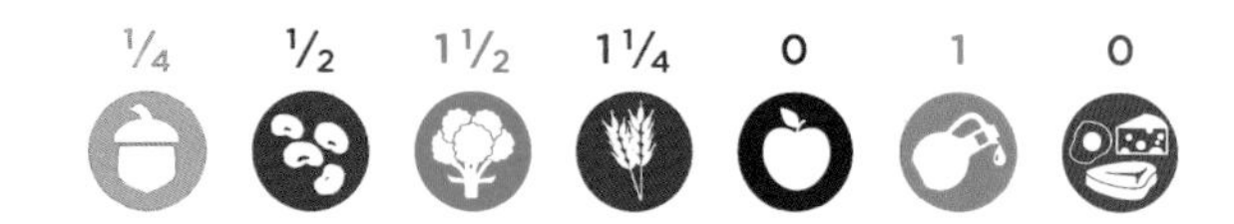

Serves 6

Whole Grain Pasta with Chard and Garlicky Crumbs

Swiss chard is loaded with antioxidant rich vitamin C and offers 33% of your daily vitamin C intake in one serving. If Swiss chard is out of season, substitute with kale, spinach or any other seasonal dark, leafy green. You will love the taste and texture of this pasta!

1 pound whole grain pasta

1 1/2 tablespoon plus 1/2 teaspoon olive oil or Earth Balance butter substitute

6 cloves minced garlic

1 onion, diced

2 cups fresh mushrooms, diced

1 teaspoon thyme

1/4 teaspoon salt

1/8 teaspoon crushed red pepper or ground pepper

1/4 cup sherry

4 cups Swiss chard, chopped

2 cups kale leaves, chopped

1 can cannellini or butter beans, drained

4 slices sprouted grain bread, diced, or 1 cup chopped walnuts

1/2 tablespoon brewer's yeast, optional

1/2 cup shredded non-dairy rice cheese for garnish

Quartered lemons for garnish

Preparation

1 Cook whole grain pasta until al dente. Drain then sprinkle with 1/2 teaspoon oil and set aside.

2 In a large wok or Dutch oven, add 1 tablespoon olive oil and heat until shimmering. Sauté 4 cloves of minced garlic, reserving 2 minced cloves for later. Cook garlic until almost browned. Add onion and mushrooms. Sprinkle with thyme, salt and crushed red pepper and continue to sauté for 5 minutes until mushrooms are cooked through. Pour in sherry then add chard and kale and cook until wilted, about 3-5 minutes. Stir in beans. Turn down heat.

3 In a small skillet, add 1/2 tablespoon olive oil, 2 cloves minced garlic and cook garlic until fragrant. Toss in bread or walnuts and roast until fragrant, about 3-5 minutes. Remove from heat and sprinkle with brewer's yeast, if using.

4 Toss cooked pasta with sautéed vegetables. Pour onto serving dish and garnish with garlicky breadcrumbs and rice cheese. Serve warm with lemons.

Per Serving: 485 calories, 9g total fat, 84g saturated fat, 0 mg cholesterol, 465mg sodium, 514mg potassium, 84g total carbohydrate, 14g dietary fiber, 19g protein

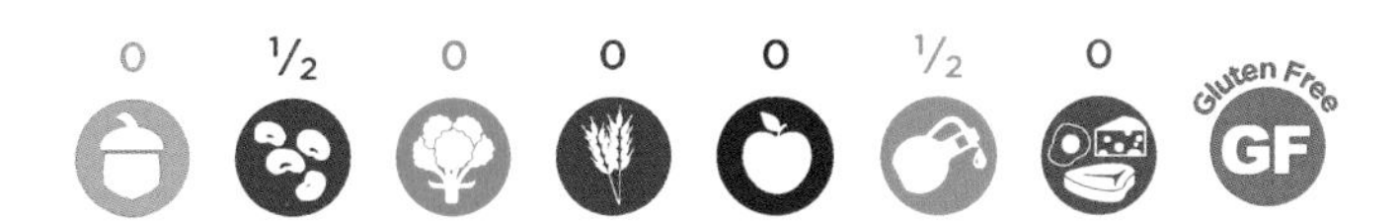

Serves 4

Zesty Mexican Bean Dip

Beans are a vegetable and an excellent source of protein. They're also rich in fiber, potassium, folate, and magnesium. Take this dip to a potluck or make it for a weekday snack. You'll love the festive flavors!

1 15-ounce can vegetarian fat-free refried or black beans

1 4-ounce can green chiles, diced

1 tablespoon Mexican spice blend, or ½ teaspoon garlic powder, ½ teaspoon cumin and 1 teaspoon chili powder

2 tablespoons olive oil

2 tablespoons water

1 teaspoon Tabasco sauce

½ teaspoon salt

¼ cup shredded non-dairy rice cheese for garnish

2 green onions, sliced, for garnish

¼ cup sliced olives for garnish

TIP

This is also an excellent base for Mexican 7-layer dip! Start with a layer of beans, then add a layer of sour cream substitute or plain non-fat Greek yogurt, followed by diced green onions, diced jalapenos, shredded romaine, and diced tomatoes. Top with rice cheese and fresh cilantro for garnish.

Preparation

1 In a blender, process beans, green chiles, spices, olive oil, water, Tabasco sauce and salt. Garnish and serve with baked corn tortilla chips.

Per Serving: 86 calories, 5g total fat, 1g saturated fat, 0mg cholesterol, 241mg sodium, 215mg potassium, 8g total carbohydrate, 3g dietary fiber, 3g protein

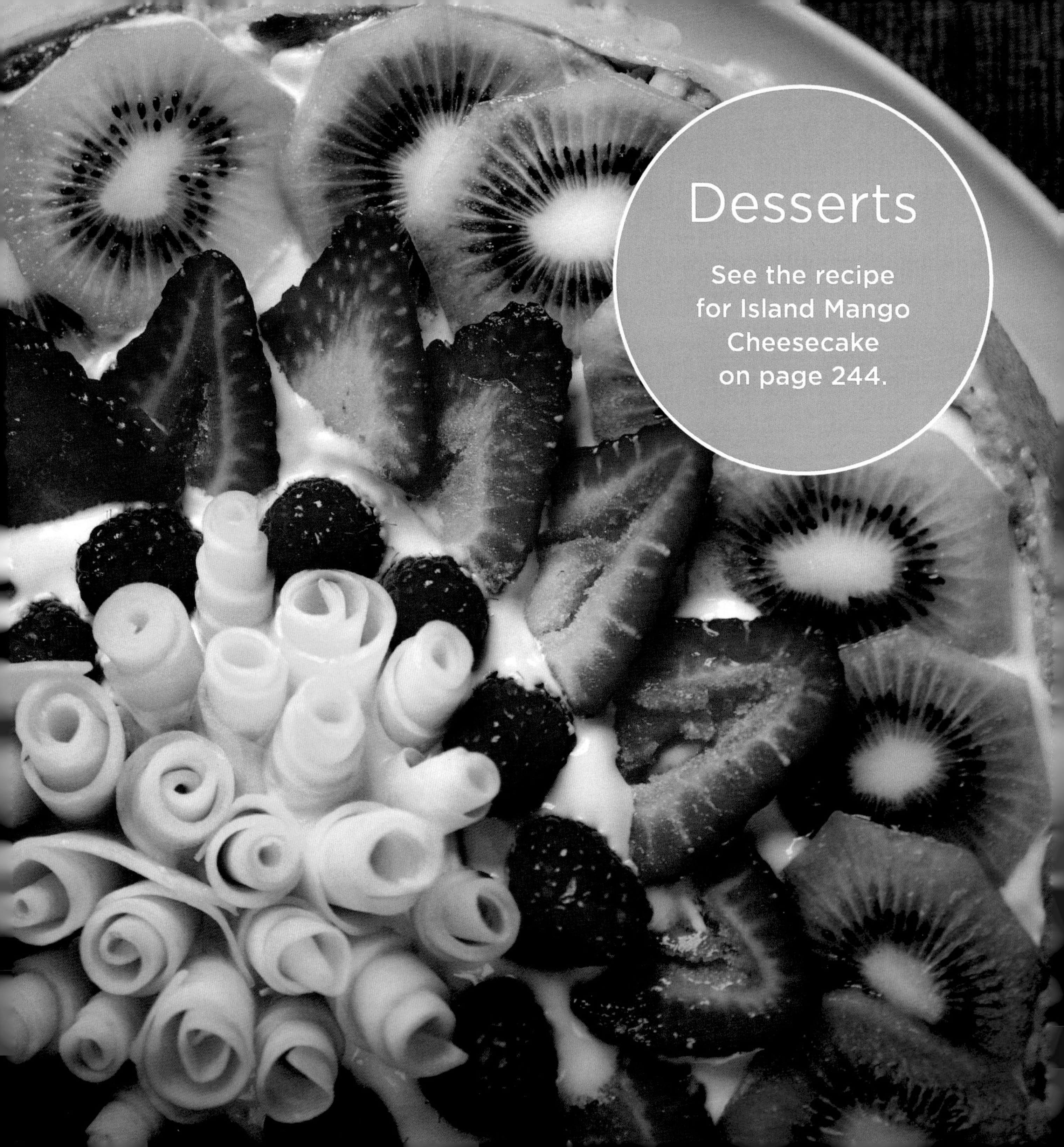

Desserts

See the recipe for Island Mango Cheesecake on page 244.

Recipe Index

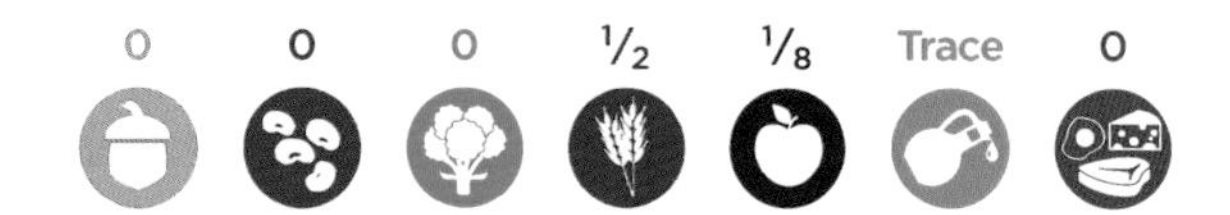

Makes 24

Apple-Cinnamon Rolls

These delicious rolls are great for the holidays or any other special occasion. Apples are a great source of vitamin C, while cinnamon is chock-full of free radical-fighting antioxidants and may help lower blood sugar by decreasing insulin resistance. This dish can be served at brunch or as a dessert!

Filling:

2 large cooking apples, peeled, cored and chopped
2 tablespoons flour
3 tablespoons honey, agave nectar or cane sugar
1/4 cup Earth Balance or Benecol butter substitute
1 teaspoon ground cinnamon
1/2 teaspoon ground nutmeg

Rolls:

5 1/2 cups unbleached wheat or spelt flour, divided
2 tablespoons honey, agave nectar or cane sugar
2 1/4-ounce packages quick-rising yeast
1 teaspoon salt
1/2 cup soy milk
1/4 cup Earth Balance or Benecol butter substitute
3/4 cup Egg Beaters

Topping:

1 cup puréed pitted dates with 1/4 cup water
2 teaspoons ground cinnamon
1/2 teaspoon ground nutmeg

Icing:

1 12-ounce container Tofutti sour cream substitute
2 tablespoons powdered cane sugar

Preparation

1 Prepare apple filling by combining apples, flour, sugar and butter substitute in a medium saucepan. Bring to a boil over medium-high heat. Cook 3 minutes.

2 Reduce heat to medium low and cook 10 minutes, stirring constantly until thick. Stir in cinnamon and nutmeg. Set aside to cool completely.

3 Make cinnamon and date topping by combining puréed pitted dates, water, cinnamon, and nutmeg. Set aside.

4 In a large bowl, combine 1 cup flour, sugar, undissolved yeast and salt. Heat 1/2 cup water with soy milk and butter substitute until warm (120-130 degrees). Gradually add one cup of mixture to dry ingredients. Beat 2 minutes at medium speed, scraping bowl occasionally.

5 Add Egg Beaters and 1 cup flour; beat 2 minutes at high speed, continuing to scrape bowl occasionally. Stir in an additional 1 1/2 cups flour to make a soft dough. Knead dough on lightly floured surface until smooth and elastic, 8-10 minutes. If dough still sticks to the sides of the bowl, add remaining 1/2 cup of flour. Cover and let rest 10 minutes.

6 Divide dough into two equal parts. Roll each dough section into a 12x8-inch rectangle. Divide cinnamon-date topping in half and spread on each rolled dough section. Divide the cooled apple filling in half and spread evenly over each dough section.

7 Beginning at long end of each rectangle, roll up dough as tightly as you would for a jelly roll. Pinch seams to seal. Cut each roll into 12 equal pieces. Place each piece, cut side up, in two greased 9-inch round pans.

8 Cover and let rise in warm, draft-free place until double in size, about 45 minutes. After dough has doubled in size, bake at 375 degrees for 25-30 minutes or until done.

9 Prepare icing and drizzle on top of warm Apple-Cinnamon Rolls and serve.

Per Serving: 273 calories, 2g total fat, 0g saturated fat, 13mg cholesterol, 335mg sodium, 145mg potassium, 55g total carbohydrate, 10g dietary fiber, 14g protein

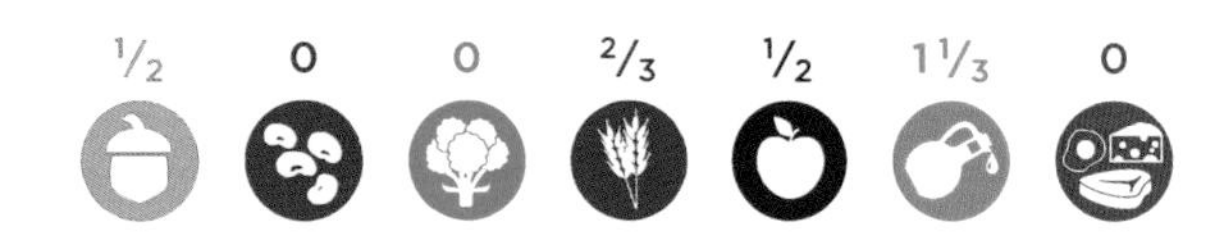

Makes 32

Chocolate-Pecan Squares

Mouth-watering and more nutritious than a cookie, these treats are sure to satisfy any sweet tooth. Pecans are a great source of manganese, which aids in carbohydrate metabolism. Try this delicious dessert today!

1 cup Earth Balance butter substitute
1/2 cup light brown cane sugar
1 cup old-fashioned rolled oats (not instant)
1 cup whole wheat flour
1 cup unbleached flour
1/2 cup wheat germ
1 tablespoon water
1 egg, beaten
2 cups pecans, coarsely chopped
1 cup chocolate chips
1 cup dates, chopped
1 cup dried apricots, chopped
2 tablespoons honey or agave nectar
1/2 cup flaxseed meal
4 teaspoons orange peel or molasses, optional

Preparation

1. Preheat oven to 350 degrees. Cream butter substitute with brown cane sugar in a large bowl until well blended. Stir in the oats, flours and wheat germ, and mix well. Add orange peel or molasses at this time if desired. (Orange peel lends a citrusy flavor while molasses offers a deeper, richer flavor.)

2. Add 1 tablespoon water to crust for moisture. Spread this mixture evenly in the bottom of a well-greased 9x13-inch baking dish and press it down to form a solid crust.

3. Combine egg, pecans, chocolate chips, dates, apricots, and honey or agave nectar in a large bowl.

4. Pour this mixture over the crust and spread evenly. Bake for 40 minutes or until browned on top.

5. Remove from oven and sprinkle with flaxseed meal and press lightly with spatula. (Optional: Add pistachios and goji berries for festive red and green holiday fare.) Allow to cool and cut into squares.

Per Serving: 324 calories, 14g total fat, 4g saturated fat, 7mg cholesterol, 63mg sodium, 144mg potassium, 26g total carbohydrate, 3g dietary fiber, 4g protein

¼ 0 0 0 ¼ 0 0

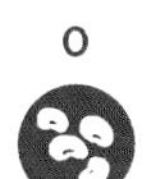
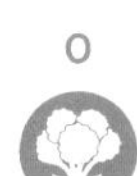
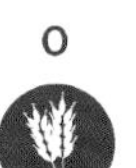
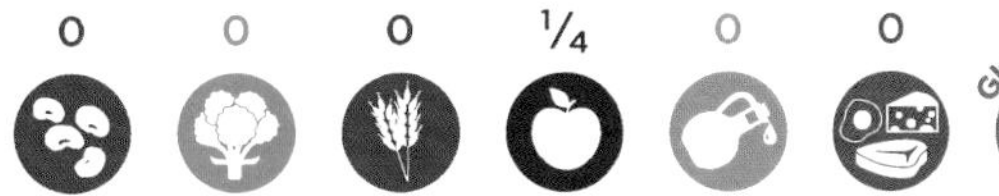
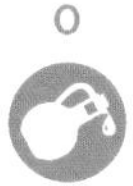
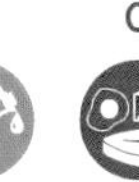
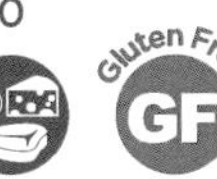

Serves 4

Coconut-Chia Seed Pudding

This pudding is a tasty dessert or snack and is a snap to make. It's made extra healthy with the addition of chia seeds, which are a good source of calcium and protein. This easy pudding also has immune-system-boosting coconut. Not a coconut lover? Substitute coconut milk with soy or almond milk.

Pudding:

1 ½ cups coconut milk

2 tablespoons of agave nectar or honey

1 teaspoon ground cinnamon

⅓ cup chia seeds

Topping:

1 cup berries or diced banana

2 tablespoons cacao nibs

2 tablespoons dried goji berries

Preparation

1. In a medium bowl, mix coconut milk, agave, cinnamon and chia seeds. Allow to set in refrigerator for 15 minutes.

2. Spoon into four bowls and top with berries, cacao nibs and goji berries, or your favorite fruit. For a sweeter pudding, add dried currants, diced mango or pineapple.

Per Serving: 179 calories, 7g total fat, 3g saturated fat, 0mg cholesterol, 12mg sodium, 93mg potassium, 25g total carbohydrate, 8g dietary fiber, 5g protein

Trace Trace 0 $^1/_4$ Trace $^1/_6$ Trace

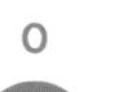
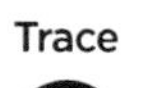
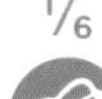
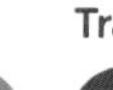
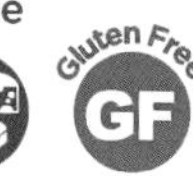

Makes 24

Double Chocolate Cookies

These decadent, rich cookies will quickly satiate your chocolate craving. Here's the best part: They can lower levels of LDL ("bad") cholesterol, thanks to healthy oats, while black beans give you a double-punch of fiber and protein.

1 box Betty Crocker Gluten-Free Chocolate Cake Mix
1 $^1/_2$ cup gluten-free rolled oats (not instant)
2 eggs
$^1/_4$ Earth Balance butter substitute
$^1/_2$ cup applesauce
$^1/_2$ cup black beans, drained and rinsed well
$^1/_4$ cup diced pecans
$^1/_4$ cup mini chocolate chips (dairy-free if available)

Preparation

1. Preheat oven to 350 degrees. In a food processor, add all ingredients except chocolate chips and nuts. Pulse mixture until thoroughly combined and scrape into a medium-sized bowl.

2. Fold in pecans and chocolate chips until mixed. Place cookie dough in the freezer for 10 minutes.

3. Line cookie sheet with parchment paper. Scoop 1 teaspoon chilled cookie dough and, using another teaspoon, drop dough onto lined cookie sheet. Bake for 8-10 minutes.

Per Serving: 132 calories, 6g total fat, 2g saturated fat, 16mg cholesterol, 146mg sodium, 35mg potassium, 18g total carbohydrate, 1g dietary fiber, 2g protein

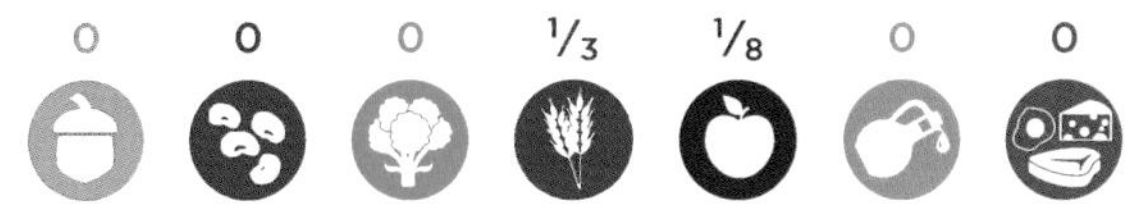

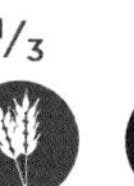

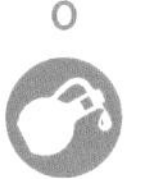
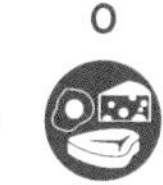

Makes 16

Fig Bars

A high-fiber fruit loaded with antioxidants, figs are a power fruit for prediabetics because they slow down digestion and absorption of sugar and help prevent spikes in blood sugar. Sweet, chewy and perfect for a mid-afternoon snack, these delicious Fig Bars are ideal for picnics and outdoor gatherings.

Filling:

10 ounces of dried figs, stems snipped
6 ounces of pitted dates
2 tablespoons honey or agave nectar
1 1/2 tablespoons lemon juice (2 lemons)
1/2 teaspoon ground cinnamon
1/4 teaspoon dried ginger or 1/2 teaspoon freshly minced ginger, optional

Crust:

1/2 cup unbleached wheat flour
1/2 cup quick oats
1 teaspoon baking powder
1/4 teaspoon salt
4 tablespoons Earth Balance butter substitute
3 tablespoons agave nectar or honey

Preparation

1 Preheat oven to 375 degrees. Grease and line an 8x8-inch cake pan with parchment paper.

2 Process figs, dates and 2 tablespoons water in a food processor. Grind into a coarse paste. Add lemon juice, honey, cinnamon, and ginger to the mixture. Pulse to combine. Scoop out mixture and set aside.

3 In a bowl, combine oats, flour, baking powder and salt. Crumble in butter substitute and add honey. Toss until mixture is crumbly. Press half of crust mixture into the cake pan.

4 Pour fig mixture onto pan and spread evenly. Top with remaining crust mixture and press top crust pieces together. Bake for 30 minutes until lightly browned. Cool completely before cutting into bars.

Per Serving: 151 calories, 3g total fat, 1g saturated fat, 0mg cholesterol, 87mg sodium, 87mg potassium, 30g total carbohydrate, 3g dietary fiber, 2g protein

0 Trace $^{1}/_{8}$ 0 0 Trace 0

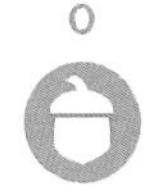  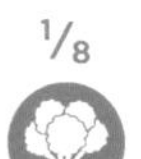 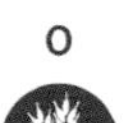  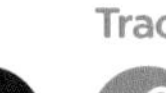  

Makes 9

Five-Star Brownies

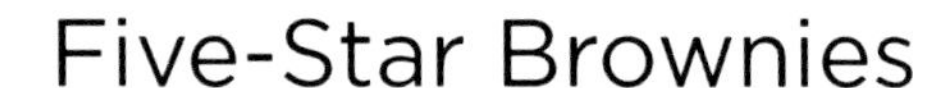

These sinful, nutrient-packed brownies include folate-rich beets, which can help boost mood. Though not common in a brownie recipe, black beans add moistness and extra depth, and also a generous serving of fiber and protein!

1 package brownie mix
¼ cup water
¼ cup cooked black beans
¼ cup cooked beets
¼ cup mini chocolate chips
¼ cup pitted cherries, optional
Cooking oil (PAM)

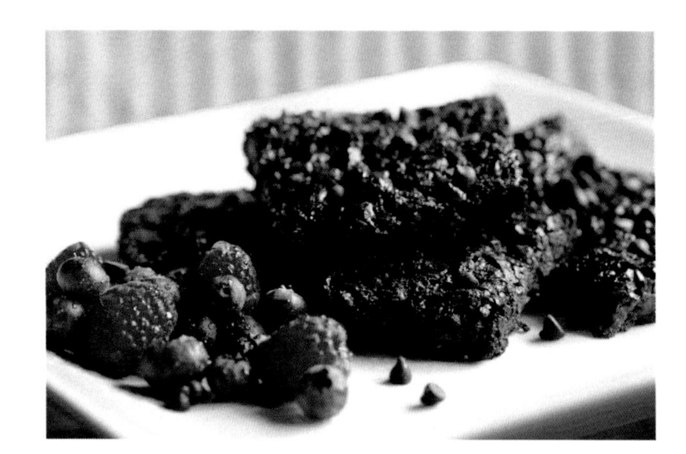

Preparation

1 Preheat oven to 350 degrees. Lightly spray bottom of pan with cooking oil.

2 Purée vegetables and water in a blender until smooth. Combine vegetable mixture with brownie mix and pour into pan. Sprinkle with chocolate chips and use a butter knife to mix chips into batter. Add pitted cherries if using.

3 Bake for 35 minutes. Cool, cut into 1x1-inch squares and serve.

Per Serving: 200 calories, 3g total fat, 1g saturated fat, 0mg cholesterol, 94mg sodium, 54mg potassium, 42g total carbohydrate, 1g dietary fiber, 2g protein

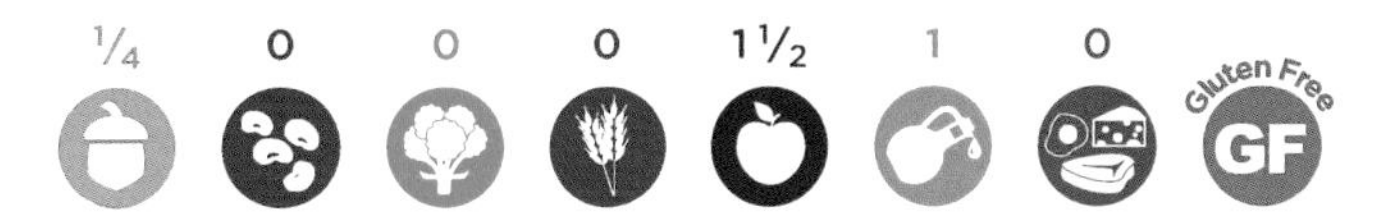

Serves 8

Gingered Fruit Salad with Coconut-Pineapple Sauce

Similar to Grandma's ambrosia salad, but tastier and more nutritious! This gluten-free salad is healthful, too, with the addition of ginger, which can help prevent glycation, the process that causes damage to organs from diabetes. Swap in soy coconut yogurt in place of coconut cream if you wish, or omit the nuts for a nut-free dessert. The beautiful colors and festive flavors will cleanse your palate and tickle your taste buds.

3 Asian pears, seeded and diced

3 Granny Smith apples, seeded and diced

5 clementine oranges, peeled and sectioned

1/2 medium pineapple, cored and diced (reserve the other half to use in sauce)

1/2 cup dried cranberries

1/2 cup diced crystalized ginger

1 pinch freshly ground nutmeg, ground cinnamon or ground pistachios for garnish

Sauce:

1 cup coconut cream

1/2 cup raw cashews

2 cups reserved pineapple, diced

1 lime, juiced and zested

Preparation

1. Combine fruit and ginger in a large bowl. Put sauce ingredients into a blender and purée until creamy and smooth.

2. Serve in small dessert cups or in a large bowl. Pour sauce over fruit and garnish with nutmeg.

Per Serving: 222 calories, 4g total fat, 1g saturated fat, 0mg cholesterol, 5mg sodium, 449mg potassium, 50g total carbohydrate, 7g dietary fiber, 3g protein

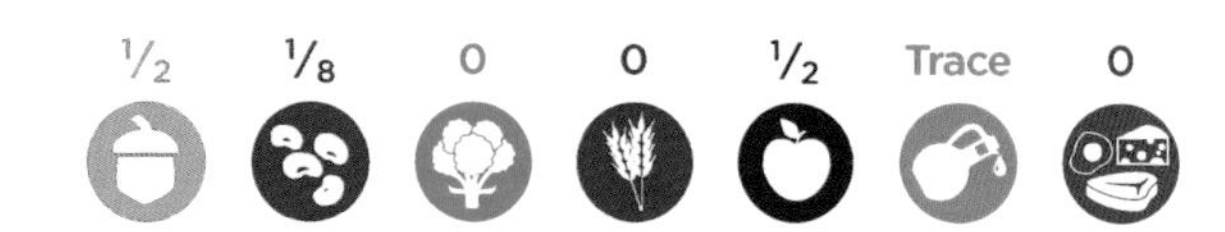

Serves 12

Island Mango Cheesecake

Perfect for any season, you can make this delicious cheesecake using either fresh or frozen mango or peaches. Mangos are rich in amino acids and vitamins C and E. Navy beans–also added to the filling–are high in fiber and can lower your risk of cardiovascular disease. Top with your favorite seasonal fruit and serve chilled.

Crust:

3 tablespoons Earth Balance non-hydrogenated shortening (preferably sticks)

1/2 cup cornflakes or Cinnamon Chex cereal

8 gluten-free snicker doodle cookies or regular graham cracker cookies

1/2 cup walnuts (pecans can be substituted)

1 tablespoon unsulfured molasses

1/2 teaspoon ground cinnamon

1 pinch salt

Filling:

2 12-ounce containers Tofutti cream cheese substitute

4 tablespoons baking powder

1 cup puréed silken (soft) tofu or 1 cup whole cashews

1/2 cup cane sugar

4 teaspoons cornstarch

1/2 teaspoon salt

2 cups canned navy beans, rinsed well

2 teaspoons pure vanilla extract or orange blossom water

2 cups mangoes, peeled and diced (reserve additional diced mango for garnish)

Topping:

1/2 of one 12-ounce container Tofutti sour cream substitute

1 tablespoon powdered cane sugar

Preparation

To prepare crust:

1. In a food processor, pulse all the crust ingredients until finely chopped like coarse cornmeal.

2. Press mixture into greased, parchment-lined 9-inch cheesecake pan. Place crust in freezer while preparing filling.

To prepare cheesecake:

1. Preheat oven to 350 degrees. In a blender, purée filling ingredients until well incorporated and smooth. Mixture should be creamy and uniform in color.

2. Pour into chilled crust and bake for 1 hour or until done. Refrigerate overnight.

To prepare topping:

1. Combine sour cream substitute and powdered cane sugar and pour on top of chilled cheesecake. Chill for 1-2 hours.

2. Unmold from cheesecake pan and slice. Garnish with additional mango, kiwi or raspberries.

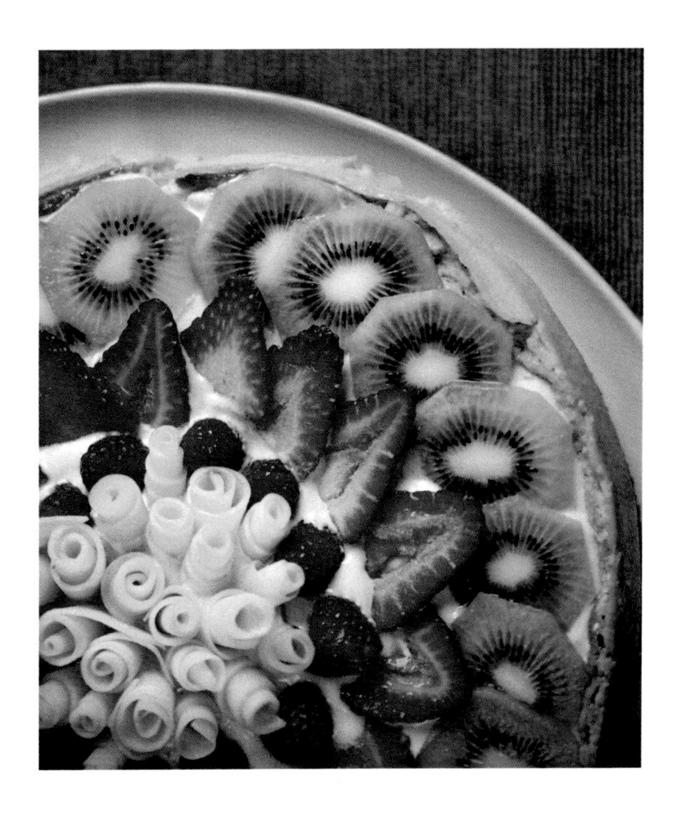

Per Serving: 285 calories, 17.1 total fat, 5.1g saturated fat, 0mg cholesterol, 512mg sodium, 29.4g total carbohydrate, 4.6g dietary fiber, 6.3g protein

1/2 1/2 0 Trace 0 Trace 0

 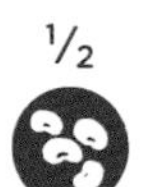  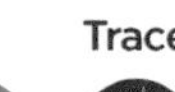 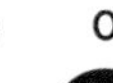 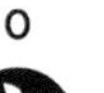  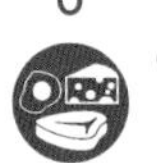 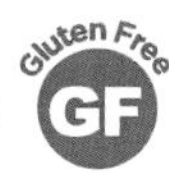

Serves 12

Mexican Chocolate Cheesecake

The medley of bold chocolate flavors is so delicious, you'll forget this cheesecake has zero cholesterol! Two cups of black beans add fiber and protein, making this dessert a health superstar. Cacao is one of the highest sources of resveratrol, the phytonutrient that gives red wine its cardio-protective properties. Serve with fresh raspberries for a boost of antioxidants.

Crust:

1/4 cup Earth Balance non-hydrogenated shortening (preferably sticks), room temperature

1/2 cup cornflakes or Cinnamon Chex cereal

10 gluten-free chocolate cookies or regular chocolate cookies

1/2 cup pecans

1 tablespoon unsulfured molasses

1/2 teaspoon ground cinnamon

1 pinch salt

Filling:

2 12-ounce containers Tofutti cream cheese substitute

1 cup puréed silken (soft) tofu or 1 cup whole cashews

4 tablespoons baking powder

3/4 cup evaporated cane juice or organic unprocessed sugar

1 1/2 teaspoons cornstarch

1/2 teaspoon salt

2 cups canned black beans, rinsed well

1 teaspoon pure vanilla extract

1 teaspoon espresso powder or instant coffee granules

2 teaspoons ground cinnamon

2 teaspoons chili powder

2 teaspoons orange zest, optional

Topping:

1 12-ounce container Tofutti sour cream substitute

2 tablespoons powdered evaporated cane sugar

Preparation

To prepare crust:

1 In a food processor, pulse all the crust ingredients until finely chopped like coarse cornmeal.

2 Press mixture into greased, parchment-lined 9-inch cheesecake pan. Place crust in freezer while preparing filling.

To prepare cheesecake:

1 Preheat oven to 350 degrees. In a blender, purée all of the filling ingredients until well incorporated and smooth. It should be creamy and uniform in color.

2 Pour into chilled crust pan and bake for 1 hour or until done. Refrigerate overnight.

To prepare topping:

1 Combine sour cream substitute and powdered evaporated cane juice and pour on top of chilled cheesecake. Chill for 1-2 hours.

2 Unmold from cheesecake pan and slice. Serve with sprinkled cinnamon, additional orange zest and fresh raspberries.

Per Serving: 285 calories, 17.1 total fat, 5.1g saturated fat, 0mg cholesterol, 512mg sodium, 29.4g total carbohydrate, 4.6g dietary fiber, 6.3g protein

0	0	0	$^{1}/_{10}$	$1^{1}/_{4}$	$^{1}/_{16}$	0	
	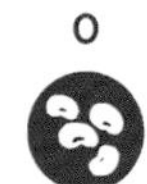	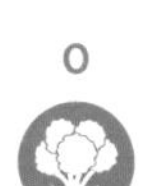	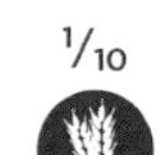	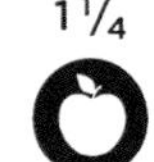		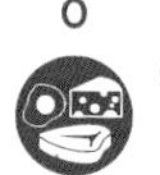	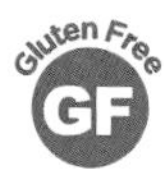

Serves 8

Mile-High Cranberry-Apple Pie

Apples and cranberries pair up to make a heart-healthy and heartwarming pie. Apples, like peaches, pears and plums, are an orchard fruit. Orchard fruits are high in fiber and low in sugar and should be eaten with the skin on. Serve with vanilla soy ice cream and sprinkle with flaxseed meal for an à la mode treat.

- 2 cups fresh or frozen cranberries
- $^{3}/_{4}$ cup agave nectar or honey
- 1 cup pitted dates puréed with 1 cup water
- $^{1}/_{3}$ cup quick-cooking tapioca
- $^{1}/_{4}$ cup water
- 2 teaspoons grated orange peel or lemon peel
- 3 cups peeled tart apples, sliced
- 1 tablespoon Earth Balance or Benecol butter substitute
- $^{1}/_{2}$ teaspoon ground cinnamon
- $^{1}/_{4}$ teaspoon salt
- 1 gluten-free or wheat pastry 9-inch double-crust pie

Preparation

1. Preheat oven to 375 degrees. In a large saucepan, combine the cranberries, agave, tapioca, water, puréed dates and orange or lemon peel; let stand for 15 minutes to thicken.
2. Bring saucepan contents to a boil, stirring occasionally. Remove from heat and stir in apples, cinnamon and butter substitute.
3. Place bottom pastry in a 9-inch pie plate. Pour filling into crust and top with remaining pastry. Cut a few slits in the top pastry to allow steam to escape.
4. Bake for 45-55 minutes or until crust is golden brown and filling is bubbly. Allow to cool.

Per Serving: 353 calories, 10g total fat, 4g saturated fat, 0mg cholesterol, 188mg sodium, 13mg potassium, 68g total carbohydrate, 3g dietary fiber, 2g protein

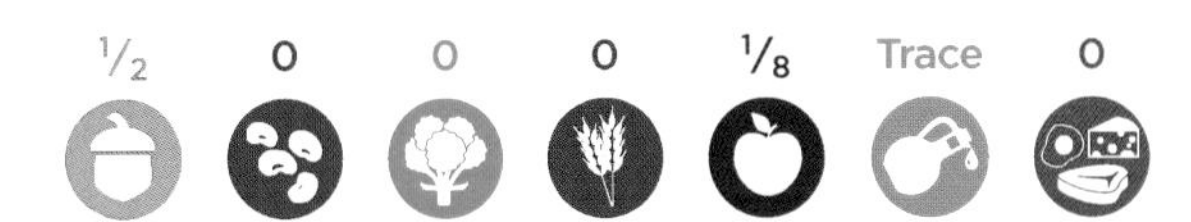

Serves 12

Pumpkin Cheesecake

Pumpkin is widely eaten around the world year-round, and with good reason! Not only is it delicious, it can help manage blood glucose levels. Serve this at your next feast for a health-smart sweet finale.

Crust:

1/4 cup Earth Balance non-hydrogenated shortening (preferably sticks), room temperature

1/2 cup cornflakes or Cinnamon Chex cereal

10 gluten-free snicker doodle cookies or 10 graham crackers

1/2 cup pecans

1 tablespoon unsulfured molasses

1/4 teaspoon ground cinnamon

Pinch salt

Filling:

2 containers Tofutti cream cheese substitute

1 cup puréed silken (soft) tofu or 1 cup whole cashews

4 tablespoons baking powder

3/4 cup cane sugar

1 1/2 teaspoons cornstarch

1/2 teaspoon salt

1 15-ounce can pumpkin purée

1 teaspoon pure vanilla extract or 1 tablespoon rum

2 teaspoons pumpkin pie spice

Topping:

1 12-ounce container Tofutti sour cream substitute

2 tablespoons powdered cane sugar

Preparation

To prepare crust:

1. In a food processor, pulse all the crust ingredients until finely chopped like coarse cornmeal.

2. Press mixture into parchment-lined and greased 9-inch cheesecake pan. Place crust in freezer while preparing filling.

To prepare cheesecake:

1. Preheat oven to 350 degrees. In a blender, purée all of the pumpkin cheesecake ingredients until well incorporated and smooth. Mixture should be creamy and uniform in color.
2. Pour into chilled cheesecake pan and bake for 1 hour or until done. Refrigerate overnight.

To prepare topping:

1. Combine sour cream substitute and powdered cane sugar and pour on top of chilled cheesecake. Chill for 1-2 hours.
2. Unmold from cheesecake pan and slice. Serve with sprinkled cinnamon.

Per Serving: 248 calories, 16.8g total fat, 5g saturated fat, 0mg cholesterol, 514mg sodium, 20.9g total carbohydrate, 2.2g dietary fiber, 3.9g protein

Sorbets

Sorbets are a tangy and refreshing low-calorie dessert that are perfect for a warm day. For added oomph and an antioxidant boost, serve with fresh fruit and berries. Each recipe serves 8.

0 0 0 0 1/4 0 0

 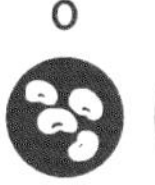  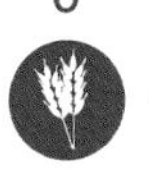   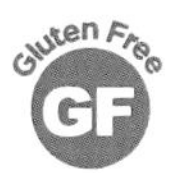 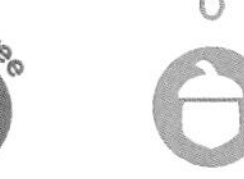

Blueberry-Pomegranate Sorbet

Blueberries and pomegranates are both high in phytonutrients, which function as antioxidants and anti-inflammatory compounds in the body, reducing inflammation and combating free radicals that cause cancer, heart disease and metabolic dysfunction. Both fruits are excellent sources of vitamin C.

1 1-pound bag fresh or frozen blueberries

3/4 cup sugar

1/2 cup pomegranate juice

2 tablespoons pomegranate liqueur, optional

Fresh blueberries and mint leaves for garnish

Preparation

1 Purée all the ingredients in a blender for 4-5 minutes until sugar is dissolved. Transfer mixture to ice cream maker. Mixture will fill a large ice cream maker. If using a smaller ice cream maker, divide the mixture in half. Process and freeze according to ice cream maker's manufacturer instructions.

Per Serving: 103 calories, 0g total fat, 0g saturated fat, 0mg cholesterol, 0mg sodium, 61mg potassium, 26g total carbohydrate, 2g dietary fiber, 0g protein

0 0 0 0 1/4 0 0

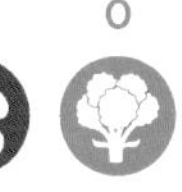 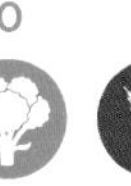 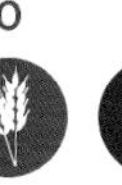 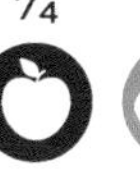 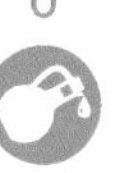  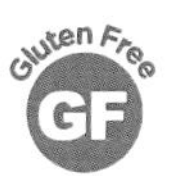

Chocolate Sorbet

This delicious chocolate sorbet will satisfy your sweet tooth without breaking the scale. Raw cacao powder and fresh raspberries bring a one-two punch of powerful antioxidants to this heart-healthy recipe. Raspberries can also help fight chronic diseases, such as type 2 diabetes, hypertension and obesity.

1 1/2 cup soy milk, coconut milk or soy creamer

2 bananas

1/3 cup sugar

1/4 cup raw cacao powder

1 tablespoon espresso powder or coffee granules

1 teaspoon vanilla extract

2 tablespoons coffee liqueur, optional

Fresh raspberries and mint leaves for garnish

Preparation

1 Purée all the ingredients in a blender for 4-5 minutes until sugar is dissolved. Transfer mixture to ice cream maker. Mixture will fill a large ice cream maker. If using a smaller ice cream maker, divide the mixture in half. Process and freeze according to ice cream maker's manufacturer instructions.

Per Serving: 115 calories, 1g total fat, 0g saturated fat, 0mg cholesterol, 27mg sodium, 147mg potassium, 27g total carbohydrate, 2g dietary fiber, 2g protein

Sorbets

0 0 0 0 1/3 0 0

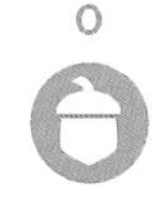
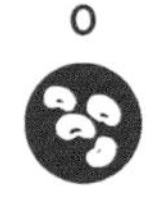

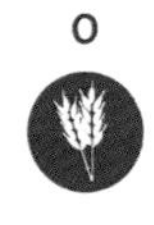

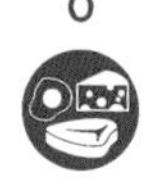
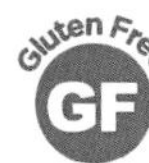

Ginger-Green Tea Sorbet

This flavorful sorbet combines ginger, green tea and lime for a light summer dessert. Ginger helps alleviate gastrointestinal problems and contains antioxidants that help fight inflammation and atherosclerosis.

2 cups water
1 inch peeled ginger, sliced
4 bags green tea
3/4 cup sugar
3 limes, 1 zested and all 3 juiced
1 pinch salt
Lime zest and mint leaf for garnish

Preparation

1. Bring water to a boil in a saucepan and add green tea, sliced ginger and sugar. Let steep for 15 minutes.

2. Pour tea through a sieve into a metal bowl and discard the solids.

3. Set bowl into an ice bath to cool and add lime zest, lime juice and pinch of salt. When mixture is cool, transfer to ice cream maker. Mixture will fill a large ice cream maker. If using a smaller ice cream maker, divide the mixture in half. Process and freeze according to ice cream maker's manufacturer instructions.

Per Serving: 75 calories, 0g total fat, 0g saturated fat, 0mg cholesterol, 19mg sodium, 18mg potassium, 19g total carbohydrate, 0g dietary fiber, 0g protein

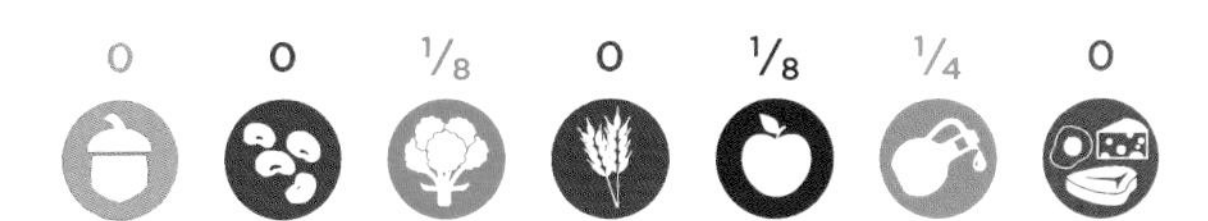

Makes 12

Strawberry Cupcakes with Creamy Vanilla Frosting

This luscious dessert is perfect for a special occasion! The phytonutrients in strawberries help reduce blood glucose levels after a starchy meal. Plus, the addition of beets can protect against heart disease. It's healthy indulgence at its best!

1 cup unbleached flour

3/4 cup wheat or spelt flour

1/2 cup cane sugar

1 teaspoon baking soda

8 ounces frozen or fresh puréed or crushed strawberries

1/4 cup canned beets

1/4 cup Smart Balance oil or melted Earth Balance non-hydrogenated shortening

1 1/2 teaspoon vanilla extract

1 tablespoon distilled white vinegar

Frosting:

1/2 cup softened Earth Balance butter substitute

1/2 cup Tofutti cream cheese substitute or 1/2 cup Earth Balance butter substitute

3 cups powdered sugar

1 teaspoon vanilla extract

Preparation

1 Preheat oven to 350 degrees. Grease and line 12 muffin tins, or grease and flour a 9-inch cake pan.

2 In a large bowl, combine flours, sugar and baking soda. In another bowl, mix vanilla extract, oil and vinegar.

3 Purée the strawberries and beets in a blender. Add the puréed mixture to the oil mixture and stir to combine.

4 Create a well in the center of the dry ingredients and add the wet ingredients. Stir gently.

5 Pour the batter into the prepared muffin tins. Bake the cupcakes for about 17-22 minutes, or until a toothpick inserted into the center comes out clean. If baking in a cake pan, bake for 35-40 minutes and check for doneness.

6 While baking, prepare frosting. Cream together butter substitute, cream cheese substitute and vanilla extract until well combined. Whip with a mixer whisking in powdered sugar 1/2 cup at a time until smooth and creamy.

7 Remove from the oven and place on a wire rack to cool. When cool, frost and garnish with whole strawberries if desired.

Per Serving: 75 calories, 0g total fat, 0g saturated fat, 0mg cholesterol, 19mg sodium, 18mg potassium, 19g total carbohydrate, 0g dietary fiber, 0g protein

0 0 0 Trace 2 1/8 0

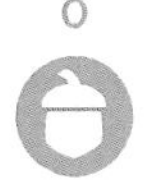 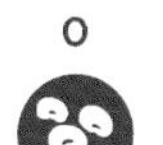  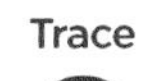 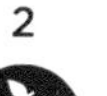 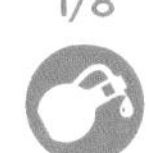 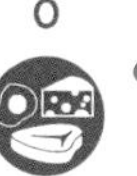 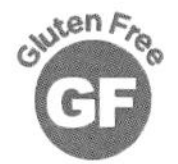

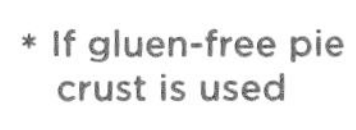

* If glueп-free pie crust is used

Serves 8

Very Berry Blueberry Pie

This traditional summer dessert features blueberries, which are high in phytonutrients and antioxidants. Fiber-rich dates are puréed to sweeten this treat. For an even sweeter taste, add more fruit purée to the filling. Enjoy this pie any time of year by swapping in seasonal fruit in place of blueberries.

6 cups fresh or frozen blueberries

1/4 cup tapioca pearls (found in baking aisle)

1 apple, peeled and grated

1 cup pitted dates

3/2 cup water

1 lemon, juiced and zested

2 tablespoons Earth Balance or Benecol butter substitute

1 teaspoon ground cinnamon

1 teaspoon cane sugar

2 frozen wheat or gluten-free pie crusts, such as Wholly Wholesome Frozen Pie Shells

Preparation

1 Preheat oven to 425 degrees. In a large bowl, combine blueberries and grated apples.

2 In a blender, add pitted dates, water, butter substitute, lemon juice, lemon zest, cinnamon, and sugar, and purée until smooth. Pour date mixture over blueberries and apples and fold in tapioca pearls.

3 Pour filling into one frozen pie shell. Take other pie shell and invert on top of pie with filling. Gently peel away crust from the pan and pinch edges to join crusts.

Cut two vent holes on top of pie. Sprinkle with additional sugar and cinnamon.

4 Place pie on foil-lined baking sheet and bake at 425 degrees for 10 minutes. Reduce oven temp to 325 degrees and bake in oven for additional 40 minutes. Watch pie after 20 minutes to make sure crust is not over-browning. Cover edges with foil if it is browning prematurely.

5 Take out and cool for 15 to 30 minutes before serving. Serve à la mode topped with vanilla soy ice cream.

Per Serving: 205 calories, 3g total fat, 1g saturated fat, 0mg cholesterol, 26mg sodium, 94mg potassium, 47g total carbohydrate, 4g dietary fiber, 2g protein

Caribbean Sunrise

Tropical Powerhouse Punch

Cantaloupe Cooler

Juices and Smoothies

See the recipes for these delicious juices starting on page 258.

Recipe Index

Juices

Smoothies

Juices and Smoothies

Juices

It can be difficult to eat the recommended 5 servings of vegetables and 3 servings of fruit every day. Here's a smart solution: Start juicing! It's a quick and easy way to maximize your intake of fruits and veggies and meet your daily dietary goals. Stronger, "greener" juices can be diluted with unsweetened coconut water as needed. Juices can also boost energy levels, making it an ideal morning beverage or afternoon pick-me-up!

The "Rise and Shine" bursts with lemonade-like flavor and makes a great introductory drink for those who have never juiced before, or for those who don't like strong vegetable flavors. The Hot Tomato Cocktail and Cantaloupe Cooler are also sweet, and as the recipes progress, more vegetables are added, increasing the nutrient value and vegetable flavor.

To prepare each juice, simply process all ingredients in the juicer and serve over ice for a cold and refreshing drink! Each recipe serves 1.

Rise and Shine

4-5 peeled carrots, ends trimmed
1 lemon, peeled
1 apple
1 handful of romaine lettuce, optional

Hot Tomato Cocktail

4 tomatoes
1 lime, peeled
1 cucumber
2 carrots
2 green onions
1 jalapeno (or bell pepper)
1 handful of spinach or kale
1 handful of cilantro

Cantaloupe Cooler

½ cantaloupe, peeled
1 lime, peeled
1 cucumber
1 handful of spinach or kale
2 carrots
12 pitted cherries

Ginger-Mint Morning

1 cucumber
2 kale leaves
½-inch piece of ginger
1 apple or 2 carrots
1 lemon, peeled
A few stems of mint and parsley

Caribbean Sunrise

½ pear
½ green apple or 1 cup blueberries or raspberries
1 handful of spinach
½ peeled beet
1 handful of parsley
2 celery stalks
½ cucumber
½-inch piece of ginger
1 slice of papaya, mango or pineapple

Tropical Powerhouse Punch

1 handful of spinach
3 kale stalks
2 carrots
½ cucumber
½ avocado
1 mango or ½ pineapple

Vim and Vigor

1 cucumber
3-4-inch piece parsnip or carrot
A few broccoli stems/spinach
2 celery stalks
A few stems of bok choy or kale
A few stems parsley

Juice these ingredients and then pour into blender and add 1 avocado.

Very, Very Green Machine

2 celery stalks
½ cucumber
½ apple
½ lemon, peeled
½-inch piece ginger
1 bok choy leaf
1 bunch cilantro
5 kale leaves
1 handful of spinach

Tips for Making Juice

- Use 60% dark, leafy greens and 40% other vegetables and fruits.
- Use fruits to sweeten and increase nutrient absorption, or eat fresh fruit whole with vegetable juice.
- For citrus fruits, peel or slice off lemon/orange/grapefruit rind, leaving some of the white pith.
- To juice small leaves such as parsley and cilantro, roll them up into a ball to compact the leaves before putting them through the juicer.
- Wash all vegetables and fruits before making juice.
- Make sure you are eating whole solid foods along with your juice regimen. Your body still needs bulk and fiber from complex carbohydrates for B vitamins, riboflavin, magnesium and other nutrients. This will help give you steady and consistent energy.

Smoothies

Smoothies are thicker and slightly less nutrient rich than juices, but they're still an excellent source of nutrition. Nutrient-dense greens and antioxidant-rich fruit make the smoothies excellent energy boosters. Use frozen fruit and vegetables for greater convenience, which also gives the drink a frosty coolness—perfect for a hot day!

To prepare each smoothie, simply process all ingredients in the blender, pour into a glass and enjoy! Each recipe serves 1.

Green Gourmet Smoothie

1/2 cup frozen or fresh baby spinach greens
1 cups blueberry-pomegranate juice, soy or almond milk
1/8 cup silken tofu, or raw cashews or almonds
1 cup frozen cherries, blueberries, berry mix, pineapple or mango
1/2 banana
1 tablespoon ground flaxseed meal
1/2 kiwi, optional
1/2 orange, optional

Tip: Purée spinach, tofu or nuts and juice or soy milk in a high-speed blender until spinach is completely dissolved. Add frozen and fresh fruit and flaxseed meal, and purée until smooth. Add more soy milk or juice if mixture is too thick. Serve immediately in a cold glass.

Almond-Cacao-Banana Smoothie

1 frozen banana
1/4 cup silken tofu or hemp seeds
1/2 cup frozen spinach
1 tablespoon flaxseed meal
1 tablespoon cacao powder
1 1/2 tablespoons almond butter or peanut butter
1 1/4 cup almond milk, soy milk, flax milk or hemp milk
1 cup ice
Cacao nibs for garnish

Get Tropical Smoothie

1/2 diced mango or 3/4 cups frozen mango
1/2 banana
1/4 cup silken tofu, 1/4 cup raw cashews or 1/4 cup hemp seeds
1/2 cup frozen carrots
1 cup frozen or fresh pineapple, or papaya
1 tablespoon flaxseed meal
1 1/4 cups coconut milk, guava nectar, or limeade
1 cup ice

Chapter **11**

Holiday Meals

Food is at the center of holidays and special occasions such as birthdays, cultural celebrations and dinner parties. These tasty affairs are wonderful to have, but they can easily derail a healthy diet. Unhealthy, high-calorie foods can be difficult to avoid, and declining food offers may offend a hardworking party host. Be proactive by incorporating delicious healthy foods into special occasions! Healthy foods can be just as exciting to eat as unhealthy foods. Once you get familiar with the recipes, you will be able to create a nutritious feast that will leave a lasting impression on friends and family.

To prepare for a special occasion meal, peruse the recipes, find one that suits the occasion and test it to make sure you like it. You can even make these dishes for non-holiday occasions, such as potlucks and workplace celebrations.

We've created menus with recipe options for several special occasion meals. You can pick one dish to take to an event or select several to serve at your special occasion. You and your fellow diners are sure to love these tasty, healthful dishes!

TIP

Get full on nutrient-dense foods before you arrive at a party. Going on a full stomach will reduce the likelihood of eating the wrong foods.

Thanksgiving Menu

Wild Mushroom Soup

Sweet Potato Biscuits

Mashed Red Potatoes with Herbs

Roasted Brussels Sprouts with Pickled Radishes

Roasted Stuffed Pumpkin with Gruyère

Roast Turkey

Mile-High Cranberry-Apple Pie

• • •

Other options:

Southern Sweet Potato and Pumpkin Soup

Triple Berry Salad with Strawberry Dressing

Haricot Vert with Mushroom Sauce and Crispy Shallot Topping

Pumpkin Cheesecake

Winter Holiday Menu

Mushroom Paté with Sherry and Thyme

Kale, Carrot and Herb Strudel

Caesar Salad with Garlicky Walnuts

Beef and Mushroom Bourguignon

Gingered Fruit Salad with Coconut-Pineapple Sauce

• • •

Other options:

Hot Artichoke-Spinach Dip

Mediterranean Tri-Color Paté

Curried Parsnip and Carrot Soup

Tri-Colored Floret Salad

Lemon-Glazed Sweet Potatoes

Moroccan Roasted Vegetable Tagine

Tarragon Chicken Potpie

Apple-Cinnamon Rolls

Fig Bars

New Year's Day Menu

White Bean Paté

Black-Eyed Pea Salad and Grilled Meat

Zesty Mexican Bean Dip

Tarragon Chicken Potpie

Chinese Cashew Chicken

Indian Chana Masala

Mexican Tamale Pie

Green Chile Chicken Enchiladas

Valentine's Day Menu

Triple Berry Salad with Strawberry Dressing

Creamy Tomato-Basil Soup

Mushroom Paté with Sherry and Thyme

Ceasar Salad with Garlicky Walnuts

Vietnamese Lemongrass Beef

Italian Chicken Cacciatore

Strawberry Cupcakes with Creamy Vanilla Frosting

St. Patrick's Day Menu

Edamame Pea Dip

Hot Artichoke-Spinach Dip

Curried Potato and Carrot Soup

Green Salad with Apples, Berries and Goat Cheese

Tri-Colored Floret Salad

Mashed Potatoes with Herbs

Thyme Potato Gratin

Haricot Vert with Mushroom Sauce and Crispy Shallot Topping

Beef and Mushroom Bourguignon

Easter Menu

Quinoa Tabbouleh

Spring Vegetable Tart

Moussaka

Moroccan Carrots

Thyme Potato Gratin

Indian Chana Masala

Baked Vegetable Risotto

Strawberry Cupcakes with Creamy Vanilla Frosting

Very Berry Blueberry Pie

Fourth of July Party Menu

Cool Garden Vegetable Gazpacho

Creamy Macaroni-Potato Salad

Lemony Chicken Salad

Whole Grain Pasta with Chard and Garlicky Crumbs

Black-Eyed Pea Salad with Grilled Meat

Very Berry Blueberry Pie

Strawberry Cupcakes with Creamy Vanilla Frosting

Mother's Day Brunch Menu

Triple Berry Salad with Strawberry Dressing

Lemony Chicken Salad

Cool Cucumber-Avocado Soup

Wild Mushroom Soup

Kale, Carrot and Herb Streudel

Spring Vegetable Tart

Quinoa Tabbouleh

Moussaka

Sake-Poached Salmon with Sesame-Ginger Sauce

Very Berry Blueberry Pie

Labor Day Menu

Corn and Summer Vegetable Chowder

Cool Garden Vegetable Gazpacho

Baked Vegetable Risotto

Roasted Brussels Sprouts with Pickled Radishes

Tarragon Chicken Potpie

Fig Bars

Coconut-Chia Seed Pudding

Halloween Menu

Caesar Salad with Garlicky Walnuts

Southern Sweet Potato and Pumpkin Soup

Roasted Stuffed Pumpkin with Gruyère

Savory Italian Meatloaf

Apple-Cinnamon Rolls

Pumpkin Cheesecake

Office Potluck Menu

Creamy Macaroni-Potato Salad

Curried Apple Chicken Salad

Quinoa Tabbouleh

Green Salad with Apples, Berries and Goat Cheese

Asian Sesame Noodle Salad

Three-Bean Salad with Almond and Lemon

Strawberry Cupcakes with Creamy Vanilla Frosting

Chocolate-Pecan Oat Cakes

Birthday Celebration Menu

Mushroom Paté with Sherry and Thyme

Thyme Potato Gratin

Tarragon Chicken Potpie

Italian Chicken Cacciatore

Oven-Roasted Halibut with Romesco Sauce

Sake-Poached Salmon with Sesame-Ginger Sauce

Beef and Mushroom Bourguignon

Strawberry Cupcakes with Creamy Vanilla Frosting

Football Season Menu

Zesty Mexican Bean Dip

Hot Artichoke-Spinach Dip

Green Chile Chicken Enchiladas

Beef Enchiladas with Hatch Rojo Sauce

Oven-Roasted Sweet Potatoes with Curry Dip

Chocolate-Pecan Oat Cakes

Five-Star Brownies

Chapter 12

Cravings, Snacks and Eating Out

Snacks are meant to be mini-meals that boost energy and help stave off hunger until the next full meal. Snacking can also help keep blood sugar steady, which is important for people with prediabetes. We recommend snacking 1-2 times a day. If you're snacking more than twice a day, try adding more filling foods to your meals so that you are able to stay satiated longer. But be sure not to snack in place of eating real meals–it can lead to poor food choices, overeating and weight gain.

Following a healthy snacking strategy starts with knowing about your personal eating habits. Think about which type of eater you are, then follow these easy tips for snacking smarter every day.

The Pleasure Eater

This type of eater enjoys food and is easily tempted to "have a little bit." Switching to a high-fiber, whole grain, protein-rich breakfast is the first order of business for the Pleasure Eater. The key is to be full, but that doesn't mean you need a calorie-laden breakfast. High-fiber, nutrient-rich foods fill you up without adding unwanted calories. As the morning progresses, your stomach will empty and you will feel hungry. Eat a satisfying lunch, and for an afternoon snack choose broth-based soups, whole grain toast with fruit, or sprouted grain energy bars.

The Efficiency Eater

This type of eater is super busy and may have an irregular schedule. Since eating is not a priority, the snacker will starve all day and reach for anything when blood sugar plummets. This snacker takes in most of the calories in the last half of the day, after vacillating between no calories to calorie overload. This is the ultimate rollercoaster for blood sugar and insulin, and requires a more steady calorie stream to get back on track. A protein- and fiber-rich breakfast is filling and provides much needed energy. The Efficiency Eater requires convenient food, so stocking the desk, car and purse with items such as individual packs of plain instant oatmeal, Cream of Wheat, nuts, whole grain crackers, almond butter, or fresh fruit will help provide nutrient-dense foods when snacks are needed. Eating a breakfast and lunch that include several servings of whole grains helps to break the starvation pattern.

The Routine Eater

This type of eater usually has specific snacks that are routinely enjoyed. It may be potato chips every afternoon or ice cream before bed every night. Routines can be difficult to change, and just the thought of having to lose these snacks may be enough to make the routine snacker quit a diet. Here's the solution: This snacker should keep the usual snack, only reduce the serving size. Also, some snacks have good substitutions–and a greater amount of nutrients–that will meet a snacker's needs. Ice cream, for example, can be traded for soy ice cream or sorbet. To reduce the frequency of snacking, be sure to eat full, satisfying meals. If you still find yourself snacking often, it may be that you are eating to fill an emotional hunger. If you are an emotional eater, you will have to learn to manage emotions in a way that doesn't involve food.

The Social Eater

The Social Eater may not intend to snack, but ends up snacking because someone offered food or because everyone in the room is eating. Eating is an important social activity, and people often feel like they've missed out or are being rude if they don't participate. That piece of cake at the office birthday party, happy hour with friends... those snacks add up! Since you're more interested in sharing social experiences, the best solution is to simply change your snack choices. Prepare healthy snacks in advance and have them available to yourself and others. This will help you avoid filling up on "empty-calorie" foods.

Smart, Nutritious Snacks

You feel hungry when you're stomach is empty. That feeling sends the signal to your brain that it's time to eat. When you reach for a snack, ask yourself first, "Am I hungry?" If the answer is "no," then pass on the snack. But if you are hungry and your next meal is hours away, then have a snack.

Not sure what to snack on? Reach for any of these healthy snacks...

- Half a whole grain bagel with 1 tablespoon almond butter, topped with dried currant, bananas and strawberries
- Smashed avocado with lemon juice on half a whole grain English muffin
- Steamed edamame
- Oven-roasted sweet potatoes (15 pieces)
- Hummus with veggies and olives
- Vegetable and fruit smoothie
- Smashed butter beans, lemon and sliced tomato on half a whole grain toast
- 16 ounces fresh vegetable juice or low-sodium V8 juice
- ½ cup low-fat Greek yogurt with 1 diced kiwi and ¼ cup mango with 1 tablespoon cashews
- Soup, hot or cold
- Raw vegetables including endive, cherry tomatoes, red/yellow/green pepper slices, carrots, snap peas, celery sticks, jicama, broccoli, cauliflower
- Steamed vegetables including green beans, broccoli, cauliflower, red potatoes, corn, squash, asparagus
- Fresh whole fruit
- Rice cake with peanut butter, coconut and dried cranberries
- Toasted whole grain bagel with 2 tablespoons cottage cheese, fresh strawberries and a drizzle of agave nectar
- Olive oil-popped popcorn
- Toasted nori seaweed sheets
- Nuts
- Dried fruit
- Sprouted grain energy bars
- Bean dip and a corn tortilla
- Veggie chicken salad on 1 slice sprouted grain toast with tomato

- Romaine fruit wrap with almond butter, sliced bananas, strawberries, dried fruit like currants and flaxseed meal
- Raw asparagus spears with Creamy Garden Ranch Dip
- Cream of Wheat or oatmeal packets with 1 cup soy or almond milk with dried fruit and coconut or walnuts
- Toasted whole wheat naan and sliced avocado roll with sprinkling of salt, red chili, tahini, lemon juice and shredded romaine
- Whole wheat or corn quesadilla with veggie rice cheese, Zesty Mexican Bean Dip and romaine leaf
- Miso soup with brown rice

Healthy Ready-Made Snacks

"Off-the-shelf" snacks aren't as healthy as foods prepared at home, but they will suffice when you're pressed for time. Not all "healthy" snacks meet the dietary criteria, and some flavors may be healthier than others. Here are a few brands (and flavors) we recommend:

- *KIND Fruit & Nut and KIND Plus bars*: Peanut Butter & Strawberry, Nut Delight, Almond Cashew with Flax & Omega 3, Blueberry, Pecan & Fiber, Pomegranate, Blueberry, Pistachio & Antioxidants
- *LARABAR*: Pecan Pie, Apple Pie, Peanut Butter Cookie
- *CLIF Bar:* Crunchy Peanut Butter, Coconut Chocolate Chip
- *Kashi Cookies*: Soft-Baked Chocolate Almond Butter
- *Kashi cereal*: *GoLEAN Original, Squares Honey Sunshine, Squares Berry Blossoms, Whole Wheat Biscuits Cinnamon Harvest*
- *Post Grape-Nuts cereal*
- *Ezekiel 4:9 Sprouted Whole Grain Cereal*
- *Uncle Sam Cereal*
- *Fiber One cereal*
- *Quaker Oatmeal Squares*
- *Quaker Instant Oatmeal Lower Sugar*: Maple & Brown Sugar
- *Weetabix Whole Grain Cereal*
- *Whole Foods 365 Raisin Bran Cereal*
- *Kellogg's Mini-Wheats, Unfrosted*
- *Post Bran Flakes*
- *Post Original Shredded Wheat*

Make Your Own Snack Mix

Trail mix is a nutritious but calorie-rich snack. Our low-calorie trail mix recipes are healthful, filling and delicious. Make several batches and store in the pantry–you'll have healthy snacks to munch all week long.

Each serving of trail mix has about 150-200 calories and has ½ a serving of whole grains.

Winter White Blend (January)
Raw cashews, walnuts, sunflower seeds, dried pineapple, dried Fuji apple crisps and Kashi Cinnamon Harvest Cereal

Sweetheart Blend (February)
Coco dusted almonds, cashews, dried strawberries, dried raspberry, sunflower seeds, Kashi Island Vanilla Cereal

Leprechaun Blend (March)
Crushed pistachios, sliced almonds, cashews, dried bananas, pumpkin seeds and Autumn Wheat Kashi Cereal

Peaches and Cream (April)
Raw almonds, pecans, dried peaches, dried strawberries, sunflower seeds and Kashi Island Vanilla Cereal

Spring Fling (May)
Walnuts, cashews, yogurt-covered raisins, cranberries, pumpkin seeds, and Kashi Island Vanilla Cereal

Tropical Piña Colada Blend (June)
Raw sliced almonds, coconut flakes, pumpkin seeds, sunflower seeds, dried banana, dried pineapple and Kashi Island Vanilla Cereal

Red, White and Blue Blend (July)
Raw cashews, almond slices, dried blueberries, dried apples, dried cranberries, sunflower seeds, Kashi Island Vanilla Cereal

Summer Medley (August)
Raw almonds, pistachio pieces, dried bananas, dried strawberries, pumpkin seeds, Kashi Island Vanilla Cereal

Harvest Blend (September)
Walnut pieces, raw cashews, dried apple, dried pear crisps, sunflower seeds, Kashi Cinnamon Harvest Cereal

Witch's Brew (October)
Raw almonds, walnut pieces, currants, dried oranges, pumpkin seeds, Kashi Cinnamon Harvest Cereal

Thanksgiving Blend (November)
Raw cashews, pecan pieces, cranberries, dried cinnamon apple, pumpkin seeds, Kashi Cinnamon Harvest Cereal

Holiday Mix (December)
Cinnamon pecans, sliced almonds, cranberries, dried oranges, sunflower seeds, Kashi Cinnamon Harvest Cereal

Preparation
Pour cereal in a large bowl. Add 1 ½ cups of each nut for a total of 3 cups of nuts. Add 1 ½ cup seeds. Add 2 cups dried fruit. Add 1 ½ cups dehydrated fruit. Add ½ cup unsweetened coconut or sesame seeds, chia seeds, hemp seeds or flaxseed meal. Mix and divide into ½-cup servings in plastic bags and store for easy grab-and-go snacks. Serves 32.

How to Deal with Cravings

Pining for a slice of your favorite pie? Don't swear off your favorite foods–include them in your diet in small amounts so that you don't feel deprived. Pay attention to the types of foods you crave: Are they sweet, salty, spicy, soft, chewy, or crunchy? After you identify your craving, try substituting with healthier versions of these foods.

CRAVING	INDULGE IN THIS INSTEAD...
Sweet	Fruit, 1 ounce dark chocolate
Salty	Nuts, edamame, dried seaweed sheets
Spicy	Wasabi peas, curry almonds, wasabi soy almonds
Soft	Peanut butter, almond butter, bread or toast, banana
Chewy	Sugar-free gum, dried fruit (raisins, apples, cherries, apricots, dates), sprouted whole grain bread or bagel
Crunchy	Apples, grapes, carrots, celery, air-popped popcorn, ice cubes

Eat foods you crave as part of a meal rather than binging on them. If you realize that your craving is unreasonable, take yourself out of your environment. Most cravings go away after 10-15 minutes. Bright lighting and warmer temperatures may decrease your food cravings, so try to keep your environment well-lit and toasty. And try to get adequate sleep; research shows that poor sleep can increase food cravings.

What About Alcoholic Beverages?

Alcohol has no nutritional value and cocktails often have too many calories when they're "mixed" with syrups, creams and juices. Try to choose alcoholic beverages that are lower in calories and mixes that have few or no calories. The body processes alcohol before carbohydrates, fats or protein, which slows down the burning of fat and, consequently, slows weight loss.

> TIP
>
> To decrease calories when drinking wine, make a wine spritzer by mixing white wine and sparkling water. In cocktails, use mixers with no calories such as water, ice and diet soda. Add a twist of lime for extra taste.

Other Beverages

Just like alcoholic beverages, non-alcoholic drinks are often a hidden source of calories and are nutrient poor. Try these drinks instead:

- Water, Perrier, San Pellegrino
- Unsweetened tea
- Green tea (try the flavored kind)
- Unsweetened black coffee
- Tomato and vegetable juice
- Fruit juice such as pomegranate-blueberry juice mixed in equal amounts with water

Full-calorie cola drinks are not recommended because they have no nutritional value and are high in calories. Diet colas may increase blood sugar levels despite having zero calories, but not all experts agree. If drinking cola is important to you, try to drink them in moderation (1-2 per day).

CALORIES IN ALCOHOLIC DRINKS

	CALORIES
Regular Beer (12 ounces)	150
Light Beer (12 ounces)	103
Champagne (4 ounces)	95
Red Wine (4 ounces)	80
White Wine (4 ounces)	80
Gin, Vodka, Rum, Whiskey, Tequila (1 shot, 80 proof)	60

TIP

Red wine is packed with antioxidants and a substance called resveratrol that may reduce inflammation in the lining of arteries and improve HDL cholesterol. This makes red wine a heart-smart alcoholic beverage!

Eating Out and How to Make Healthy Choices

Restaurants often have healthy menu options that will help keep you on your diet plan when dining out. Before you dine, visit the restaurant's website and plan what you will order. The Whole Grains Council has an excellent website that features a list of independent and chain restaurants offering meals with whole grains. Check it out at www.wholegrainscouncil.org/find-whole-grains/eating-away-from-home.

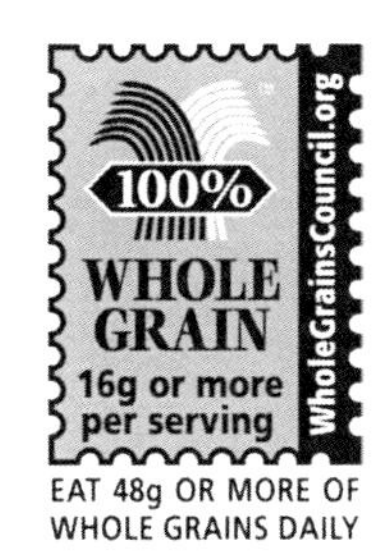

When shopping for food, choose products that have the Whole Grain stamp.

Here are more ways to ramp up your nutrition when dining out:

- Never leave the house starving. Have a light snack such as raw veggies or fruit before going out.
- Look for nutrient-dense foods on the menu and ask for modifications and substitutions. Ask for whole grains, such as whole wheat bread, corn tortillas and brown rice.
- If you're drinking alcohol, have thirst-quenching water or seltzer first.
- Restaurant portions are usually twice the standard portion. Split meals, order appetizer portions or plan on taking it home so you keep portions in check.
- Order sauces on the side.
- Grilled or broiled foods are usually brushed with oil and butter. Request them dry or prepared with olive oil.
- Request the starch to be replaced with a second vegetable.
- Have the bread basket at the table removed, or eat only one roll with dinner.
- Order fresh fruit.
- Chew slowly and savor the environment, your company and the flavors of the food. Enjoy your meal for at least 20 minutes and stop eating when you're full. Remove uneaten food promptly.
- Drink a full glass of water and get it refilled during the meal.
- If eating family-style, eat only one plate and do not have seconds.

Many restaurant menus offer plenty of healthy selections and others have very few. Always ask your server how menu items are prepared and if they are able to go light on butter and oil. Choose or ask for whole grains.

International cuisine offers plenty of healthy options. Here's what to order at each type of restaurant:

At an Italian restaurant, choose spaghetti marinara, minestrone soup, pasta fagioli, healthy salads, tomato-vegetable pizza, broccoli, and spinach. Since their foods are made to order, ask the chef to leave off the cheese and minimize the oil. Ask for whole grain pasta.

At a Mexican restaurant, choose black bean and vegetable burritos or salads topped with avocado and salsa. Pass on the cheese and food items with lard (like refried beans).

At a Latin American restaurant, opt for black bean dishes, brown rice, plantains, salads, salsa, and fruits.

At a Chinese restaurant, choose vegetable springrolls, vegetable potstickers and non-meat soups. Choose the vegetable dishes, ask for tofu or mushrooms instead of meat, and request extra vegetables. Most restaurants offer brown rice.

At a Japanese restaurant, choose sushi made with brown rice, edamame, miso soup, salads, seaweed, and vegetarian dishes.

At a Thai or Vietnamese restaurant, most all dishes on the menu can be prepared with extra vegetables and no meat. Substitute with tofu and enjoy dishes with rice, noodles or soups with nut sauces. Be sure to ask for brown rice or whole wheat noodles.

At an Indian restaurant, choose vegetarian soups, rice dishes and curries. Avoid dishes that are deep-fried or made with cream.

At an American restaurant, choose salad bars (without salad dressing), vegetable plates, baked potatoes with the skin on, whole grain pasta and brown rice dishes. Beware of sauces.

How to Navigate the Fast-Food Trap

It's best to avoid fast food altogether, but when you have no other options, choose wisely. Many fast-food chains have healthy menus. Visit their website ahead of time so that you're well prepared when you arrive. Choose foods that have as many whole food ingredients as possible. When healthy doesn't seem to be an option, choose foods that are the right amount of calories for you. You may be surprised to learn that a steak and egg breakfast sandwich, for example, has almost double the calories of a steak breakfast burrito!

Chapter 13

Nourish Your Body with Nutritional Supplements

We emphasize a natural approach in the prevention and treatment of prediabetes. Eating unprocessed, natural food will help boost your health and prevent chronic illness, including prediabetes and many of its associated conditions. But sometimes healthy food isn't enough. To nourish your body and protect against disease, you must add nutritional supplements to your diet.

Replenishing stores of vitamins and minerals can aid in disease prevention and treatment, studies say. It can help boost your heart health, immune system and energy levels, and replenish the body with essential vitamins, minerals and nutrients.

In some cases, medication is necessary to treat prediabetes and its associated conditions. However, supplementing with key nutrients is still necessary and may help minimize your medication needs over time.

Why You Need to Take Supplements

Harmful metabolic processes occur when the body is in a prediabetic state. A deficiency of nutrients in the body over many years can prevent proper body functioning, including the processing of blood sugar.

You can boost your nutrient levels with a daily regimen of nutraceuticals, which are food or food products that have health benefits. Examples of nutraceuticals include oats, bran and canola oil and also nutritional supplements, such as omega-3 fatty acids, vitamin B12 and folic acid.

Like most Americans, you probably aren't eating the right kinds of foods and are deficient in certain dietary categories. Consider these statistics: Each American consumes an average of 142 pounds of sugar annually, according to the U.S. Department of Agriculture. This intake includes sweets, sugar added to processed foods, and sweeteners such as high-fructose corn syrup. This intake has increased 19% since 1970 and accounts for 18% of caloric intake. Additionally, Americans are eating 30% or more grains than is recommended, the majority of which is refined grain, such as white flour. Nearly 20% of calories come from white flour, which quickly breaks down to sugar in the body.

It's clear that a significant portion of the diet provides no nutritional benefit and prevents intake of foods that provide high nutrient content. In fact, it lowers vitamin and mineral intake by up to 35%.

Processed foods, which are common in an American diet, lose much of their nutritional benefit during processing, and adding substances to the food often blocks critical nutrient function in the body. For example, fluoride and bromide are added to many bread products. These minerals can compete with iodine for binding sites in the body, thereby blocking adequate thyroid production and conversion.

Because of over-farming and soil depletion, many fruits and vegetables have not been exposed to adequate soil minerals, reducing their own nutrient content over time. This means that many foods may not deliver the same levels of nutrients as they did 100 years ago.

Absorption of nutrients may also be decreased because of the high prevalence of gastrointestinal disorders in our population. Some of these include gastroesophageal reflux disease (GERD), irritable bowel syndrome (IBS), celiac disease/gluten sensitivity, and lactose intolerance. Some of these processes result from dietary intake and some, like GERD, can be worsened by increased weight, chronic stress and poor nutrition.

It's critical that you take supplements to ensure you have adequate levels of nutrients to help your body function and metabolize sugar.

Key Nutrients for Prediabetes

Key nutrients for prediabetes include vitamins, minerals, acids (both fatty acids and amino acids), herbal (plant-based) therapies and other substances. Many nutrients in these categories play important roles in helping individuals with prediabetes reverse or slow the progression to diabetes. You may feel overwhelmed as you read over the several types of nutrients you might need. Keep in mind that the PreDiabetes PATHFinder Program incorporates key nutrients into clients' regimens in a simplified, efficient way. To help you meet your nutraceutical needs, we've designed formulas containing multiple key nutrients that minimize the number of capsules and pills consumed every day.

Vitamins

Vitamins are nutrients the body needs for optimal health and development. They can be classified as either water- or fat-soluble.

Vitamins help keep the body working, protect you from disease and play a key role in glucose metabolism.

B-complex vitamins

- *Vitamin B1 (thiamine)*: This vitamin is important for brain and heart function. Individuals with diabetes tend to have lower serum thiamine levels, a deficiency which may also be related to the development of nerve problems in patients with abnormal glucose.
- *Vitamin B2 (riboflavin)*: Riboflavin plays a key role in energy production in cells of the body.
- *Vitamin B3 (niacinamide)*: Niacin is one of the most effective treatments for dyslipidemia (an abnormal amount of lipids in the blood). It has been shown to help increase "good" HDL cholesterol and lower "bad" LDL cholesterol and triglycerides. This can offer significant protection against atherosclerosis.
- *Vitamin B5 (pantethine)*: Pantethine and pantothenic acid have many key roles in the body including supporting healthy adrenal (stress) gland function. It also helps convert carbohydrates, fats and protein into energy, a critical process in someone with prediabetes.
- *Vitamin B6 (pyroxidine)*: Levels of vitamin B6 drop sharply after age 50, when risk for type 2 diabetes increases. Daily supplementation with this vitamin can reduce insulin needs and improve basic health. Vitamin B6 can also offer protection against

diabetic neuropathy (nerve disease) and decrease the risk of heart disease.

- *Folic acid*: Supplementation of folic acid and vitamin B12 can assist in lowering homocysteine levels, one of the biomarkers for cardiometabolic disease risk.

- *Biotin*: A B-complex vitamin that works with insulin to help in glucose utilization, biotin can also help relieve symptoms of peripheral neuropathy.

- *Choline*: This critical nutrient prevents fatty liver, a common co-existing problem in patients with prediabetes or insulin resistance due to increased abdominal fat. There is some evidence to suggest that choline is anti-inflammatory.

- *Vitamin B12 (cobalamin)*: This vitamin is essential for many critical functions in the body including metabolism, iron absorption, energy production, and mental clarity. Vitamin B12 also can be helpful in lowering homocysteine levels, which reduces your risk of cardiovascular disease.

Vitamin A

Vitamin A plays a role in stimulating insulin release from the pancreas.

Vitamin C

Deficiency of vitamin C can cause degeneration or breakdown of the cells in the pancreas that produce insulin. Vitamin C is an antioxidant, a substance that protects your cells from the damaging effects of free radicals.

Vitamin D

Vitamin D is both a fat-soluble vitamin and a hormone. You can get vitamin D from your diet and in supplement form, but the body also makes substantial vitamin D following exposure to ultraviolet sunlight. Vitamin D also boosts bone health by promoting calcium absorption. It's central to cell growth, immune function and inflammation control, promotes heart health, and helps control obesity and diabetes. Researchers have discovered that vitamin D receptors are located all over your body, including in the pancreas, which produces insulin and is a key player in the onset of diabetes.

Recent studies show that most prediabetics are vitamin D-deficient. People with low vitamin D tend to have higher fasting blood sugar levels, impaired glucose tolerance, higher rates of metabolic syndrome and a higher incidence of prediabetes. These findings suggest that supplementation with vitamin D among prediabetics improves insulin secretion, insulin sensitivity and insulin resistance. Restoring vitamin D levels to normal, healthy levels is key to preventing the progression to type 2 diabetes.

Vitamin E

Vitamin E is a powerful antioxidant and an essential part of a diabetes-prevention regimen. It helps break down blood clots, protects from vascular damage and lowers hemoglobin A1C levels and high triglyceride levels.

Minerals

The next important category of nutraceutical is minerals. Like vitamins, minerals are necessary for the body's proper function. Unlike vitamins, which are organic compounds, minerals are chemical compounds. In addition to other important functions in the body, several minerals are important in keeping blood glucose levels under control.

Chromium

Chromium plays an important role whenever glucose and insulin enter the bloodstream. Stores of chromium are immediately mobilized in response to blood sugar and insulin, and even a slight deficiency of this mineral can impair glucose tolerance. Chromium deficiency is common among Americans for two reasons: The lack of adequate chromium in the diet and the high amounts of refined sugar, which robs the body of stored chromium. Chromium levels may also be increased through exercise.

Chromium has been shown to support normal insulin function in patients with type 2 diabetes. Without chromium, insulin's action is blocked and glucose levels rise in the blood. Emerging evidence shows that chromium supplementation improves cholesterol balance by lowering total cholesterol and triglyceride levels, while increasing HDL cholesterol.

Copper

Copper is involved with insulin binding, with deficiency possibly resulting in increased glycosylated hemoglobin, indicative of chronically raised blood sugar levels.

Magnesium

Decreased magnesium levels in the cells may lead to abnormal insulin response, which contributes to the development of obesity and type 2 diabetes. Magnesium supplementation may contribute to an improvement in both islet beta-cell response (the cells in the pancreas that produce insulin) and insulin action in non-insulin dependent diabetics, resulting in improved glucose tolerance. People with high magnesium intake had a 33% lower chance of developing both metabolic syndrome and type 2 diabetes, according to a study published in the journal *Diabetes Care*.

Manganese

Deficiency of this mineral can lead to impaired glucose tolerance. Manganese is a compound involved in the metabolism of carbohydrates. Diabetics have been shown to have only half the manganese of normal individuals.

Selenium

Selenium is an antioxidant that is critical for proper immune system function. Low levels appear to be associated with higher risk of type 2 diabetes. Selenium supplementation is also important in patients with hypothyroidism or Hashimoto's thyroiditis (an autoimmune thyroid condition).

Vanadium

This trace mineral has been shown to decrease fasting blood sugar levels and liver insulin resistance. It also assists to block cholesterol accumulation in blood vessels and aids in fat metabolism. Studies have confirmed that vanadium has a blood sugar-lowering effect in non-insulin dependent diabetes.

Zinc

Zinc is essential for the normal production of insulin and is involved in all aspects of insulin metabolism: synthesis, secretion and utilization. Zinc also protects against beta cell destruction and has well-known immune-boosting effects. Diabetics typically excrete too much zinc in the urine and therefore require supplementation.

Fatty acids

Fatty acids comprise the next category of key nutrients for prediabetes. They are a powerful source of energy production in the body when metabolized.

Alpha-lipoic acid

Alpha-lipoic acid (ALA) is a potent antioxidant that enhances the activity of vitamins C and E. It also helps the body produce insulin, use glucose and detoxify the liver.

Evening primrose oil

Extracted from the seeds of the North American evening primrose (Oenothera biennis) plant, this oil is an excellent source of essential fatty acids, particularly gamma linolenic acid. In addition to anti-inflammatory properties, evening primrose oil can aid in weight loss and blood pressure control.

EPA/DHA (fish oil)

The two key omega-3 essential fatty acids, EPA and DHA, are found in fish oils, particularly in salmon and other cold water fish. These fatty acids are used as energy by cells and can aid in the reduction of heart disease and reduce inflammation. These omega-3s can be helpful in patients with dyslipidemia through effects of lowering LDL, VLDL, lipoprotein(a), and triglycerides.

Amino Acids

These acids are the building blocks of proteins that make the body work properly and assist in metabolizing proteins.

Arginine

The amino acid arginine has been shown to improve insulin sensitivity, lower blood pressure and decrease CRP. L-arginine has been shown to improve both beta cell function and insulin sensitivity, increasing the likelihood of a return to normal glucose tolerance.

Carnitine

Carnitine is an amino acid made in the body from the essential amino acids lysine and methionine. It has been shown to decrease fat mass, increase muscle mass and improve energy, which has a positive effect on weight loss, which is known to decrease insulin resistance.

Carnosine

Carnosine is an amino acid compound found primarily in red meat. It's important to supplement in patients who are decreasing the amount of red meat in their diets.

N-acetyl-cysteine (NAC)

A derivative of the amino acid cysteine, NAC reduces oxidative stress and free radical damage and is critical for making the potent key antioxidant glutathione. It also helps to keep vitamins C and E in their active forms and can improve insulin sensitivity.

Taurine

Taurine works by increasing the action of insulin, improving glucose tolerance and enhancing antioxidant levels—which are important functions to balance the negative effects of high-sugar diets.

Important Compounds

Coenzyme Q10

CoQ10 is a potent antioxidant that plays a key role in energy production in every cell in the body by converting food into cellular energy. CoQ10 also boosts heart health and stimulates the production of insulin in the pancreas. The amount of CoQ10 in the body naturally declines with age, making it especially important to supplement after age 50, or if a patient is on medications which may cause its depletion (such as statin drugs).

Inositol

This chemical compound can decrease fasting insulin levels and improve insulin resistance, particularly among patients with metabolic syndrome associated with polycystic ovary syndrome.

Quercetin

Quercetin is a flavonoid, a compound that provides potent antioxidant defense. Quercetin may reduce blood pressure and LDL cholesterol, and also reduce the effects of free radicals in the body.

Herbals

Many herbal remedies have medicinal properties that have been used by healers for thousands of years. Several herbs and spices can help treat prediabetes and its associated conditions.

Berberine

Berberine is the active ingredient in the Chinese herb golden thread. It can reduce blood sugar levels by increasing glucose uptake and glycolysis, raising insulin production, and promoting beta cell regeneration.

Bitter melon

This herb lowers fasting and postprandial (post-meal) glucose levels.

Cinnamon

Cinnamon has been shown to lower the average level of blood glucose by 0.83% when added to a treatment regimen. It enhances insulin release and sensitivity and increases glucose disposal and uptake in skeletal muscle. Cinnamon extract can help reduce fasting blood sugar and systolic blood pressure, and improve body composition in men and women with metabolic syndrome, according to a study. The results suggest that cinnamon supplementation can reduce risk factors associated with diabetes and cardiovascular disease.

Curcumin (turmeric)

Studies show that curcumin has anti-inflammatory, antioxidant, wound-healing and anti-cancer effects.

Fenugreek

This herb improves blood glucose control and insulin resistance in diabetic patients. Some studies show that fenugreek can decrease triglycerides and VLDL cholesterol levels. It appears to work by increasing insulin secretion and sensitivity, as well as inhibiting carbohydrate digestion and absorption from the GI tract.

Garlic

Garlic's main active ingredient is allicin, an antibacterial compound produced when garlic is crushed or chopped. Garlic has a long list of health benefits and can help manage prediabetes by balancing blood sugar, decreasing LDL cholesterol, lowering blood pressure, lowering triglycerides, and increasing HDL cholesterol.

Ginkgo biloba

This herbal extract comes from the leaves of the ginkgo tree that grows in China. Although it is best known for boosting cognitive ability, it also increases the uptake of glucose from the blood.

Ginseng

Ginseng has been shown to significantly reduce insulin resistance and fasting blood glucose levels in patients with type 2 diabetes. It can also reduce post-meal blood sugar in both non-diabetic patients and those with type 2 diabetes.

Grape seed extract

This extract is another potent antioxidant that can protect the health of cells and blood vessels by significantly reducing the effects of free radicals.

Green tea

Green tea can fight obesity by blocking the creation of fat cells by reducing glucose uptake in fat tissue while stimulating glucose uptake in skeletal muscle.

Policosanol/octacosanol

Policosanol and one of its breakdown products, octacosanol, are natural substances purified from sugar cane wax that can lower cholesterol. In fact, one study of postmenopausal women on a lipid-lowering diet found that 10mg daily of this nutraceutical decreased LDL cholesterol levels by 26% and total cholesterol by 19%, and also increased protective HDL cholesterol by 7%. These results were achieved without significant adverse effects. This nutraceutical component can be a valuable addition or alternative to standard medication therapy.

Red yeast rice

Red yeast rice is a fermented product of rice and is used to make rice wine and as a food preservative for maintaining the color and taste of fish and meat. It's also known for its medicinal properties.

Studies report that red yeast rice can lower cholesterol concentrations. A University of California, Los Angeles, study found that red yeast can significantly reduce LDL cholesterol, total cholesterol and triglyceride levels beyond the effects of dietary changes alone.

How to Supplement

Key nutraceutical therapies for prediabetes include vitamins, minerals, acids (both fatty acids and amino acids) and herbal, plant-based therapies. Each nutraceutical category plays an important and integrated role in helping patients with prediabetes reverse or slow the progression to diabetes.

Nutraceuticals have few side effects and are easily incorporated into your dietary, fitness and pharmaceutical plan. A nutraceutical regimen may even minimize the number and length of time that prescription medications are used.

The PreDiabetes Centers treatment program has specifically formulated several nutraceutical options to target improving overall health and metabolic function of the body, glucose and insulin levels, as well as common problems that accompany prediabetes such as lipid/cholesterol abnormalities, stress and poor sleep.

The quality of materials and production of these nutritional supplements incorporate Good Manufacturing Practice (GMP). To achieve the best results, PreDiabetes Centers designed nutrients that the body can easily absorb and utilize.

PreD Foundation

The cornerstone nutraceutical in the program is the PreD Foundation formula. Each pack consists of five capsules to take in the morning and evening. It includes many of the key nutrients listed in this chapter and was made as a multivitamin, eliminating the need to take each vitamin, mineral or nutrient separately.

The contents of each PreD Foundation pack include:

Vitamin A (beta carotene and Acetate)	10,500IU
Vitamin C (calcium ascorbate)	400mg
Vitamin D3 (cholecalciferol)	400IU
Vitamin E (d-alpha tocopherol succinate)	160IU
Thiamin (vitamin B1)	20mg
Riboflavin (vitamin B2)	20mg
Niacin (niacinamide)	60mg
Vitamin B6 (pyridoxine HCL)	20mg
Folate (calcium folinate)	315mcg
Vitamin B12 (methylcobalamin)	425mcg
Biotin	400mcg
Pantothenic Acid (calcium pantothenate)	100mg
Calcium (ascorbate/pantothenate/folinate/citrate)	80mg
Magnesium (citrate)	160mg
Zinc (citrate)	15mg
Selenium (selenomethionine)	70mcg
Copper (lysinate)	1mg
Manganese (manganese gluconate)	3mg
Chromium (polynicotinate)	400mcg
Inositol	160mg
Berberine Sulfate	100mg
Vanadium	40mcg
Cinnamon Extract	40mg
Gymnema Sylvestre Extract (leaf)	40mg
Alpha Lipoic Acid	40mg
Grape Seed Extract	30mg
Quercetin	30mg
Turmeric Root Extract	30mg
N-Acetyl L-Cysteine	20mg
Choline	12mg
PABA (para-aminobenzoic acid)	10mg
Fish Oil Omega 3	1,000mg
Evening Primrose Oil	1,000mg

The PreDiabetes Centers physicians recommend that most clients take this formulation twice daily to ensure adequate levels of each nutrient and herb throughout the day.

In many cases, additional deficiencies or needs may be identified through medical history and biomarker evaluation. These associated conditions may be treated with nutraceuticals as well as prescription drug therapy. The PreDiabetes Centers physician will guide clients and develop an individualized nutraceutical plan that best integrates with drug therapy, nutrition and fitness plans, and the most pressing needs.

Other abnormalities may include an abnormal lipid profile, suboptimal vitamin D levels, elevated homocysteine levels or low B12/folate levels, increased stress, poor sleep, hormonal imbalances, and gastrointestinal disorders. Additional formulas have been developed for clients who need extra support lowering glucose and insulin levels.

PreD Vitamin D

People with suboptimal vitamin D levels may be prescribed PreD Vitamin D, which contains 5,000 IU of vitamin D. This high-dose Vitamin D3 supplement was formulated to allow flexibility in dosing dependent on patient needs. The vitamin D tablet should be taken with a meal containing fat for best absorption.

PreD Omega 3

People with an abnormal lipid (cholesterol) panel may be prescribed PreD Omega 3. Each capsule contains 1,000mg of DHA/EPA. This nutraceutical provides additional support to your nutrition plan. It also may eliminate the need for cholesterol-lowering prescription drugs or decrease the amount of these drugs needed. They are a great natural complement to any lipid-lowering interventions.

PreD Cardio Health

PreD Cardio Health can also help improve an abnormal lipid panel. This specialized, powerful lipid-lowering formula contains the following nutrients in three capsules:

- Vitamin C 50mg
- Vitamin B5 50mg
- Red yeast rice 600mg
- Guggul extract 10% 320mg
- Bromelain (2,400 GDU) 100mg
- Taurine 100mg
- Pancreatin 8x 100mg
- Policosanol 22mg
- Coenzyme Q10 15mg
- Octacosanol 15mg

Guggul extract has anti-inflammatory effects, reducing the levels of C-reactive protein. The formula also contains bromelain, an extract from pineapple stem, which decreases the ability of the blood to stop platelets from clumping together, an effect that's enhanced by the inclusion of pancreatin (digestive enzymes). Appropriate dosing is individualized and should be determined under the guidance of a PreDiabetes Centers physician.

PreD Co-Q10

This nutraceutical also helps improve HDL cholesterol and lower LDL cholesterol. Each capsule of the PreD Co-Q10 formulation contains 100mg. It's critical that any person taking lipid-lowering medications, or even red yeast rice, include Co-Q10 as part of the nutraceutical regimen.

PreD Restful Nights

People with sleep issues may be prescribed this nutraceutical. Sleep is a key factor in insulin metabolism, stress management and overall well-being. You should try to avoid or decrease the need for prescription sleep aids, if possible, and opt for supplements. To help you get better sleep, the PreDiabetes Centers team has specially formulated a natural sleep nutraceutical designed to relax, calm and improve the quality of sleep. Your physician will recommend the best dosing to meet your needs. The nutraceutical formula includes the following in one capsule:

- Melatonin 3mg
- Taurine 360mg
- L-theanine 100mg
- 5-HTP 30mg
- GABA 100mg

This nutraceutical works by combining nutrients and melatonin, which work together to help clients achieve a restful sleep. Melatonin is a hormone produced and released by the pineal gland in the brain. It signals the brain that it is time for sleep and can help improve the quality of sleep. L-theanine, an amino acid derived from green tea, improves deep sleep and relaxation and plays a role in the formation of GABA (gamma-aminobutyric acid), another component of this formula. Through its ability to block excitation in the brain, GABA induces sleep and relaxation. The body uses 5-HTP to make serotonin, a neurotransmitter that improves the quality of sleep and may also aid in weight loss.

For those of you who require additional support to lower blood sugar and insulin levels, you may also be prescribed targeted formulas by your physician. Targeted formulas for glucose control will be incorporated into your treatment plan to complement your medication regimen or to possibly avoid the need for medications.

Nutraceuticals for Specific Health Conditions

Elevated Homocysteine Levels

Elevated homocysteine levels may increase risk of cardiac or other vascular diseases like stroke and peripheral vascular disease, all problems that are potential complications of prediabetes or diabetes. Vitamin B12 and folic acid can help lower the level of homocysteine in the blood. Although the Foundation Formula nutraceutical contains adequate doses of vitamin B12 and folic acid for most clients, some clients may have persistently elevated homocysteine levels. For these clients, a PreDiabetes Centers physician may recommend additional dosing with vitamin B12 and folic acid.

Excess Stress

Stress plays a role in the development of prediabetes and progression to diabetes. Although it's not possible to lead a stress-free life, you can decrease your stress response from the adrenal glands, which secretes adrenaline and cortisol in response to stressors, by taking nutraceuticals. Components of our stress-reducing nutraceutical formula include phosphatidylserine, an amino acid derivative that reduces the release of cortisol from the adrenal glands. In addition, the amino acid theanine and the herbals ashwaganda and magnolia (both adrenal adaptogens) help regulate the adrenal stress and cortisol response. Your PreDiabetes Centers physician will work with you to reduce increased cortisol levels.

Hormonal Support

Many patients with prediabetes have underlying hormonal imbalances that contribute to or exacerbate their condition. These abnormal hormone levels may include suboptimal thyroid function in men and women. In women, a condition called polycystic ovary syndrome (PCOS) may lead to insulin resistance and increased testosterone levels. Also, the decline in female estrogen levels at menopause may affect the body's sensitivity to insulin and the ability to process glucose. In men, falling testosterone levels during andropause, or aging-related hormone changes in men, can impair glucose and insulin systems. Your physician may recommend nutraceuticals to treat a hormonal imbalance.

Suboptimal Thyroid Function

Thyroid disorders can influence a prediabetic state in several ways, particularly when the thyroid is underactive, known as hypothyroidism. This occurs when the thyroid gland is not producing enough hormone to regulate energy and metabolism, which can lead to a lower metabolic rate. Low thyroid levels worsen high cholesterol, elevate homocysteine levels and cause changes in blood vessels that can lead to vascular disease. Patients with low-grade hypothyroidism (often referred to as "borderline") are more likely to suffer from coronary artery disease and cardiovascular death than people with normal thyroid function, according to studies.

Hypothyroidism may be caused by an autoimmune condition called Hashimoto's thyroiditis, particularly in women. This occurs when the body's immune system loses the ability to differentiate between "self" and "not self," and antibodies are formed which attack the thyroid gland and lead to its gradual destruction. Stress and hormonal and dietary factors contribute to this disorder.

PreDiabetes Centers will test you for underactive thyroid function and Hashimoto's thyroiditis. Your physician will discuss options for thyroid treatment. The PATHFinder Program's dietary and fitness guidelines are also beneficial for thyroid function, as are any efforts to improve sleep and reduce stress. In addition, some nutraceutical options can improve thyroid hormone levels in the body. These nutrients include the minerals selenium, zinc and iodine. Also, iodine supplementation may be recommended to help improve production of the thyroid hormone as well as conversion to its most active form in the body.

Some clients will require extra supplementation to optimize thyroid function. In these cases, the PreDiabetes Centers physician will discuss how and when to initiate thyroid hormone therapy.

Female Hormonal Imbalance

PCOS is an endocrine disorder caused by insulin resistance and hormonal imbalance. It affects 5%-7% of women and may have serious health consequences. Symptoms of this disorder include irregular menstrual cycles (or lack of menstrual cycle), elevated levels of testosterone, obesity, excess facial or body hair, and acne. Ovarian cysts may or may not be present. Lack of ovulation can expose patients to higher levels of estrogen that are not balanced by progesterone, increasing the risk of certain cancers, such as uterine cancer. All women entering the program will have an evaluation to assess risk for PCOS.

A comprehensive program with aggressive medical intervention can treat PCOS. The PreD Foundation formula also supports medical therapy, as it includes many nutrients, including D-chiro-inositol, which can improve the symptoms and underlying insulin resistance associated with PCOS. Clients who are also experiencing irregular menstrual periods may also benefit from nutraceuticals such as indole-3-carbinol–found in low levels in cruciferous vegetables like broccoli and cauliflower–which can help metabolize estrogen; evening primrose oil to help improve progesterone production; and chasteberry to balance the effects of too much estrogen. Additionally, natural progesterone supplementation may be recommended to provide further protection from the imbalance between estrogen and progesterone. Your PreDiabetes Centers physician will determine whether you need nutraceuticals for PCOS.

Perimenopause and Menopause

Menopause is the end of a woman's menstruation and fertility, occuring 12 months after the last menstrual period. The time leading up to the final menstruation is known as perimenopause. During perimenopause and menopause—which occurs around the age of 51—the female hormones estrogen and progesterone are produced at much lower levels. Women may experience symptoms including hot flashes, night sweats, anxiety, mood swings, weight gain, and headaches. Decreases in hormone levels can cause other changes in the body that affect prediabetes. For example, estrogen improves the body's sensitivity to insulin, decreases inflammation—when used topically—and increases HDL and decreases LDL. These changes are why postmenopausal women have a higher cardiovascular risk. Improving hormone balance can reduce these effects in women.

A healthy diet low in saturated fats, sugar and refined carbohydrates can improve the symptoms of menopause. Regular exercise, stress management and restful sleep can also help. Nutraceutical options for supporting symptoms during menopause/perimenopause include the herbs black cohash, Don Quai, chasteberry and phytoestrogens (soy). Estrogen therapy balanced with natural progesterone may be needed in some cases. A PreDiabetes Centers physician will discuss the risks and benefits of potential treatment options.

Male Hormonal Imbalance

Just as women experience declining estrogen levels with age, men experience declining testosterone levels. This "male menopause" is called andropause. Levels of testosterone in men begin to decline in their mid- to late 30s and continue to decline with age. Symptoms of declining testosterone levels include fatigue, depression, changes in muscle tone, and decreased libido and sexual function. Reduced testosterone levels can lead to a rise in insulin resistance and increased fat tissue. The PATHFinder program tests all men to determine if any testosterone deficiency exists.

In cases of low testosterone, treatment with bioidentical testosterone can increase muscle mass, decrease LDL and total cholesterol, improve insulin sensitivity and blood sugars, and decrease incidence of cardiovascular disease. Men using testosterone therapy may take nutraceuticals that include saw palmetto and lycopene to support prostate health, and also indole-3-carbinol to support healthy estrogen metabolism.

Some men with prediabetes may experience higher than normal circulating estrogen levels (yes, men have small amounts of the female hormone estrogen). These elevated estrogen levels can lead to breast enlargement and fat retention, and a possible worsening of insulin resistance (the opposite effect than what occurs in women). The PreDiabetes Centers program checks men for elevated estrogen levels and will help regulate estrogen levels in men on testosterone therapy.

Indole-3 carbinol is a good nutraceutical to alleviate any negative effects of estrogen. PreDiabetes Centers physicians will assist clients in developing a customized plan for addressing suboptimal testosterone levels.

Gastrointestinal Problems

Some prediabetics suffer from gastrointestinal problems, including irritable bowel syndrome and gastroesophageal reflux disorder (GERD). These disorders can decrease absorption of various nutrients from the intestines. To improve GI irregularities and nutrient absorption, you may be given probiotics, beneficial bacteria that reduce the growth of harmful bacteria and promote a healthy digestive system. Nutraceuticals can complement and enhance your efforts to reverse prediabetes and are best used in combination with Concierge Nutrition, the personalized fitness plan and prescription therapies under the guidance of a PreDiabetes Centers physician. Your physician will work with you to ensure that you take the safest and most effective levels and combinations of nutraceuticals.

Medications

Sometimes medication is necessary for people with prediabetes. The pancreas is overworked when the body overproduces too much insulin and C-peptide. Medication can help the pancreas work more efficiently, and also lower blood sugar levels into a healthier range. The ultimate goal is to discontinue medication after the body no longer needs medicinal assistance.

Metformin is a popular diabetes drug that can lower blood sugar levels. It works by reducing production of glucose by the liver (a process called gluconeogenesis) and also encourages peripheral tissues to utilize insulin more effectively. Metformin can decrease fasting blood sugars by 20% and hemoglobin A1c levels by 1.5%. We recommend a slow escalating dose of metformin to diminish potential side effects, which may include nausea and diarrhea. However, few patients have to discontinue the medication due to intolerable side effects. Metformin therapy should eventually be discontinued after the body stabilizes.

High Cholesterol (Dyslipidemia)

A vertical analysis profile (VAP) will be performed. The VAP will examine various components of the lipid panel and help your physician determine which course of treatment to pursue. Your doctor may prescribe lipid-lowering medication to treat high cholesterol.

One commonly prescribed medication for the condition is nicotinic acid (niacin), a natural B vitamin that can increase HDL cholesterol while also lowering LDL cholesterol and triglycerides. It is available in immediate-release, sustained-release and extended-release formulations. We avoid the immediate-release medication because it may cause flushing, or redness of the skin. We look to avoid this side effect by slowly increasing the dose of niacin over a period of four weeks. Also, taking niacin with an apple, or aspirin 30 minutes before, can decrease the side effects. If flushing occurs, it will likely improve after 7-10 days. This medication also requires liver function monitoring, as there have been rare cases of liver toxicity at high doses. Niacin should also be avoided in patients that have elevated levels of uric acid or homocysteine, as niacin may further increase these levels. Niacin can also produce low blood pressure in people taking vasodilator medications such as nitroglycerin, and it can sometimes worsen chest pain (angina pectoris).

Statins are the most powerful drugs for lowering LDL cholesterol and preventing coronary heart disease, heart attack, stroke, and death. These medications work by blocking the action of a chemical in the liver that is necessary for making cholesterol, and can reduce levels of LDL cholesterol by 30%-60%. They also reduce triglyceride levels an average of 20%-40% and increase HDL cholesterol by 5%. Side effects of statins may include elevation of liver enzymes or myopathy, a muscle disease resulting in muscle weakness that usually occurs during the first few weeks of treatment.

Your doctor may also prescribe fibrates, which can lower triglycerides up to 50%, reduce total LDL cholesterol and slightly raise HDL cholesterol. Although generally well-tolerated, side effects can include myopathy and an increased risk of gallstones. Myopathy may result if fibrates are taken after statin therapy.

Sleep

There are many medications available for the treatment of sleeplessness and insomnia. We prefer natural treatment with the use of melatonin, a naturally secreted hormone that can regulate circadian, or sleep and wake, cycles. Side effects are uncommon.

Hypothyroidism

Hypothyroidism occurs when the body produces too little thyroid. It requires lifelong treatment that consists of supplementing the thyroid hormone with a thyroid hormone replacement drug called "dessicated thyroid," which combines T3 and T4. The most common type is called "Armour

Thyroid." Clients with absorption issues or high-fiber diets—recommended for most prediabetics—should use combination therapy, as T3 is more readily absorbed from the GI tract, compared to T4. Dessicated thyroid has the same potential side effects as the thyroid medication Synthroid but must be used more cautiously in older clients and those with heart disease because of the rapid absorption of T3.

Testosterone Deficiency

To treat low testosterone, a condition commonly associated with prediabetes, your PreDiabetes Centers physician may prescribe medication in the form of an injection, gel, patch or mouth lozenge. We recommend treating testosterone deficiency with use of a once-daily gel. The gel dries quickly and testosterone levels increase within two hours and are stable for 24 hours. Side effects are uncommon and the medication is easy to administer.

Personalized
Fitness

Personalized
Fitness

Chapter 14

Your Personalized Fitness Plan

Have you avoided the gym for years? Maybe you work out occasionally, but need a little help getting back into a consistent exercise routine. Whatever your previous experience with fitness may be, one thing is for certain: It's time for you to get moving!

Fitness is a crucial part of your treatment plan. Research shows that a combination of regular cardiovascular exercise and strength training can help manage blood glucose levels and lower insulin resistance. The body burns blood sugar during aerobic activity, and strength training builds muscle that will, in turn, use greater amounts of sugar in the blood for energy, which can stabilize your blood glucose. Exercise can also reduce stress on the pancreas, as insulin-producing cells don't have to work as hard to maintain blood sugar levels.

The Dangers of Not Exercising

Inactivity is one of the 10 leading causes of death and disability, according to the World Health Organization. It also may cause your body to become less responsive to the hormone insulin, which can lead to the development of type 2 diabetes.

Many prediabetics have other health conditions—such as obesity, arthritis or gout—that can make standard exercise programs difficult to start or maintain. When designing your individual fitness plan, your PreDiabetes Centers health team will consider these special circumstances and any functional limitations you may have.

Your fitness goal is simple: You need to burn fat–especially visceral fat, which is the fat that accumulates in your abdomen, surrounds your organs and puts you at greater risk for diabetes and other health conditions. You also need to build lean muscle to increase your overall strength.

Combined with comprehensive treatment, regular exercise can help improve your biomarkers, reverse the progression to diabetes, and decrease your risk of other diseases including heart disease, cancer and Alzheimer's disease. Soon, you will enjoy greater strength and flexibility, increased stamina and a better quality of life.

A Personalized Fitness Program

Before increasing your physical activity level, your body needs time to respond to new therapies, start correcting imbalances and re-energize. Building and incorporating your fitness plan will take time. To ensure that your body is ready for the Personalized Fitness Plan, you will be evaluated by a personal trainer approximately 3-4 months after you begin your program. This evaluation will be pre-approved by your physician. Your health team will slowly integrate increased exercise into your treatment plan, and evaluate and re-evaluate your program.

The PreDiabetes Centers personal trainer will review the fitness questionnaire you completed at the time you joined the program. This review along with a detailed conversation at the time of your evaluation will be considered to assess your fitness experience, preferences and what you hope to accomplish over the next several months. In addition, your physician will complete a Fitness Prescription based on your medical history, comprehensive physical exam and biomarker results. The trainer will use this information to develop a specific program that meets your needs and helps you become healthier and stronger.

During your fitness consultation, our personal trainer will evaluate your ability to perform basic movements. The trainer will demonstrate each exercise and have you repeat the moves to assure proper form and technique. You will leave this one-hour appointment with your own Personalized Fitness Plan that you can perform at home. Depending on the recommendations, you may need to purchase a few inexpensive pieces of workout equipment, including a set of resistance bands with various tensions and dumbbells. A stability ball and yoga mat are helpful accessories, though may not be required.

Incorporating fitness into your daily life is key to establishing new healthy habits. Your health coach will focus on helping you adjust to daily exercise and customized strength-building and flexibility workouts.

You will be re-evaluated by the trainer approximately 60 days after starting your Personalized Fitness Plan. Adjustments are recommended based on your response and abilities since your initial evaluation. For many, this second phase of the fitness plan focuses on building your strength and increasing the intensity of workouts. Your plan will be customized to your needs and abilities. For others, an advanced level of intensity is not possible or recommended. If it's recommended, the personal trainer will examine your fitness progress and add interval training and higher weights to your workout, which help build lean muscle and boost your metabolism. (Yes, high-intensity workouts can increase the number of calories you burn in the hours after a workout!)

Starting Your Fitness Regimen

Starting and maintaining a cardiovascular exercise regimen in your daily life is a critical goal. It will help prevent diabetes and move your biomarkers in the right direction.

Almost any form of movement can be considered cardiovascular exercise, as long as it's sustained for at least 15 minutes and it gets your heart rate up. Also called aerobic exercise, it will increase your stamina and improve your body's ability to use oxygen, which helps strengthen your heart and lungs. Such exercise can include brisk walking, jogging, swimming, bicycling, dancing, step classes, rowing machines, elliptical trainers, housework, mowing, washing the car, and other physical activities.

You'll gain the most benefits when you exercise in your target heart rate zone. To calculate this range, you must first find your maximum heart rate, which is your age subtracted from 220. Your target heart rate should be 50%-70% of the maximum heart rate for moderate-intensity exercise. For vigorous-intensity exercise, your target heart rate should be 70%-85% of the maximum heart rate.

Based on your fitness evaluation results, you will start either a beginner, intermediate or advanced fitness regimen. This will be phase I of your fitness program.

Here are the different cardiovascular regimens you may perform:

Beginner workout:

- 30 minutes of cardiovascular activity a day, five days a week. This can be broken down into two 15-minute workouts throughout the day. You may even extend your workouts past 30 minutes, as long as you have at least 150 minutes a week of aerobic activity.
- Take at least 3,000-4,000 steps per day (1.5-2 miles), which can be achieved through a variety of activities. It's important to mix up what you do to avoid boredom and burnout. It will help keep you motivated!

You will be given an activity tracker that counts your walking or jogging steps and keeps you on target for reaching your daily goal. Other cardiovascular activities also can be keyed into the tracker. Taking into account your weight and activity level, the tracker can estimate how many calories you burn during each activity.

Intermediate workout:

- 30-45 minutes of cardiovascular activity a day, five days a week
- Take at least 6,000-8,000 steps a day (3-4 miles)

Advanced workout:

- 45 minutes of cardiovascular activity a day, five days a week. This can be broken down into 15-20 minute increments throughout the day.
- Take at least 10,000 steps per day (5 miles)

Build Lean Muscle with Strength Training

Strength training, also referred to as resistance training, involves movements that use resistance, such as dumbbells or your body weight, to build lean muscle and strengthen your body. It can also help reduce body fat—especially in the abdominal region—and increase bone density, caloric burn and improve overall blood glucose control.

Your personal trainer will increase the intensity of the strength-training exercises as you progress in the fitness program. Additionally, your workout will include pushing and pulling exercises, which work the major muscle groups of the upper and lower body. Your trainer will create three primary groups, or circuits, of strength-training exercises that target different parts of the body. Each will be performed once weekly.

Here are a few strength-training exercises you may perform:

- Dumbbell Biceps Curl
- Push-Up (modified or traditional)
- Seated Row with Resistance Band
- Lunge
- Chair Squat

Beginner workout:
3 times a week, perform 2 sets (7 reps of each exercise) of one circuit

Intermediate workout:
3 times a week, perform 2 sets (11 reps of each exercise) of one circuit

Advanced workout:
3 times a week, perform 2 sets (11 reps of each exercise every 90 seconds) of one circuit

Improving Your Core Strength

Building your core muscles, which includes muscles in your abdomen, back and around the pelvis, will help keep your spine in alignment and your body more stable. Doing a variety of core-strengthening exercises will enable you to strengthen all 29 of your core muscles.

Our program focuses on two components of core strength: rotation and resistance to rotation. Rotation exercises will strengthen hip, abdominal and back muscles, and include oblique crunches and single-leg planks. Resistance to rotation exercises target different muscles and include crunches, back extensions, sit-ups, leg raises, and planks.

Core-strengthening exercises will target one of five areas: your trunk, arms, legs, back, and gluteal region. Targeted core-strengthening workouts should be performed at least twice a week. Plan to do two different targeted groups each week. Give your body ample time to recover after a core-strengthening set; we recommend waiting 2-3 days between each circuit.

While performing the specific exercises, concentrate on doing them slowly and correctly. Quality of the movement is more important than how many you are able to complete.

Here are a few core-strength workouts you may perform:

- Plank on Stability Ball
- Side Plank
- Back Bridge
- Standing Crunch
- Twisted Crunch

Drink H_2O

Ditch the caffeinated beverages and sports drinks! Instead, drink water before, during and after workouts. Aim to consume 8-12 ounces of water every 10-20 minutes during exercise, though you may need to drink more if you've increased the intensity of your workout or if it's hot outside. Be sure to rehydrate after the workout too!

Beginner workout:
Twice a week, perform 4 sets (7 reps of each exercise)

Intermediate workout:
Twice a week, perform 4 sets (11 reps of each exercise)

Advanced workout:
Twice a week, perform 4 sets (11 reps of each exercise every 90 seconds)

Improving Balance and Flexibility

Balance and flexibility are critical to maintaining full range of motion and preventing injury. Flexibility training stretches and elongates muscles and helps tone your body. Stretching exercises also increase blood flow to your muscles, joints and surrounding tissue, resulting in greater pliability and better performance.

The benefits of balance and greater flexibility don't end there: It can also reduce stress, improve your sense of well-being and raise your quality of life.

If you're not a very flexible person, it's okay. Flexibility improves over time. Here's a tip: Stretch your upper and lower body muscles (on each side of the body) three days a week. It will help build and maintain flexibility.

Get More Zzz's

Experts recommend getting at least 7-8 hours of uninterrupted sleep a night. It will help your body repair muscle and prepare for the physical and mental demands of exercising.

Flexibility Dos and Don'ts

- Do use a full range of motion when stretching
- Do hold each stretch for 15-30 seconds and complete at least one stretch for each major muscle group
- Do stretch both sides of your body or joint
- Do perform flexibility and balance exercises 2-3 times per week
- Do breathe deeply during each stretch to relax your muscles and increase oxygen flow
- Don't bounce while performing exercises–it can tear muscles and injure the joints
- Don't stretch to the point of pain or extreme discomfort

Here are a few stretches you may perform. Perform the following stretches on each side of the body 3-5 times each with a 10-second hold:

- Hamstring Stretch
- Quad Stretch
- Chest Stretch
- Shoulder Stretch
- Calf Stretch
- Lower Back Stretch

The PreDiabetes Center personal trainer may recommend that you perform this balance exercise for 30 seconds 3-5 times on each leg:

- Single-Leg Balance

Advancing Your Fitness Regimen

Your personal trainer will re-evaluate your level of fitness and determine your progress in the Personalized Fitness Plan approximately 60 days after beginning your fitness regimen.

Based on your progress and comfort level, you will move forward to an advanced fitness regimen, called phase II, or stay in your current regimen. The goal of phase II is to increase the intensity of the workouts and add interval training to your fitness plan. Recent studies have shown that exercising at a higher intensity can help make the body more sensitive to insulin.

Advanced Cardiovascular Exercise

Increase to 10,000 steps per day (5 miles) at least 5 days a week or more. To advance your fitness regimen, you will add interval training to your workout. Interval training is a simple form of exercise that alternates bursts of intense activity with intervals of lighter activity. You can perform any type of exercise when interval training: walking, biking, jogging, rowing, or any other cardiovascular activity of your choice. Just make sure you regularly increase the intensity throughout the workout. For example, if you're taking a walk, incorporate short bursts of fast walking or jogging. Repeat this sequence at regular intervals and try to increase the amount of time you spend at this faster pace. You'll notice that your stamina increases and you are able to walk longer distances without tiring.

Advanced Strength Training

To intensify your strength training, your trainer will increase the weight of the resistance or tension of the resistance bands. You will move to more complex exercises that target all major muscle groups, including the arms, shoulders, back, chest, abdominals, buttocks, and upper and lower legs. Your workout should be moderate to vigorous, and the last set you complete should be somewhat difficult. For recovery, rest for 2-5 minutes between each exercise.

Here are a few exercises you may perform:

- Traveling Lunge
- Triceps Dip
- Push-Up (progression)
- Overhead Chop
- Straight-Leg Raises (lying face-up on mat)

As you get stronger, you can increase the amount of weight lifted or increase the intensity of each session. Go slow and make sure you continue to use correct form.

Beginner workout:
Three days a week, perform 4 sets (11 reps of each exercise) of one circuit

Intermediate workout:
Three days a week, perform 4 sets (11 reps of each exercise) of one circuit

Advanced workout:
Three days a week, perform 4 sets (11 reps of each exercise every 90 seconds) of one circuit

Advanced Core Strength

To increase your core strength, you will perform a core workout twice a week, one day focusing on rotation and the other day focusing on resistance to rotation.

Here are a few exercises you may perform:

- Side Touches or Russian Twists
- Ins and Outs
- Crunches on stability ball
- Single-Leg Stretch
- Side Kicks
- Plank (progression)

Beginner workout:
Twice a week, perform 4 sets (11 reps of each exercise)

Intermediate workout:
Twice a week, perform 4 sets (11 reps of each exercise)

Advanced workout:
Twice a week, perform 4 sets (11 reps of each exercise every 90 seconds)

Advanced Balance and Flexibility

Your personal trainer will add additional exercises to increase your balance and flexibility. You will learn how to perform gentle exercises that stretch your muscles. Many of these exercises are performed in Pilates, yoga and tai chi. These moves should be for at least 5-10 minutes three or more days per week. Perform each exercise slowly and deliberately to maximize your results.

Many find balance and flexibility routines enjoyable and relaxing. Stress reduction is often experienced when you allow yourself to relax and breathe deeply through each exercise.

Here are a few exercises you may perform:

- Triceps Stretch
- Doorway Shoulder Stretch
- Outer Hip Stretch
- Leg Hover Step-Up
- Closed-Eyes Single-Leg Balance

Your Weekly Workout Schedule

Need help scheduling the different types of exercise? Use this weekly fitness schedule to help keep you on track!

Monday:	Cardio / Strength
Tuesday:	Core / Balance & Flexibility
Wednesday:	Cardio / Strength
Thursday:	Core / Balance & Flexibility
Friday:	Cardio / Strength
Saturday:	Cardio / Balance & Flexibility
Sunday:	Cardio

A New Lifelong Healthy Habit

Maintaining a lifetime fitness habit can be a challenge. Exercise often falls to the bottom of our to-do list. We tend to focus on reasons why we can't exercise. "I don't have time," "I'm overweight," "I'm in pain," and "I'm not in the mood" are just a few of the excuses we give ourselves. Here's the bottom line: You must set aside time to exercise and follow through on it, no matter what.

Consciously focusing on the benefits of exercise will help you turn fitness into a lifelong habit. Be sure to discuss any concerns you may have about your fitness regimen with your health coach or PreDiabetes Centers physician. They're here to assist you as you improve your health and empower yourself to live a fit, healthy life.

As a bonus, we've rounded up top exercises that your personal trainer may ask you to perform. In the pages that follow, we explain how to do them correctly and offer modified versions of exercises that might be difficult to perform. Remember, your health team members are committed to your success. Reach out to them immediately if you have any trouble adhering to your Personalized Fitness Plan.

Push-Up

Push-ups can help build your chest muscles, including your pectoral minor and major. If you have trouble performing a traditional push-up, do a modified push-up with your knees on the floor. Or, perform the push-up standing up while facing a wall; simply push away from the wall with your hands.

1 Place your hands on the floor so they are slightly wider than shoulder-width apart and point your fingers forward. Rise up on your toes with your legs and back straight. Press up to the starting position keeping your abs tight.

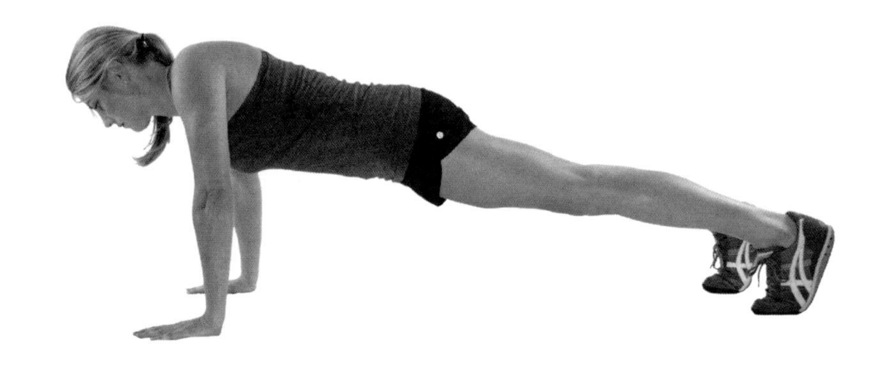

2 Bend your elbows and lower your chest toward the floor. Push your body back to the starting position.

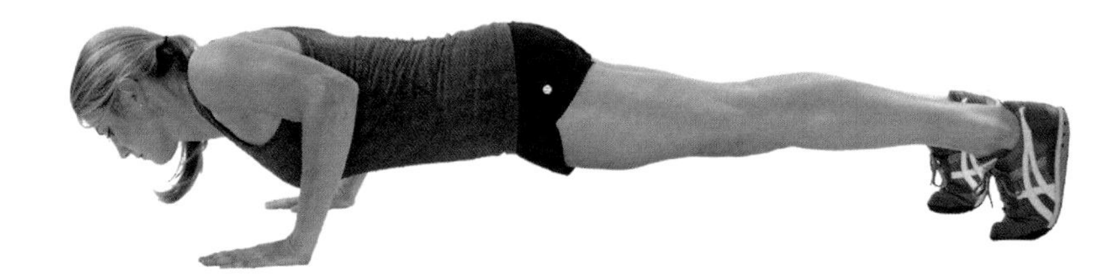

Seated Row with Resistance Band

1 Sit on the floor and wrap the resistance band around your feet in front of you. Extend your legs, keeping your knees together and slightly bent. Hold the resistance band with both hands and extend your arms in front of you with the palms facing each other.

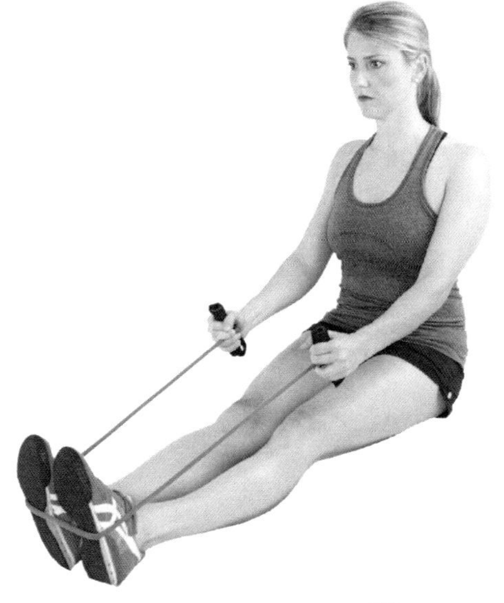

2 Pull the elbows in towards the torso in a rowing motion. Keep your shoulders relaxed. Return to the starting position.

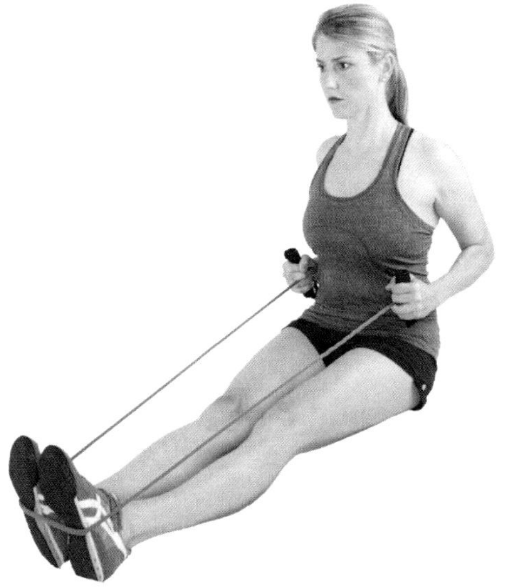

Lying Triceps Extension

1 Lie on your back with knees bent and feet flat on the floor. Grip two equally weighted dumbbells and extend your arms straight above your chest, with the dumbbell shaft in the horizontal position.

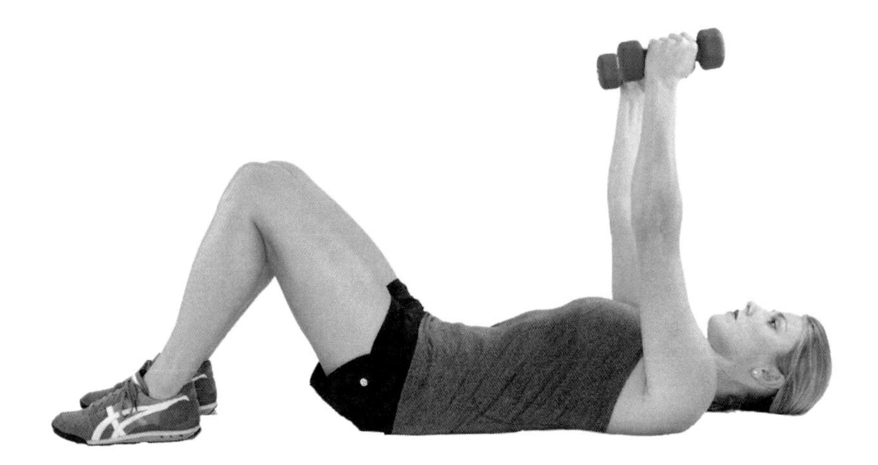

2 Take a breath, bend your elbows and lower the weights towards the back of your head until the dumbbell heads are about an inch from the floor, or the lowest point that is comfortable for you. Exhale and lift the dumbbells back to the starting position.

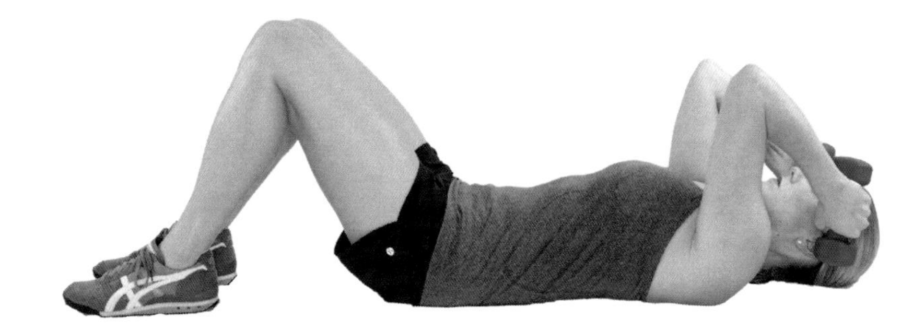

Dumbbell Biceps Curl

This exercise, which works your biceps, should be done in a calm, fluid motion. Try not to move your shoulders, hips, legs, or back when performing this exercise.

1. Hold a pair of dumbbells and stand or sit with your feet shoulder-width apart. Relax your knees and let the dumbbells rest in front of your thighs.

2. Bend your elbows and curl the weights up to shoulder level. Hold for 3 seconds and return to the starting position.

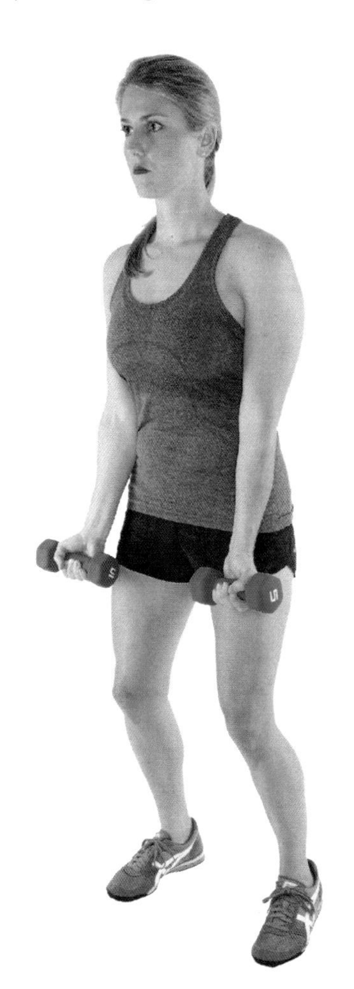

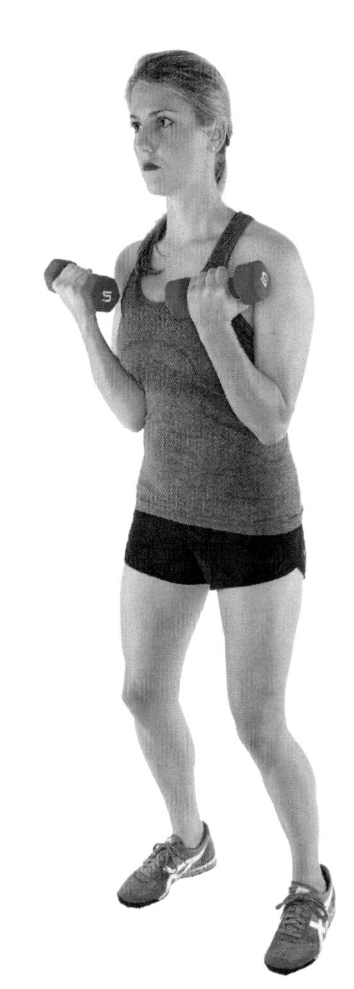

Squat

Squats help build several muscles in your legs, including your quadriceps, hamstrings and buttocks. When performing a squat, don't bend at your lower back; try to keep your back straight.

1 Stand with your feet shoulder-width apart and bend your knees. Keep your weight back on your heels, not on the balls of your feet. Extend your arms straight out in front of you.

2 Push your hips back and slowly squat down. Continue lowering until your knees are at a 90-degree angle, keeping your knees behind the toes. Hold for 3 seconds. Push through your heels and return to the starting position.

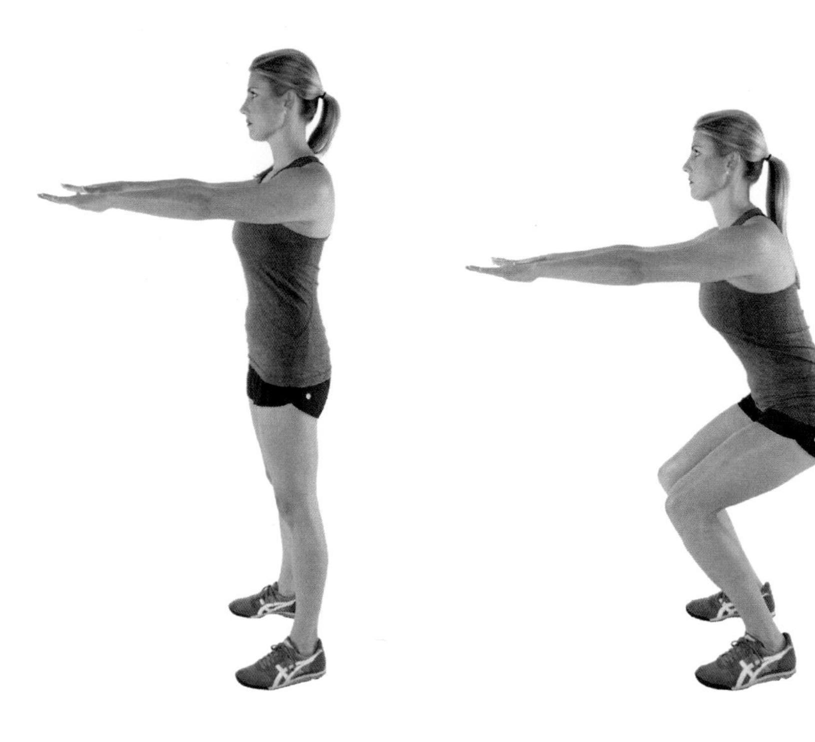

Open Clamshell (Side-Lying Hip Abduction)

1 Lie on your side with your legs stacked one on top of the other. Tuck your knees forward about 45 degrees. Rest one hand on the floor in front of you and use the other hand to support your head.

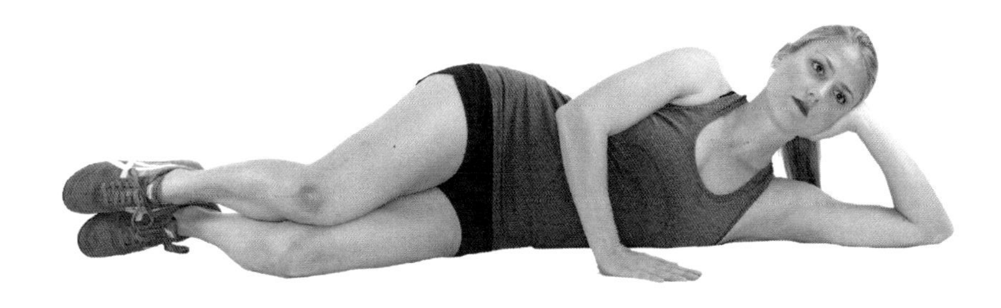

2 Exhale as you slowly lift the top knee up, keeping your toes and heels stacked. Your legs should look like an open clamshell. Do not allow your pelvis to rotate. Inhale as you close your legs and return to the starting position.

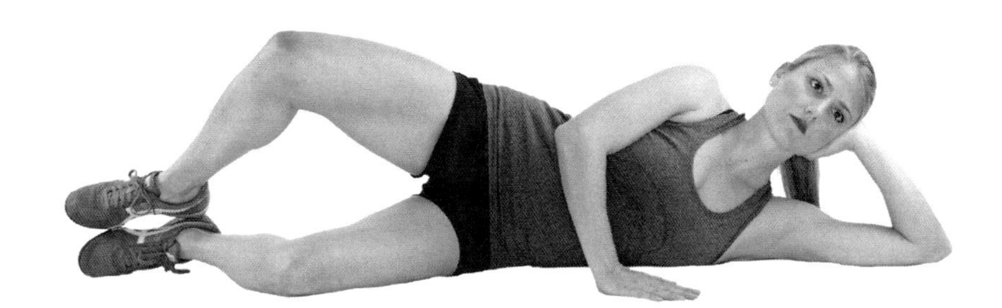

Short Crunch

1 Lying on your back, place the feet flat on the floor with knees bent at a 45-degree angle. Lift the arms off the ground, keeping them parallel to the torso.

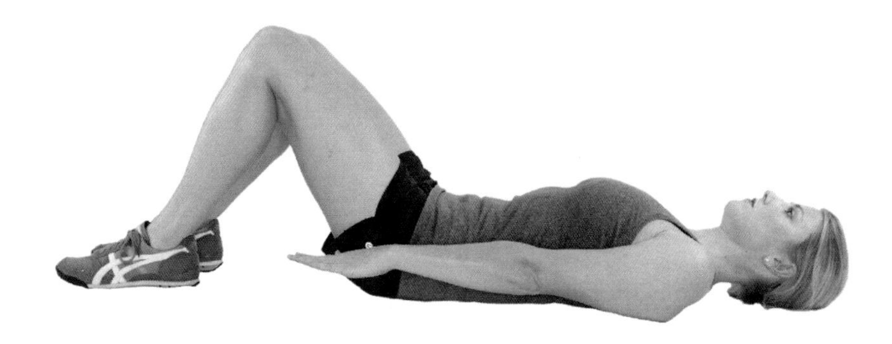

2 Push your chest and head up towards the ceiling, pushing your lower back flat onto the floor. Keep your head and neck in line with the spine. Don't let your chin touch your chest. Return to the starting position.

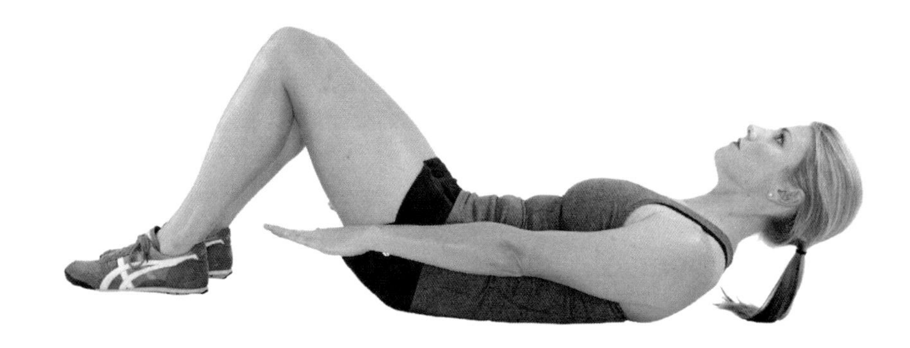

"V" Sit-Up

1 Sit on the floor with your arms slightly behind you, elbows bent, palms down and fingers pointed toward your body. Extend your legs out, keeping your knees together, and raise your heels off the ground.

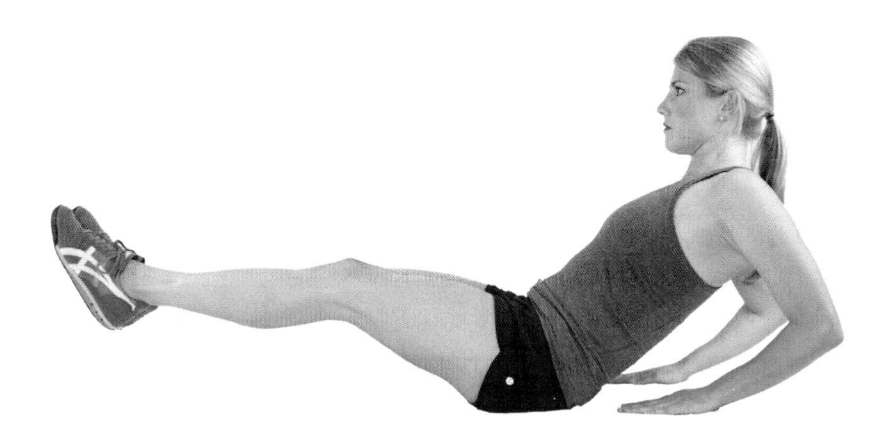

2 Pull your knees into your chest and create a "V" with your upper legs and torso, keeping your heels elevated. Hold for 3 seconds. Return to starting position.

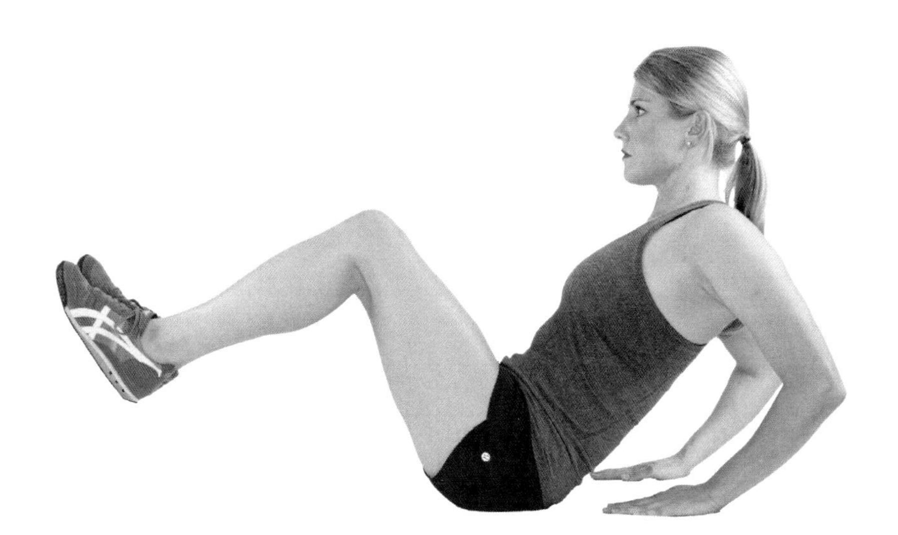

Plank

The Plank builds strength in your abdominal and hip muscles. If it's difficult for you to perform, modify the exercise by resting your knees on the mat.

1 Lie face down on an exercise mat. Raise your chest so that only your forearms and toes touch the floor. Make sure your elbows are directly under your shoulders. Keep your torso straight and your body in a straight line from ears to heels with no sagging or bending. Your head should be relaxed and you should be looking at the floor.

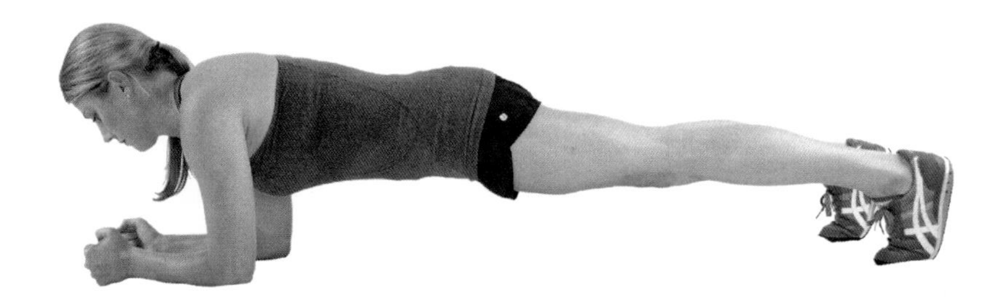

Hold the position for up to 20 seconds to start.

Russian Twist

1 Sit on the floor with your knees bent and feet together. Keeping your feet flat on the floor, hold your arms straight in front of you with your fingers intertwined.

Lean back approximately 45 degrees and twist side to side.

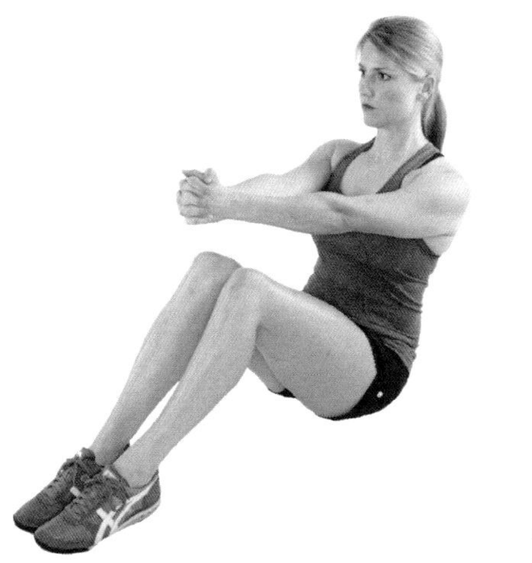

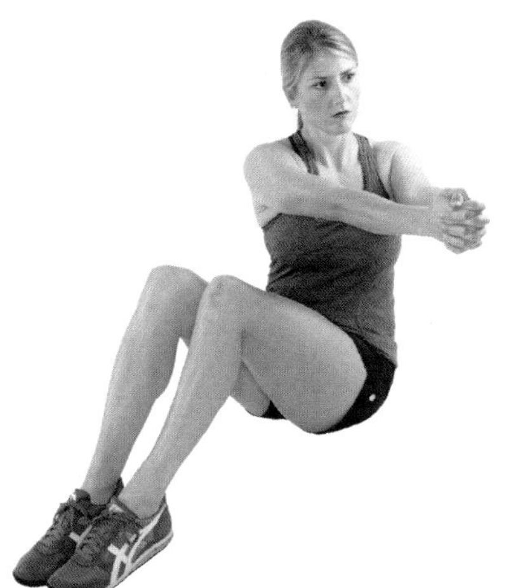

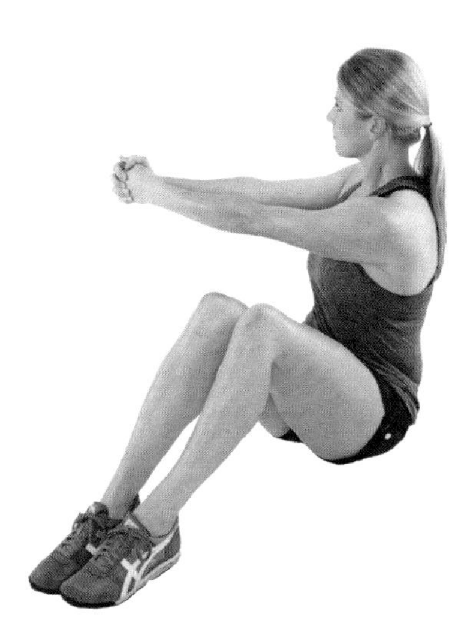

Lying Bridge

1. Lie on your back with arms by your sides, palms down. Keep your knees bent and feet flat on the floor under your knees. Tighten your abdominal and buttock muscles.

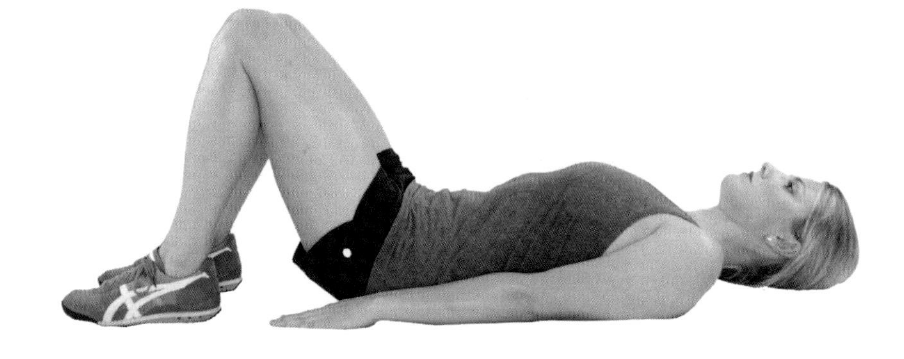

2. Raise your hips to create a straight line from your knees to your shoulders. Squeeze your core and try to pull your belly button toward your spine. Hold for 20-30 seconds. Return to the starting position.

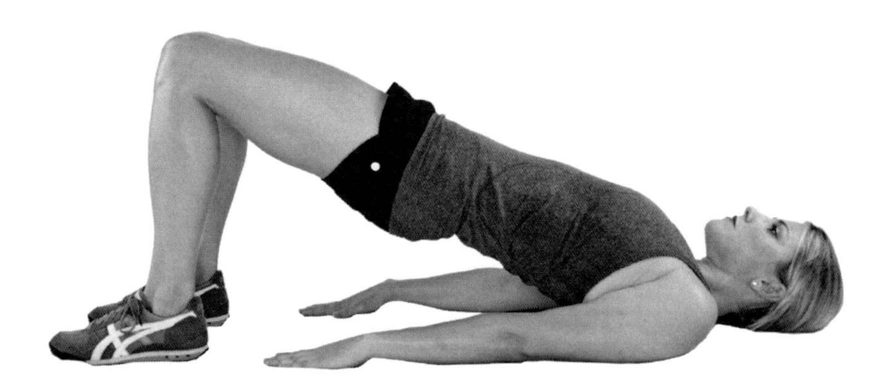

Single-Leg Plank

If you can perform a regular plank for 20 seconds, then you're ready for the Single-Leg Plank.

1 Lie face down on an exercise mat. Raise your chest so that only your forearms and toes touch the floor. Make sure your elbows are directly under your shoulders. Keep your torso and body in a straight line from ears to toes with no sagging or bending. Your head should be relaxed and you should be looking at the floor.

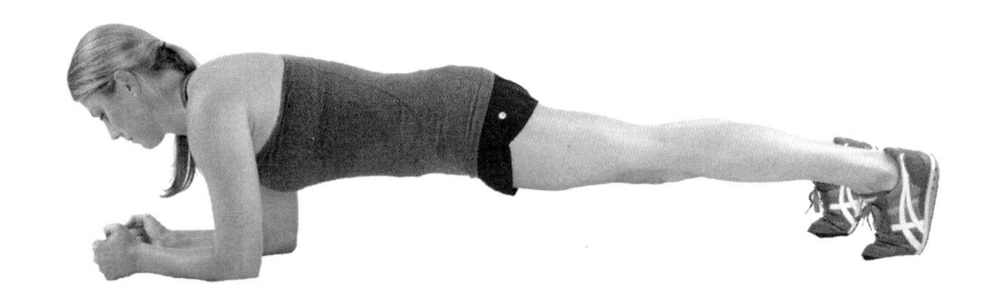

2 Raise one leg a few inches off the floor and hold the plank for up to 20 seconds. Lower leg back to the floor and repeat with the other leg.

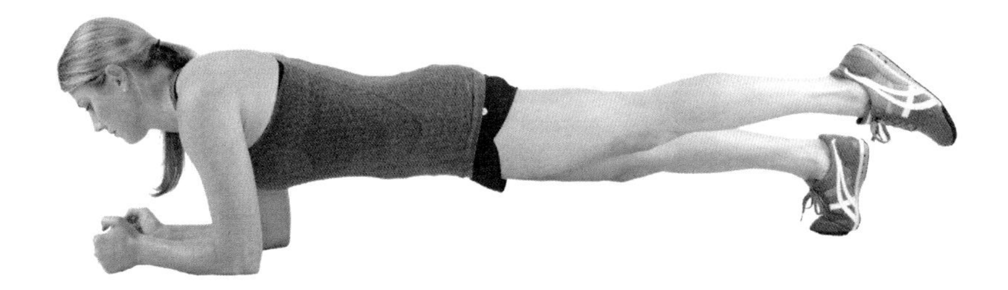

Wide-Legged Forward Bend

1 From a standing position, place the feet shoulder-width apart with legs straight and knees locked.

2 Reach the hands gently toward the toes. Be sure not to bounce. Return to the starting position.

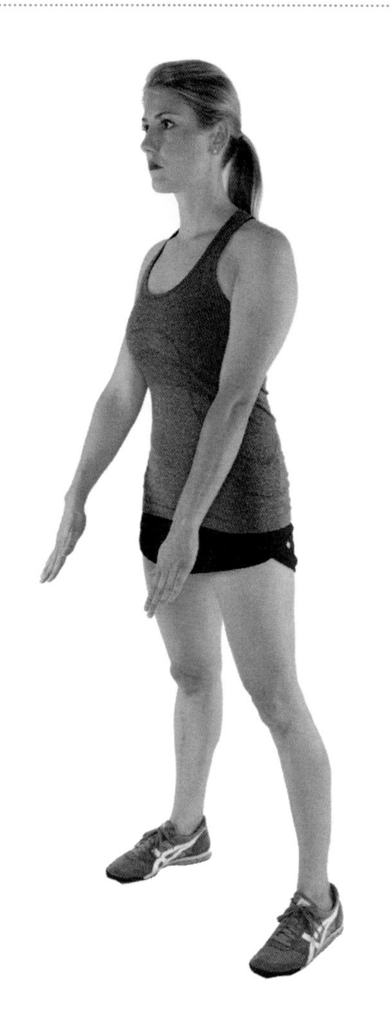

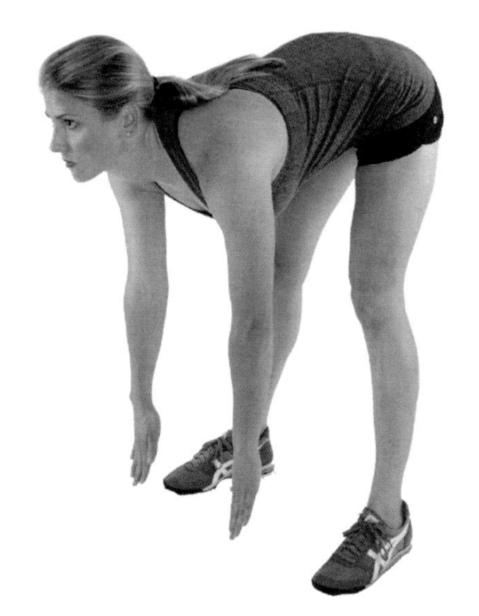

Standing Quad Stretch

1. Stand and touch the wall or a stationary object for balance. Grasp the top of the left foot with your left hand and pull it toward the buttocks.

2. Hold for 10 seconds. Repeat with right leg.

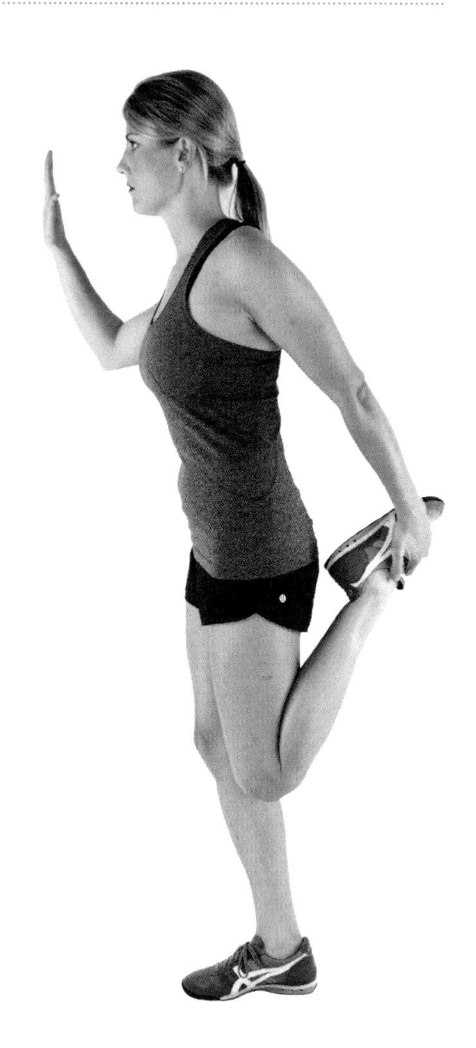

Total Back Stretch

Kneel on a mat and sit on your heels.

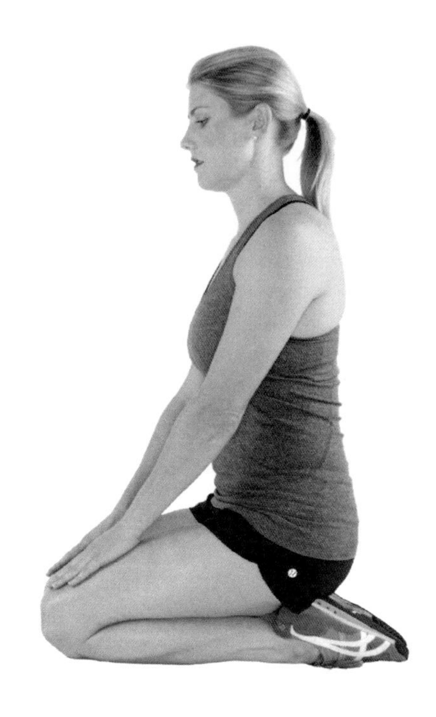

2 Extend your arms out as far as you can reach. Lean forward and plant your hands on the floor with palms down. Tuck your head toward your chest and keep your elbows and forehead off the mat and your hips close to your heels.

Breathe deeply and hold position for 15-30 seconds.

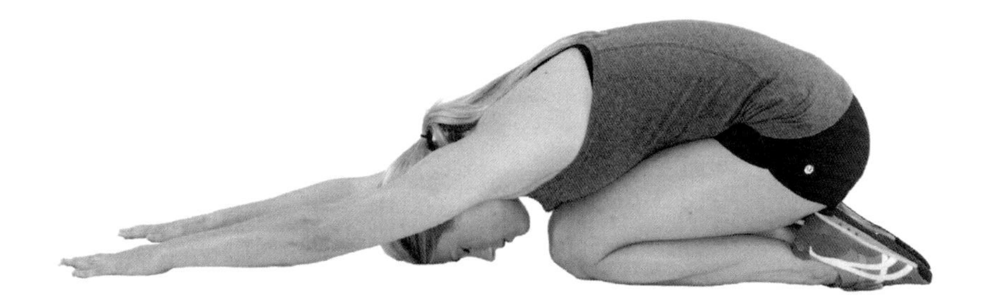

Sleep and
Stress

Sleep and Stress

Chapter 15

The Connection Between Sleep and Prediabetes

A good night's rest is vital to your health. It boosts your immunity and promotes physical and mental health, and also plays an important role in the development of prediabetes.

Getting adequate sleep is key to reversing the prediabetes process. Lack of sleep can prevent your body from using glucose for energy and result in high blood sugar, which raises risk for diabetes. One study shows that people who suffer from sleep deprivation (less than 6 hours of sleep per night) were almost five times more likely to progress from normal blood sugar levels to impaired fasting glucose, compared to people who sleep for 6-8 hours a night. That's why it's important for you to get good sleep–it'll help prevent the development of diabetes.

Your prediabetes team will examine your sleep habits and identify whether you have a sleep disorder, such as obstructive sleep apnea, or another health condition that is causing loss of sleep. You will answer questions about the quality of your sleep several times throughout the program, including during meetings with your health coach and physician. Learning more about your sleep patterns will help your prediabetes team develop a more personalized treatment plan.

Experts say that most adults need 7-8 hours of sleep a night for good health. However, some people are "short sleepers" and need 6 or fewer hours of sleep a night. "Long sleepers" require 9 or more hours of sleep to feel well-rested.

It's not just the quantity of sleep that matters–the quality of sleep is important too. Each stage in the sleep cycle has benefits, but deep sleep is vital to your health. Deep sleep, also known as the slow-wave, non-REM stage of sleep, can last for about 90 minutes to 2 hours, and helps the body repair and regenerate tissues, builds bone and muscle, and strengthens the immune system.

Here's the question you have to ask yourself, "Are my sleep habits making me feel exhausted and unable to function properly throughout the day?"

If you're tired throughout the day, then you are most likely not getting enough sleep.

Sleep affects just about every aspect of our health:

- ***Emotional health.*** Lack of sleep can cause you to become more irritable and decreases your ability to cope with stress.
- ***Intellectual health.*** Sleep loss affects cognition and is linked to dementia. Your ability to make crucial judgments may be impaired.
- ***Immunity.*** The cumulative effect of not getting enough sleep makes you more vulnerable to illness.
- ***Energy levels.*** Fatigue and loss of motivation are common side effects.
- ***Motor skill impairment.*** This is especially dangerous when driving or operating machinery.

Loss of sleep every once in a while is not that harmful. But chronic sleep loss causes a big sleep deficit that reduces your body's ability to cope with emotional and physical stressors.

Types of Sleep Disorders

Insomnia is a serious sleep disorder that can sap your energy level and hurt your health. Studies show that insomnia can lead to insulin resistance and raise your risk for diabetes. People with insomnia have difficulty falling asleep and staying asleep, and usually wake in the morning feeling unrefreshed.

Insomnia generally falls into two categories: sleep-onset insomnia, which occurs when a person has difficulty falling asleep at bedtime, and sleep-maintenance insomnia, when a person wakes up and cannot fall back asleep. Some people suffer from both types of insomnia.

Insomnia can cause daytime sleepiness and impaired performance at work. One study reports that people with insomnia who slept for 5 or fewer hours had the highest risk of diabetes. Insomniacs who slept for 5-6 hours also had an elevated risk of diabetes.

Half of insomnia cases are attributable, at least in part, to psychological factors including stress, depression and anxiety.

Sleep apnea is another sleep condition. It's characterized by breathing that repeatedly stops and starts during sleep, with episodes of breathing cessation lasting 10 seconds or as long as 2-3 minutes. Often, people don't know they have the condition because it occurs during sleep, causing them to awaken repeatedly during the night and experience excessive daytime sleepiness. Chronic snoring may be a sign of the condition. The condition is more common in men, older or overweight people and women with polycystic ovary syndrome (PCOS). A sleep apnea diagnosis puts a person at higher risk of cardiovascular disease, since the cessation in breathing causes oxygen levels in the blood to drop, which makes the heart work harder.

Sleep apnea is the most common type of sleep disordered breathing (SDB), which is linked to decreased insulin sensitivity and other prediabetic conditions. One study showed that SDB was strongly associated with a decrease in the three major metabolic pathways that the body uses to metabolize glucose: insulin sensitivity, glucose effectiveness and pancreatic cell function.

If your physician finds you are at risk for sleep apnea or if you have previously been diagnosed with sleep apnea, it will be recommended that you consult with a Sleep Specialist for further evaluation. Those findings and recommended treatments will be incorporated into your PreDiabetes Centers treatment plan.

Research shows that women with PCOS who also suffer from obstructive sleep apnea are at least three times more likely to develop prediabetes, compared to women without the condition. Scientists believe that the low progesterone levels seen with PCOS may contribute to obstructive sleep apnea. Also, lower levels of the female hormone progesterone can cause higher blood sugar levels, according to research.

Health Problems Associated with Sleep Loss

There are medical disorders that have close ties to sleep problems. Many of these disorders coexist with prediabetes, such as cardiovascular disease. Too little sleep has been linked to high blood pressure and may contribute to calcium deposits in the arteries. Poor sleep can also promote inflammation and is linked to both cardiovascular disease and diabetes. Chronic sleep problems can also be related to depression and anxiety.

Lack of sleep may lead to weight gain and obesity. Loss of sleep can cause your body to make more of the hormone ghrelin, which signals your brain to eat more, and make less of the hormone leptin, which tells your body to stop eating. In response to sleep deprivation, your body may also produce more cortisol, which can increase your appetite. Sleep loss can also compromise judgment and willpower, leaving us more vulnerable to making poor food choices and overeating.

Conditions like leg cramps, allergies, and restless legs syndrome are health conditions that may be linked to sleeplessness. Other disorders may be impairing your ability to get a good night's sleep without your knowledge, such as periodic limb movement and grinding teeth. A sleep disorder, such as insomnia, could also be a sign of medical problems related to kidney or thyroid health. People with prediabetes are at greater risk for these conditions, which are screened in the comprehensive initial lab testing.

Periodic limb movements (PLM) may cause sleep problems too. The condition occurs when your arms and/or legs twitch or jerk, with episodes lasting from a few minutes to several hours. This not a harmful condition but it may disrupt your sleep. More often than not, you are unaware of these PLMs as the twitch occurs while you are still asleep. A possible sign of this condition is finding your sheets and blankets in disarray in the morning.

Many individuals who experience PLM also have restless-legs syndrome (RLS), characterized by a crawling or tingling sensation deep within the leg muscles, causing a powerful urge to move the legs. The leg discomfort makes it difficult to fall asleep. Scientists are not entirely certain what causes this disorder, but treatment is available. The combination of stress and obesity may put you at risk for another potentially sleep-stealing condition called gastroesophageal reflux disease (GERD). Most people who suffer from GERD experience a burning sensation in their upper chest, sometimes in the middle of the night. However, some people may have the disorder and never experience symptoms. If you think GERD may be a problem for you, try sleeping with your head elevated and discuss the possible use of medication with your physician.

Techniques to Improve Your Sleep

PreDiabetes Centers will create a customized approach to help you address the particular sleep problem you might be facing.

Having a regular bedtime schedule is vital to getting good sleep. An irregular sleep pattern can disrupt sleep. It seems logical to want to stay in bed longer after a poor night's sleep, but sleeping late actually makes it harder to fall asleep at bedtime. Conversely, going to bed early to catch up on sleep can also backfire. Ideally, you should pick a time to go to sleep and a time to wake, and then stay within a half hour of those times.

It's also important to use your bed for sleep. And if you can't sleep, get out of bed.

Create a sleep-friendly environment.

Light is an important stimulant to keep you awake during the day, and lack of light tells your body it's time to sleep. When we are exposed to bright light, particularly sunlight, our body's production of the hormone melatonin slows down thereby promoting wakefulness. The absence of light increases melatonin levels and helps gear the brain's internal clock towards sleep.

Create an Optimal Sleep Environment

- Keep your bedroom dark and the temperature cool—between 60°and 66°F.
- Ban electronic devices (cell phone, computer, tablet) from the bedroom.
- Invest in quality bedding, replacing pillows every year and the mattress every 7 years. Wash your sheets often.
- For many, a time-free bedroom environment equals a stress-free environment. If you need an alarm clock, place it out of sight.

It is not uncommon for people who suffer from sleep disturbance to remain indoors during much of the day, working in rooms without windows. This promotes a feeling of drowsiness during the day. Try to get outside in natural sunlight for at least 30 minutes each day, and get a good night's rest in a dark environment.

Electronics is another sleep-stealer. Many people use electronic devices in the evening, when the darkness of night is supposed to be signaling the brain to downshift toward dreamland. Research shows that the light from electronics like laptops, tablets and cell phones can prevent your body from producing melatonin, especially handheld devices, which are held close to the face and emit a larger amount of light into the eyes. The American Medical Association recommends avoiding exposure to excessive light at night, including extended use of some electronic devices to prevent disruption of sleep or further worsening of sleep disorders, especially in children and adolescents.

Don't worry, watching television before bedtime is fine. Television tends to be a passive activity, unlike other forms of electronic media–such as playing games or reading engrossing texts, e-mails or blogs–that are more stimulating.

Change your thoughts about sleep.

It is not uncommon for people with sleep problems to lie awake in bed, frustrated that they're unable to fall asleep. You cannot "force" sleep to come. Often, the harder you try to snooze, the harder it becomes to fall asleep. If you are unable to fall asleep within 20-30 minutes, don't continue to lie in bed. Instead, go to another room and engage in a relaxing activity until you feel drowsy, then return to bed. Reading a book, listening to soothing music or playing a repetitive game like Sodoku are a few activities that can help induce sleep.

Negative thoughts is another sleep-stealer. Many people form irrational thoughts about sleep–they tell themselves "I'm never going to fall asleep" or "If I don't fall asleep right now, I'll be a wreck tomorrow." Negative sleep thoughts and worrying before bedtime cause stress and can make falling asleep even more difficult, if not impossible.

Your health coach and physician will ask you questions about your attitude toward sleep. Assessing and correcting bad habits and false beliefs that contribute to sleep problems, called sleep hygiene education, can be a powerful ally in your treatment plan.

How do you counteract these negative thoughts and deal with the anxiety that frequently accompanies restless nights?

You have to change your sleep attitude! Formulate positive thoughts when you're lying in bed and keep your mind focused on activities not related to sleep. Think about a relaxing vacation you took or an enjoyable movie you recently watched. Occupying your mind with positive thoughts can help you doze off much faster.

Relaxation techniques can also help. To learn ways to relax, see Chapter 16.

Stress less.
Many sleep problems are caused by stress. Your responses to stress throughout the day may feel effective, but once you hit the sheets stress can consume your mind and body. Stress hormones, especially cortisol, are elevated earlier in the day and help you respond to the truckload of daily responsibilities. The levels of these hormones are supposed to decrease later in the day as you approach bedtime, but when faced with chronic stress these hormones can remain elevated at night.

To reduce the odds of bedtime stress, avoid thinking about workplace dilemmas, engaging in heated debates or watching an adrenaline-pumping movie. Wind down with a serene nighttime ritual. Watching TV or reading a book can help relax you before bed. And be sure to practice relaxation techniques during the day and at night before bed.

Exercise regularly.
Regular exercise also makes it easier to get a good night's sleep. It helps you manage stress and promotes feelings of relaxation and overall well-being. A warning: Don't exercise within 3 hours of bedtime—it can raise your body temperature and cause alertness, making it more difficult to fall asleep. Before you jump in the sack, try stretching, meditation and gentle yoga instead.

Factors Contributing to Insomnia

Stress
Depression
Anxiety
Hormone imbalance
Pain
Snoring
Diet
Smoking
Alcohol use
Poor sleep habits
Nightmares/night terrors
Leg cramps
Indigestion
Allergies
Restless-legs syndrome
Frequent urination during the night
Sleep apnea
Teeth grinding
Sleepwalking

Avoid tobacco and limit consumption of alcohol and caffeine.

Smoking is not just bad for your health, it also robs you of sleep! The nicotine in tobacco is a stimulant, raising blood pressure, speeding up heart rate, and keeping the mind wired. Smokers often experience difficulty falling asleep and even wake up in the middle of night due to withdrawal symptoms.

Many people use alcohol as a way to unwind and help them sleep, but it actually can prevent you from getting a good night's rest. Alcohol invokes a lighter sleep pattern and suppresses deep, restorative sleep. Doctors advise limiting yourself to one drink at least two hours before bedtime.

Caffeinated drinks may also contribute to sleep loss. People who suffer from sleeplessness or insomnia usually feel tired during the day because of lack of sleep and turn to caffeine to wake up. This can perpetuate an unhealthy cycle of caffeine-loading and sleeplessness.

Drinking caffeinated beverages early in the day is fine, but avoid drinking them later in the day.

What about energy drinks? These caffeine bombs contain large amounts of caffeine and sugar and can make you feel anxious, jittery and tired at the same time. Plus, the sugarload in these drinks will cause blood glucose levels to spike-which is exactly what you're trying to avoid as a prediabetic.

If you're addicted to energy drinks or any other form of caffeine, aim to cut back on these drinks gradually. You will find that your ability to fall asleep—and stay asleep—will improve.

How to Cut Back on Sleep-Stealing Beverages

- Avoid all caffeinated beverages after noon.
- Enjoy a cup of hot herbal tea an hour before bedtime. Chamomile is an excellent choice to promote relaxation and sleepiness.
- Avoid alcohol after dinner. Alcohol can initially make you sleepy, but when the depressive effect wears off, it can actually wake you up.

Take supplements.

Melatonin supplements also promote sleep by regulating the sleep-wake cycle. Melatonin, which is produced in the body in response to darkness, helps prepare the body for sleep. Melatonin is a major ingredient in the PreD Restful Nights nutraceutical, along with the sleep-promoting amino acids taurine, theanine, 5HTP, and GABA.

Eat nutritiously.

A balanced dietary plan is vital for a good night's sleep. This plan should not include eating large, heavy meals late in the evening. Snacking until bedtime can also contribute to sleep problems. These habits make your digestive system work hard and can keep you awake during the night.

Ask your doctor about prescription medication.

PreDiabetes Centers promotes a natural, customized approach for the prevention of diabetes. However, we do understand that some clients may have extenuating health needs that require pharmaceutical intervention. Prescription sleep medication can be an excellent short-term treatment for sleeplessness or insomnia. Your PreDiabetes Centers team can determine whether a prescription sleep aid is right for you.

Sleep Well Every Night

With guidance from your health coach and physician, you should be on the road to better sleep habits. For some, sleeplessness has been a long-term problem and will not go away quickly. It may take several weeks for sleep to improve. In combination with a nutritious diet and vigorous exercise routine, enhanced sleep habits will help you get better quality sleep and boost your overall wellness.

7 Tips for Better Sleep

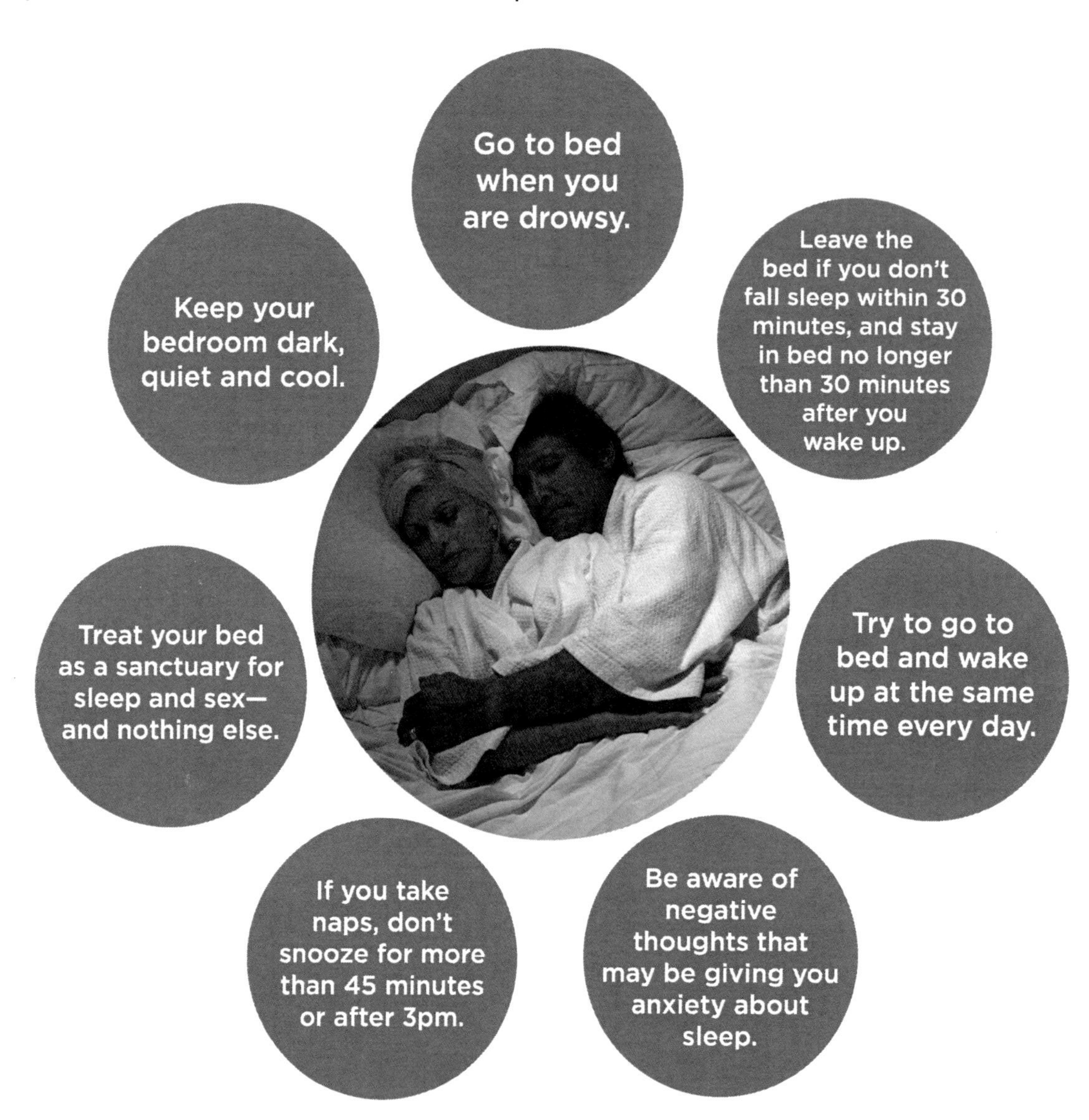

Chapter 16

The Stress and Prediabetes Link

Stress can affect your body, mind and behavior. Physical or mental stress stimulates the nervous system, a network of nerves that manages and controls the body's reaction to stress. Both acute and chronic stress have significant effects on our bodies. Unmanaged stress leads to low energy levels and decreased motivation to exercise and eat nutritiously, which has a negative impact on your health. Experts agree that reducing chronic stress can help prevent the onset of chronic diseases.

Stress management, a key part of the PATHFinder program, is critical to warding off diabetes. Your treatment plan includes an emphasis on pinpointing stressors, successful relaxation techniques, and stress-eating response education.

So how does stress affect processes in the body? Here's how it works: The autonomic nervous system is comprised of the sympathetic nervous system, which activates the fight-or-flight system in response to stress, and the parasympathetic system, the division that is responsible for stimulation of "feed and breed" activities that occur when the body is at rest. The two systems work in opposition to each other. When a person experiences stress, the body works overtime to help the body cope. The sympathetic system reacts and releases hormones—including adrenaline, epinephrine and cortisol—to give you added energy and concentration. Adrenaline breaks down stored glucose, releasing it into the bloodstream, resulting in higher blood glucose levels. Cortisol decreases the ability of insulin to function normally. This makes insulin resistance worse, especially in people with prediabetes.

Stress may also cause emotional eating and, consequently, weight gain, which can contribute to the development of diabetes. During times of stress, people often turn to foods that are high in "bad" fats, simple sugars and low in fiber.

Reactions to external stressors can lead to feelings of anxiety or depression and can impair your ability to take care of yourself. Stress may lead to other unhealthy behaviors, such as smoking, which is linked to poor blood glucose control and increased risk for diabetes-related complications.

Stress can promote other activities that heighten your risk of prediabetes. It can cause you to:

- Stop exercising
- Use poor judgment
- Stop eating nutritiously
- Avoid contact with others who can provide help

In addition to releasing hormones, your body also releases glucose from your liver, muscles and stored fat reserves. Stressful stimuli may also spike blood glucose levels through several different hypothalamic pituitary pathways. Cortisol causes enhanced glucose production by the liver and diminished cellular glucose uptake. This mechanism may lead to both obesity and a predisposition to diabetes if individuals are exposed to chronic stress. Stress-induced release of growth hormone and beta-endorphin can also decrease glucose uptake, suppress insulin secretion and elevate glucose levels.

Glucocorticoids are "stress" hormones produced by the adrenal glands. They affect glucose metabolism and are involved with inflammatory, cardiovascular and behavioral processes. Cortisol is an essential hormone that protects and prepares the body for daily challenges. It's the principal active glucocorticoid in humans and is released when the brain senses stress or tissue demand.

Excessive stress has significant effects on the body. It causes an overproduction of glucose in our liver and signals the body to retain more blood sugar in the circulation.

Chronic stress also affects the metabolism of carbohydrates. With chronic stress, cortisol levels can be elevated or high-normal. In a normal sleep-wake cycle, cortisol levels are most elevated after waking up in the morning, as the hormone helps get the body going and prepare for the day. Cortisol levels tend to decline as the day progresses. (Cortisol is usually measured in a blood test in the morning.)

Elevated cortisol levels are a precursor for insulin resistance and prediabetes. The chronic stress release of this hormone can start a vicious cycle: Cortisol stimulates glucose production, salt retention and triglyceride production. Excess glucose is typically converted into fat, which ends up as stored fat. These fat cells are dysfunctional and begin releasing inflammatory hormones that tell the body to eat more. A person will then increase caloric intake, produce more fat cells and eventually develop the full features of metabolic syndrome–insulin resistance, obesity, elevated lipids, and hypertension.

Types of Stress

Stress can occur in several forms. Life stress, or major stress, is triggered by life events and can include marriage, divorce, death, the birth of a baby, or job loss. Daily stress results from ongoing unresolved situations. Also known as chronic stress, daily stress can include feeling stuck in a bad job or marriage.

Stressful situations and events can also be thought of as changeable or unchangeable. Changeable stressors can be rectified and may include a stressful daily commute or ongoing financial stress. Death and natural disasters are examples of unchangeable stressors.

Each person is unique and has different symptoms and intensity of stress. Signs of stress can include:

Physical: Jaw clenching, teeth grinding, sweating, increased heart rate, headache, rapid and shallow breathing, oversleeping, undersleeping, fatigue, increased infections, gastrointestinal symptoms such as diarrhea or constipation, a flare-up of existing diseases (high blood pressure, acne, eczema, irritable bowel syndrome)

Emotional: Nervousness, depression, feeling overwhelmed or trapped, sadness, irritability, moodiness, anger, frustration, feeling hopeless

Behavioral: Overeating, undereating, binge eating, increased use of alcohol or drugs, increased or decreased physical activity, increased smoking, reckless behavior

Cognitive: Worrying, obsessive thoughts, anxiety, decreased ability to concentrate or make decisions, poor judgment

Coping with Stress

Stress is the interaction between an event or situation and our perception of it. It is not so much the event, but rather the interpretation of the event that determines our stress level.

The perception and interpretation of stress is dependent on two variables: a person's thinking style and explanatory style, the way in which a person explains events experienced in his or her life. People who have a rigid, inflexible or pessimistic thinking style are more vulnerable to stress.

Long ago, our ancestors developed the ability to respond quickly to threats by discharging the fight-or-flight response. This rapid release of adrenaline and cortisol serves us well when people face an immediate life-threatening situation, but is not very effective when it comes to chronic, complex problems we face in the modern world. These problems require the use of higher-level thinking and problem solving. It also requires cognitive action, thinking that involves identifying and challenging negative thinking styles, and behavioral action, which are actions to deal with events.

Practicing relaxation techniques can have an immediate impact on high levels of stress. Being conscientious of the signs of stress will aid in early identification. Understanding types of stress, their symptoms and how to manage them will allow a person to be more successful when faced with stressful situations. Through individualized assessment and approach, the goal is to reduce chronic stress and prevent the onset of chronic diseases.

Managing your stress starts by accepting responsibility for the role you play in creating and maintaining your stress. Implementing solutions to stress is the best way to ensure that you relieve stress quickly and prevent the serious health problems associated with stress.

Are you ready to increase your ability to cope with life's challenges? Here are nine surefire ways to manage stress:

1. Take charge of your schedule.

Include time in your schedule to take care of yourself. Use a calendar and enter all activities and events.

2. Get organized.

Spend time each evening organizing for the next day. Make a list of tasks that must get done and do the most important things first. Minimize "should do" items so that you can focus on the "must do" items.

3. Learn to say "no."

If your plate is full, say "no" to requests for your time and energy. If "no" doesn't work in a particular situation, find a compromise by letting people know what's on your plate and when you could reasonably expect to meet or have something done.

4. Express your feelings.

When you feel overwhelmed, talk to a confidant, friend or loved one. Sometimes just venting is all you need. Other times, your friend may be able to help put things in perspective. Train yourself to find and express the emotion that you're experiencing. Annoyance and frustration, for example, are forms of anger. Ask yourself why you're angry and if the situation really warrants the emotion. If it doesn't, then adjust your expectations of both the situation and your response. If it does, ask yourself what you can do about it.

5. Evaluate your stressors.

Have a heart-to-heart discussion with yourself about what is causing your stress, what you can do about it and what you want to do about it. Make a list of your stressors and make a plan to deal with each one. Some things aren't changeable. Make a decision to accept the things you can't change, and avoid, eliminate or alleviate stressful situations. If traffic causes you stress, consider a different route or, if possible, alter your work hours. If you have a family member that you find stressful to be around, consider seeing him or her less frequently.

6. Eat right.

Stress can cause us to eat poorly. Most people reach for sugar-filled foods and crunchy foods, studies say. Try to get your fix from healthier choices such as apples, nuts, carrots or celery. Sugar-free gum can also satiate a craving for something sweet.

7. Take care of yourself.

When faced with a stressful life event such as death, try to stick to a strict healthy living schedule. Eat three healthy meals a day, get 8 hours of sleep, exercise for at least 30 minutes, and take time to reflect on your feelings. Taking care of yourself will help you get through it.

8. Manage technology.

Cell phones, computers and iPads are convenient tools that can help organize your life. But these devices may become a burden if they are a distraction and take time away from real social interaction or make you less productive. Are you constantly checking email and taking calls no matter where you are and what you're doing? Are you unable to "unplug" from devices at the end of the day? Don't let your devices rule your life, and limit usage of them if they do.

9. Avoid competitive thinking.
We often create our own stress by wanting to outdo others. That may mean trying to be the best employee, doing the most for the PTA or looking the best. Envy and jealousy can cause stress and are not beneficial to your health. Adjust your standards and focus on the positive aspects of yourself and your life.

De-Stress with Relaxation Techniques

Excessive stress can cause loss of sleep and lead to several health problems, including heart attacks, cancer and disabling accidents. That's why it's important to practice relaxation techniques every day.

Relaxation has many health benefits, including relieving emotions such as stress, anxiety and anger. It also decreases muscle tension, lowers blood pressure, slows the heart rate, slows breathing, and helps improve sleep. Relaxation does not always come easy: It takes training and experimentation, since different methods work for different people. There is no right or wrong way to relax. You will have to find an activity, or a few activities, that works for you and incorporate it into your daily life.

Here are a few activities that can help you relax and reduce stress:

Exercise: Exercise improves mental and physical health, releases stress stored in the body and increases circulation. Rhythmic exercises that incorporate repetitive movements–such as kayaking, rowing, walking, cycling, skating, and swimming–can also help.

Meditation: A mind-body contemplative exercise that helps increase tranquility, meditation is a useful and practical relaxation technique. To meditate, sit in a comfortable place, close your eyes, relax your body, and focus your concentration on something for a period of time. By meditating, you rest your body, allow stress hormones to subside, and occupy your mind so that unpleasant, stressful thoughts do not intrude.

Visualization: Visualization, or guided imagery, is a variation of traditional meditation that requires you to employ not only your visual sense, but also your sense of taste, touch, smell, and sound. Visualization is an inner process that invokes and uses all five senses.

Deep breathing: This activity sends messages to the body to relax. By focusing on full, cleansing breaths, deep breathing is a simple yet powerful relaxation technique. Deep breathing is the cornerstone of many other relaxation practices and can be combined with other relaxing elements, such as aromatherapy and music.

Deep breathing from the abdomen allows you to get as much fresh air as possible in your lungs. When you take deep breaths from the abdomen, rather than shallow breaths from your upper chest, you inhale more oxygen. The more oxygen you get, the less tense, short of breath and anxious you feel. Here's how to deep breathe:

- Sit comfortably with your back straight. Put one hand on your chest and the other on your stomach.
- Breathe in through your nose. The hand on your stomach should rise. The hand on your chest should move very little.
- Exhale through your mouth, pushing out as much air as you can while contracting your abdominal muscles. The hand on your stomach should move in as you exhale, but your other hand should move very little.
- Continue to breathe in through your nose and out through your mouth. Try to inhale enough so that your lower abdomen rises and falls. Count slowly as you exhale.

Mindfulness: Becoming aware of and comprehending what is going on in the physical, emotional and perceptive sense. Mindfulness is often combined with meditation.

Massage: This technique involves the rubbing and kneading of muscles, joints, skin and lymphatic tissue. There are many kinds of massage, including acupressure, deep tissue, shiatsu, hot rock or stone, Swedish and Thai.

Some studies show that massage can help relieve stress, manage anxiety and depression, ease pain, reduce stiffness, control blood pressure, heal sports-related injuries, and boost immunity.

Positive thinking: This technique is centered on self-talk that approaches stressful thoughts and events in a positive and productive manner. Positive thinking allows you to get more done and is typically infectious among those around you. Positive-thinking exercises, like affirmative self-talk, suppresses the release of cortisol from the adrenal glands and can help you feel calm and peaceful.

Deep muscle stretches: These stretching exercises aim to stretch muscles, particularly muscles that are difficult to reach by massage. Here's how to do it: Tense all your muscles for 10 seconds and then let go. You can also purchase a stress ball for tensing/releasing activity.

Yoga: This practice combines mental focus with stretch and strength-building movement.

Qigong: This Chinese practice combines breathing, martial arts-type movement and mental awareness.

Tai chi: A Chinese martial art that uses slow movements, tai chi is sometimes described as "meditation in motion" because it promotes serenity through gentle movements—connecting the mind and body. Originally developed in ancient China for self-defense, tai chi evolved into a graceful form of exercise that's now used for stress reduction and aids in a variety of other health conditions.

Acupuncture: Small needles are placed in specific acupuncture points with the goal of improving health. During a typical acupuncture treatment, the needles are left in for about 20-30 minutes. During this time the body temperature may lower; organ systems, heartbeat and respiration may slow down; and muscle tension dissipates. In most cases, the patient will sink into a very relaxed state.

Research shows that acupuncture causes the body to release neurotransmitters such as endorphins and serotonin. Endorphins are the body's natural opiates, which relieve pain and increase the patient's relaxation response.

Endorphins and serotonin also stimulate the adrenal gland, which secretes cortisol. Cortisol is the body's stress-fighting and anti-inflammatory hormone. It helps regulate immune functions, blood pressure and glucose metabolism. Over the course of treatments, patients experience physical, emotional and mental well-being.

Take a time-out: Remove yourself from a stressful situation for a few minutes to get your thoughts, emotions and perspective together. The goal is to de-escalate the stress and to improve your functioning in the midst of a stressful event.

Music: Listening to music has a calming effect. Try putting together a selection of music that you find calming and play it during stressful times of the day, such as during a daily commute.

Hobbies: Hobbies can be relaxing, but it's important to ask yourself if you truly feel relaxed or if your hobby sometimes becomes stressful for you. Avoid leisure activities that are competitive, involve a lot of running around or that can become frustrating. Again, avoid activities that are competitive. Examples of relaxing hobbies include painting, photography, gardening, bird watching, reading, cooking, dancing, model building, car restoration, creative writing, scrapbooking, woodworking, fishing, knitting, jewelry making, collecting, billiards, and astronomy.

Games: Choose games that allow you to relax and enjoy yourself. If the game is frustrating or too competitive you may want to choose a different relaxation tool. Examples of games include cards, bridge, chess, darts, mahjong, Scrabble, bocce, croquet, board games (such as Monopoly), dominoes, and craps.

Baths: Taking a long, hot bath can be relaxing. Consider adding bath salts for added relaxation.

Pets: Pets can lower stress levels and relax you. Before deciding to get a pet, consider the type of pet you would enjoy and whether or not getting a pet is right for you.

Take a walk: Consider different routes such as walks in the city or countryside, by the water, with a beautiful view, or at sunrise or sunset, to add to the relaxing effect.

Go to bed early or take a power nap: If you are stressed, you may need extra rest. Consider heading to bed a little earlier if you feel particularly stressed. Cool cucumbers placed over your eyes can add to the relaxation effect.

Professional sports game: If you have a favorite sport, consider going to a few games versus watching them on TV.

Comedy: Laughter is the best medicine, as they say. Tune into a comedy channel on TV or radio, or check out a local live comedy show.

The type of relaxation method is not important, but rather it is the act of relaxation that produces the benefits. Relaxation takes practice. If you can master the art of relaxation, you'll reap the benefits on a daily basis and be better armed to deal with life's stressful events.

Assess Your Stressors

Your health coach will ask you to complete two surveys that will help your health team identify stress triggers and determine your risk of serious illness due to chronic stress.

First, take the Day-to-Day Stress Assessment. The survey will give insight on common daily actions that could be stress triggers. The Life Stress Survey evaluates your risk for health problems based on major stress, since research shows that stressful life events can raise the risk of disease and illness. After you complete the surveys, your health team will review the results and develop personalized techniques for stress management.

Maintaining Your Success

Chapter 17

Your Life Strategy

Whether you're beginning the 12-month program or are halfway through it, you need to begin thinking about your long-term care plan.

Your personalized treatment plan employs a variety of targeted treatment to correct imbalances and optimize your overall health. It also provides you with tools for healthy living, nutritious eating, meal preparation, sleep, and fitness. Your ability to avoid diabetes requires you to adjust these fundamental concepts and habits in your daily life.

To achieve your best health, you need to stick with the VITALITY Plan and commit to eating whole, nutrient-dense food and avoiding or limiting intake of harmful foods. You will need to stay physically active, continue a supplement regimen, and regularly nourish your body with deep, refreshing sleep. All of these healthy practices should be top priorities.

Why Focusing on Maintenance Is Important

Prediabetes simmers in your body for many years and increases in severity week after week. Because of your proactive steps, you will gain control of your body and dramatically improve your health. But before you reach the end of the 12-month program, it's critical that you put safeguards in place.

Every year, minor changes occur in the body that may affect your state of wellness. These changes occur at the cellular level and, over time, could significantly affect your prediabetic state. Other medical issues may also arise that can impact your ability to sustain your health improvements–unless, with guidance from your physician and health coach, new treatment plan recommendations are implemented in your long-term care.

For example, if your metabolism slows, you may require a thorough reassessment and possible hormone balancing, nutrition plan changes, or adjustments to your nutraceutical regimen. Or, you may experience arthritis changes that are affecting your ability to maintain a consistent exercise or activity schedule. You may also develop new sleep problems. These are just some examples of medical issues that may cause changes in your health, impact your ability to remain free of diabetes and require you to take action quickly.

Many of our clients will want to join a maintenance plan after completing the 12-month program. The goal of these plans is to ensure you remain on track. Should you struggle in any particular area, your PreDiabetes Centers health team is ready to respond. We want to help identify any problem areas early on, implement changes and bring you back to good health as soon as possible. Around the ninth month of your program, you will begin discussing long-term maintenance of your personalized treatment plan with your physician and health coach, which will include minimum requirements for sustaining your progress. These discussions will occur frequently, and together you will determine your maintenance needs.

Tips for Maintaining Your Progress

✓ Stay committed to maintaining your improved health and wellness.

✓ Get your family and friends involved in your wellness regimen! Ask your kids or spouse to help with meal preparation and invite your pals out for a jog or brisk walk. Creating an active, nurturing support system is key to sustaining your new healthy lifestyle habits.

✓ Be prepared to make adjustments to your maintenance plan. As your health changes in the future, your diet, fitness habits and recommended treatment will change too.

✓ Monitor your health during the program, in the months following and for the rest of your life. To ensure sustained good health, you may need continued reassessment by your PreDiabetes Centers health team through physical examination, biomarker testing, analysis and readjustment to your maintenance plan.

✓ Ask for help if you have difficulty establishing and maintaining your health. Your friends and family can support you during tough times and motivate you to stay committed to healthy lifestyle habits. Your health team is also available for long-term support and guidance. Your physician and health coach want to ensure you stay healthy and maintain lifelong success.

Your success is always measurable: You can see and feel the results in your daily life. Your success also will impact the rest of your household, which makes your success even more important and beneficial!